Advanced Nursing Practice

Edited by Thomas David Barton
and Douglas Allan

Advanced Nursing Practice

Changing Healthcare
in a Changing World

 macmillan education palgrave

First published 2015 by
PALGRAVE

Palgrave in the UK is an imprint of Macmillan Publishers Limited,
registered in England, company number 785998, of 4 Crinan Street,
London, N1 9XW.

Palgrave Macmillan in the US is a division of St Martin's Press LLC,
175 Fifth Avenue, New York, NY 10010.

Palgrave is a global imprint of the above companies and is represented
throughout the world.

Palgrave® and Macmillan® are registered trademarks in the United States,
the United Kingdom, Europe and other countries.

ISBN: 978-0-230-37813-1

This book is printed on paper suitable for recycling and made from fully
managed and sustained forest sources. Logging, pulping and manufacturing
processes are expected to conform to the environmental regulations of the
country of origin.

A catalogue record for this book is available from the British Library.

A catalog record for this book is available from the Library of Congress.

Typeset by Cambrian Typesetters, Camberley, Surrey.

Printed in China

Contents

List of illustrations

Figures

Boxes

Tables

Foreword

It has taken four years to bring this book to completion, a long journey with many hurdles, setbacks and successes along the way. The work is a product of the input of many individuals, not only the editors and authors. It has relied on advice, experience and wisdom from colleagues and practitioners far and wide.

The book provides a detailed review of the evolution of advanced nursing, its practice, theory and concepts, and the contemporary clinical, strategic, educational and research developments. It focuses primarily on developments in advanced nursing practice in the UK over the last 20 years and aims to offer the most up-to-date picture. While no text could comprehensively present the full global context, it is our intention to allude to developments that compare or contrast with the UK experience, which has been replicated in many countries.

We acknowledge from the outset that advanced nursing is now widely regarded as requiring a master's level of preparation, so the book's content will reflect this, exploring the current level of evidence, its quality, and the gaps in knowledge that need to be addressed. Thus it takes a critical approach, being evaluative and interrogative as well as descriptive.

Our target audience is primarily student advance nurse practitioners and their educators and mentors. However, we see the text as also offering a resource to undergraduate student nurses who have exposure to areas of advanced nursing practice, and to registered nurses, educators and service managers with an interest in the development and current status of advanced nursing.

Issues that relate to research and evidence-based practice, service design, service delivery and education are all themes that are developed throughout the book. Contributors highlight features that draw out the role of, or impact on, the patient within any one of these themes. Indeed, the book draws from a wide range of authors, and that diversity brings a rich context. In many ways the chapters are all individual missives from acknowledged experts across the UK. As such, you may find common themes being raised in several chapters, but from the distinctive perspective of each individual author.

There are two particularly noteworthy features of this book. First, it is edited by David Barton and Douglas Allan, both of whom have a national profile in the development of advanced practice. Secondly, the contributors come from the member universities of the Association of Advanced Practice Educators (AAPE UK, formerly AANPE), a nationally influential body that has lobbied widely on advanced practice to government and regulators.

We hope you will find this text useful in developing your understanding and development of the ever-growing world of advanced practice.

David Barton and Douglas Allan

Acknowledgements

The author and publisher would like to thank Skills for Health for permission to reproduce Figure 4.3 'The Career Framework for Health' from http://www.skillsforhealth.org.uk/index.php?option=com_mtree &task=att_download&link_id=163&cf_id=24; The Royal College of Nursing for permission to reproduce Table 5.2 'Threads of arguments put forward by proposers and supporters of the resolution' from Royal College of Nursing Congress (2010) *Resolution: Advanced regulation for advanced nursing* [accessed 2015] Available from: http://www.rcn. org.uk/newsevents/congress/2010/archive_webcast; Skills for Health and Public Health Resource Unit for permission to reproduce Table 8.1 'Core areas of public health activity' from the Public Health Skills and Knowledge Framework: http://www.phorcast.org.uk/page.php?page_ id=313; American Psychological Association for permission to reproduce Figure 8.1 'The transtheoretical stages of change model' from J.O. Prochaska and C.C.D. DiClemente (1982) 'Transtheoretical therapy: toward a more integrative model of change'. *Psychotherapy: Theory Research and Practice* 19: 276–88; John Wiley & Sons Ltd for permission to reproduce Figure 9.1 'The Ethical Grid' from D. Seedhouse *Ethics: The Heart of Healthcare* (1991); The Royal Bournemouth and Christchurch Hospitals NHS Foundation Trust for permission to reproduce Figure 10.1 'A local framework for advanced practice career progression' (2012).

CHAPTER 1

The evolution of advanced nursing practice

David Barton and Linda East

Chapter outline

- Introduction
- The historical and international context of advanced nursing practice
- The contemporary status of advanced nursing in the UK
- Advanced nursing practice in context today
- Conclusion

Introduction

This introductory chapter seeks to set the scene and the guiding principles that will structure the rest of this book. It will review the foundations of advanced nursing, both internationally and in the United Kingdom (UK). It will consider sequentially the historical basis of advanced nursing practice, its potential contributions to modernization and service improvement, the mechanisms by which it may be governed and its potential for the future. The aim is to give some provisional early clarity to this topical, controversial and emergent area of developing health practice. Of course, all of these points will be covered in far more detail in the later chapters of the book.

Our book sets out with a challenge to all its readers. It is our belief, our challenge, that there is no single unified formula that will embrace and explain all that is advanced nursing practice. This book will certainly not strive to achieve that end, and if you are looking for ultimate answers and conclusions you will not find them here. It is clearly our contention that no one book, no single text, no individual competency set, governance framework or definition can adequately capture

1

the entirety of advanced nursing practice. If we accept this premise, then we can also accept the extraordinary diversity and potential of advanced nursing practice and the multiplicity of ways in which it may contribute to healthcare in the future.

It is our hope that this book will stimulate your thinking and thirst for advanced nursing practice, and will pave the way to a greater understanding of the developing cultural healthcare paradigm that it represents. We hope that it will help you to look towards how you may respond and utilise the principles, diversity and totality of what we know as advanced nursing in your own practice and career.

The historical and international context of advanced nursing practice

The expansion, growth and understanding of the concept of advanced nursing practice have been a long and complex journey. Advanced practice has already given rise to extensive innovation, and holds considerable promise for future development of the nursing profession. Yet equally, the emergence of advanced nursing practice has resulted in confusion and misconceptions about what it actually is, exactly what benefits it can bring to patient care and how that can be measured. Perhaps more importantly, the emergence of advanced nursing practice has illustrated how slowly the traditions of healthcare organizations and their constituent professions have responded to the demands of new ways of thinking and delivering healthcare. Many barriers have been encountered along the way, affecting how the implementation of advanced nursing practice has actually happened. It is the analysis of these barriers, and how they might be overcome, that is central to the future of advanced nursing practice.

What is certain is that reservations over advanced nursing practice have manifested themselves in different ways among not only the nursing profession, but also the medical and allied health professions, and indeed patients. Certainly there has been tension between the more traditional view of fundamental nursing and a concern that advanced nursing practice may be undermining that professional foundation. We, the authors, clearly do not see it that way – we believe that advanced nursing is a natural career evolution for our profession. What perhaps best illustrates this wide concern and interest in advanced nursing is the vast literature that has explored its meaning and enactment (AANPE 2011).

The foundation of advanced nursing: The registered nurse

Advanced nursing is all about being a nurse! This is one of our fundamental beliefs. With that in mind, and before we can further the discussion of advanced nursing, we must first consider the foundation of all modern nursing practice – the registered nurse. It is not the remit of this book to present a detailed review of the history of the campaign for nursing registration (Helmstadter 2007; Borsay and Hunter 2012). However, we would be remiss if we did not allude to the significance of that history to the modern-day development of advanced nursing. It is crucial to understand that the framework for regulation and the process of education to attain a fundamental, first-level standard of nursing skill were not always givens. Shaw (1993) addresses the complexity of the foundations of modern nursing in the late nineteenth and early twentieth century:

> The discipline of nursing slowly evolved from the traditional role of women, apprenticeship, humanitarian aims, religious ideals, intuition, common sense, trial and error, theories, and research, as well as the multiple influences of medicine, technology, politics, war, economics and feminism. (Shaw 1993: 1651)

Into this mix of social issues came the reformers of the time, seeking to establish a baseline of education and skills for nursing, something that today people take for granted. It is difficult to appreciate now that when Mrs Bedford Fenwick founded the British Nurses' Association in 1887, along with her contemporaries in the UK and United States of America (USA) she had to fight for education and registration to ensure a professional and dependable nursing labour force (Birnbach 1985; Griffon 1995).

However, after the ambition for educational standardization and registration was gradually achieved in many countries, and since nurses through the twentieth century refined their technical and practical ability within a regulated professional framework, it was inevitable that this would lead to the emergence of new nursing skills, new roles and new hierarchies. That the development and acknowledgement of these new nursing roles would be as prolonged and complex as the road to registration could perhaps not have been so easily predicted.

Specialist nurses

Specialist nurses are the first evidence, and the first product, of that professional evolution of nursing, and are the foundation of today's advanced nursing practice. Such nurses have been identified in practice as long ago as the late nineteenth century (Manton 1971). In the 1930s and 1940s, the number of nurse specialists multiplied, particularly in the USA (Peplau 1965; Storr 1988), and by the 1960s, clinical nurse specialists were firmly established in the nursing profession internationally (Storr 1988; Hamric and Spross 1989; Fenton 1992).

However, a significant feature of this evolution must be noted. Even though their skills often extended beyond those expected at initial registration, the health professions (most importantly medicine) and patients alike perceived the clinical activity of this developing resource of nurse specialists to lie comfortably within the traditionally understood domain of nursing practice (Hamric and Spross 1989). Thus, the clinical nurse specialist role initially offered enhanced patient care at the same time as not presenting a significant threat to the established professional order. This meant that the development of the clinical nurse specialist role was able to proceed unhindered, and was even arguably enabled.

In contrast, today's clinical nurse specialists have become commonly identified as practitioners of advanced nursing. This leads us on to the next significant development in advanced nursing practice, which would more visibly challenge the status quo.

Nurse practitioners: The American origins

In contrast to the comparatively lengthy emergence of specialist nurses and their embedding into the nursing profession, the new concept of 'nurse practitioner' developed quickly as a result of service pressures within the primary healthcare paediatric service in the USA in 1965. Two Americans, one a physician and the other a nurse (Ford and Silver 1967), initially extended the role of the clinical nurse specialist. However, the new role also clearly incorporated traditional medical diagnostic and clinical management skills, thus inaugurating a 'substitution' model, whereby the nurse practitioner takes on many aspects of the role of the junior doctor. The urgent need for this development arose from the social health issues of the time: severe and irresolvable shortages of paediatricians and family practice physicians, fuelling a lack of primary healthcare for rural and urban deprived and poor populations, compounded by escalating healthcare costs (Marchione and Garland 1980).

However, the establishment of such a role inevitably led to unease over the implications of transgressing the professional boundaries between traditional medicine and nursing practice (Marchione and Garland 1980; Fondiller 1995). This was particularly significant at a time when the nursing profession in the USA was preoccupied with establishing its professional identity. Nursing was achieving greater autonomy from the traditional dominance of medical authority, thus enhancing its claim to independent 'professional' status (Shaw 1993). The wish to distance nursing materially from medicine underpinned much of the prevailing nursing ideology (Walby and Greenwell 1994). However, paradoxically, this ideology conflicted with the introduction of new clinical roles such as the nurse practitioner, which included a significant component of traditional medical skills while simultaneously promoting the development of more advanced clinical careers in nursing. Thus, the introduction of nurse practitioners was a controversial and challenging development affecting nursing and its relationship with other healthcare professions, most specifically the interface with medicine (Fondiller 1995).

Despite this tension, support for the nurse practitioner concept gained considerable momentum in the USA in the 1970s. Marchione and Garland (1980) found evidence of this in the state-by-state proliferation of educational programmes for nurse practitioners, although the expansion of the role was unregulated and fragmented, which led to a lack of uniformity. Nevertheless, by the 1990s a greater degree of regulation and standardisation of nurse practitioner education was emerging in the USA (Campbell-Heider et al. 1997), facilitated by the creation and growth of the National Organisation of Nurse Practitioner Faculties (NONPF). By the early 2000s, the role of the nurse practitioner was firmly established, with state-wide licensure systems in place (Hodnicki 1998; Styles 1998; Ponto et al. 2002), which provided more clarity to the conceptualisation and utilisation of advanced nursing.

Today the USA has integrated advanced nurses not only into its healthcare system, but also into the heart and soul of the nursing profession. This has enabled professional acknowledgement, clinical innovation, governance and regulation (Center for Health Workforce Studies 2004; Morgan 2010). That integration has provided a foundation for appropriate education, regulation and licensure, and wide acceptance and use of advanced nursing (Hodson and Sullivan 2001).

Nurse practitioners and advanced practice: The UK experience

It is perhaps unsurprising that many of the US experiences concerning the development of nurse practitioners were mirrored in the UK during the 1990s and early 2000s. This included the influence of complex social demographics, increasingly restricted health service resources, and a lack of coordinated education and regulation (Hunt 1999, Carnwell and Daly 2003).

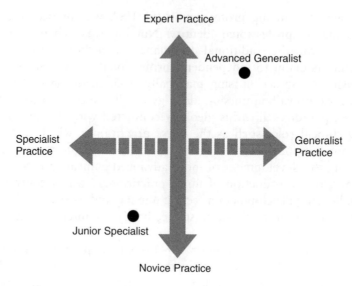

Figure 1.1 The cross diagram

The origin of the nurse practitioner in the UK is attributable to the pioneering work of Barbara Stilwell (1988), who introduced the role into primary healthcare in the late 1980s. Stilwell's vision of a nurse practitioner was an experienced front-line clinical nurse, using well-developed nursing skills in combination with equally well-developed health assessment and diagnostic skills to deliver autonomous patient management. Subsequent to her landmark work, during the late 1990s nurse practitioner roles in primary care slowly, but progressively, emerged in clinical practice (Hunt 1999; Carnwell and Daly 2003). Their emergence into secondary care settings would be somewhat later, in the early 2000s, when nurse practitioners found themselves in new relationships with clinical nurse specialists, and the distinction between specialist and generalist became more clearly articulated (Figure 1.1).

It was in the early 1990s that the Royal College of Nursing (RCN), in conjunction with the University of London, established the first formal training/education programme for nurse practitioners in the UK. The two-year, part-time diploma-level programme was based on a curriculum that required an assessed measurable advancement of skills in physical health assessment, deriving differential diagnosis and patient management skills; that was underpinned by detailed study of anatomy and pathophysiology. The diploma was based on a traditional apprenticeship model, with collaborative mentorship in practice provided by a clinically active doctor. This arrangement enabled students' skills to be gained, tried and tested in the clinical environment (Stilwell 1988).

The modular curriculum was initially franchised, with the modules made available to other educational institutions on a commercial basis. Later, this model of education developed into an RCN accreditation system, allowing interested universities to run accredited nurse practitioner programmes. It should be noted, however, that there were other universities which quickly created their own independent programmes, albeit along very similar lines.

It was during these formative years that the first UK educational competencies for nurse practitioners emerged. The RCN, in collaboration with UK universities, adapted the established American NONPF competencies for UK use and guidance (RCN 2008). Those competencies were founded on consultancy skills, disease screening, physical examination, chronic disease management, minor injury management, health education and counselling. This development was a major milestone, setting as it did a benchmark by which clinical outcomes and curriculum content could be assessed and, more importantly, compared and contrasted across educational institutions. As momentum gathered in the late 1990s and early 2000s, new curricula proliferated. The RCN competency framework (2008) meant that new courses could be structured on clear criteria, against which existing courses could also be evaluated. That said, the use of competencies was often complex, as the RCN framework was not the only option. During the 2000s, many other competency frameworks were developed and tailored to a multitude of new roles and services. Educationalists well remember spending endless hours mapping competency frameworks from one to another. Nevertheless, the baseline competencies were established, and the RCN competency framework provided a 'gold standard' for nurse practitioner practice outcomes.

Universities around the UK have worked industriously to develop and progress programmes of nurse practitioner education. Initially at an academic diploma level, these programmes evolved to undergraduate- and then master's-level programmes of study. Indeed, the current strategic drivers state that master's-level education is a requisite for the advanced nurse (SGHS 2008; NLIAH 2010; DoH 2010).

The expectation of an increasing level of academic education has resulted in an important new distinction in nomenclature. Until this point, specific roles and titles were being discussed, such as clinical nurse specialist and nurse practitioner. However, as the 2000s progressed, the educational and policy discussions became increasingly focused on the level of practice that could be described as advanced. This was clearly significantly above that normally expected of a new registrant, or even an experienced nurse. However, the notion or paradigm of advanced practice encompasses a plethora of titles and job descriptions that range across practice sectors, from the most acute to primary and community care. Thus, academic/apprenticeship clinical programmes are increasingly referred to as educational preparation for 'advanced practice' rather than for any particular role.

At the same time, a glaring inconsistency emerged between the fairly progressive developments in advanced nursing practice education in the UK and the students these were preparing, and their place and use in the health service. Although it was evident that UK healthcare services employers needed and wanted advanced nurses to enable and facilitate service redesign, they had at the same time a limited understanding of the organizational constraints that had to be overcome to achieve this (Fulbrook 1995). There were many possible reasons for this situation. It was perhaps due to the lack of a structured clinical nursing career framework to accommodate and position advanced practice nurses at that time (1990s and early 2000s). It was also, perhaps, due to the long history of organizational and professional traditions that were resistant to new ways of working. Finally, and perhaps inevitably, service providers wanted 'right here, right now' quick fixes to skills shortages and struggled with the notion of two- or three-year academic programmes that took experienced nurses out of the workplace, albeit on a part-time basis. What they wanted was rapid, tightly focused skills training packages that would meet their needs in months, or even weeks.

Thus, while internationally a clear concept of advanced nursing was emerging (Offredy 2000; Ketefian et al. 2001; Pearson and Peels 2002), in the UK the debate was less sophisticated, focused on titles and job descriptions, specific areas of clinical practice, and 'extended' tasks and competencies (Spitzer and Sackett 1990; Maylor 1997). One consequence of this was that advanced nursing from a service delivery perspective was not articulated by diversity, clinical role, competency or innovation, or most importantly by the urgency of service redesign. Instead, it was dominated by endless debate on the meaning of the varied titles that nurses used to describe their advanced role in an attempt to establish their identity and status in health organizations.

A key contributor to this problem was the long-undeveloped career structure of the nursing profession in the UK. There have been many efforts to restructure clinical nursing, notable among which was the clinical regrading exercise in 1988 (Holliday 1995). This was a government-led initiative to provide a clinical hierarchy based on role and responsibility, using a hierarchical system of alphabetical grades (D, E, F etc.). Arguably, this initiative failed first because employers manipulated it to control costs, and second because no one at that time had been able to articulate adequately a clinical career progression for nursing. The introduction of the Knowledge and Skills Framework (Agenda for Change) in the 2000s was more significant and far reaching (DoH 2004). Yet even this comprehensive competency-based model has not fully described a clear career framework for nursing and other professions, which are still essentially service driven as opposed to professionally conceived.

Five other significant professional developments paved the way for advanced nursing in the UK:

- Introduction of the *Scope of Professional Practice* document (UKCC 1990).
- Introduction of the Specialist Practice Award (UKCC 1997).
- Exploration of the Higher Level of Practice (HLP) framework (UKCC 1998).
- Government-led introduction of consultant nurses (Waller 1998).
- Legislative introduction of non-medical prescribing (DoH 2005).

Each of these contributed in varying but important ways to the slow and purposeful evolution of advanced nursing, and to a more refined awareness of the need for a clinical career structure for nurses (Read et al. 2000; Carnwell and Daly 2003). Each issue warrants considerable critique, and will be explored in later chapters in this book.

From an educational perspective, it is also important to note the emergence in the UK during the early 2000s of the Association of Advanced Nursing Practice Educators (AANPE 2011). This is an influential lobby of 40 or more UK universities that represents a collective view of the education of advanced nurses. Its terms of reference point to collaborative curriculum development and standard setting, as well as advising on and establishing the role and status of advanced nursing through interface with other professions, professional and statutory bodies, commissioners, employers and relevant government bodies. AANPE has established close links with the RCN, the RCN Nurse Practitioner Association, the Nursing and Midwifery Council (NMC) and the International Council of Nurses' (ICN) International Nurse Practitioner/Advanced Practice Nursing Network. It has evolved into a powerful educational voice in the world of advanced nursing.

The critique of advanced nursing

It is our contention throughout this book that the evidence points to advanced nurses playing a central role in resolving future health resource issues and service redesign imperatives. In many countries around the world, advanced nurse practitioners, if deployed appropriately either individually or in teams, are not only cost effective but can also improve patient outcomes (Dunkley and Haider 2011).

However, it is important that we acknowledge the challenges and questions regarding motivation that advanced nursing practice faces. Are advanced practitioners really 'pioneers', facilitating service redesign and enabling new roles that lead to improved patient outcomes? Or are they a cost-effective response to health service cuts, shortages of junior doctors and medical recruitment problems (McKenna et al. 2003)? These are important issues to which advanced nursing needs to respond, and they will receive further consideration elsewhere in this book. Our contention at this juncture is that a degree of pragmatism is needed here. If our ultimate goal is service delivery and patient care, then we must ask whether such questions matter. A more useful perspective is that professional boundaries are constantly moving (Barton et al. 1999; Barton 2006) and that all health professionals draw on a common toolkit of theoretical knowledge and clinical skills. Thus, what is critical is the governance of advanced practice, the practical application and outcome of health and illness knowledge and clinical skills in the context of patient care.

The contemporary status of advanced nursing in the UK

There are two significant and intimately connected issues that define and challenge the future of advanced nursing in the UK:

- Ongoing concern for the regulation and governance of the advanced nurse.
- Major structural changes to the National Health Service and resource restrictions that demand innovative service redesign.

Let us consider first the issue of regulation. In an international review by Pulcini et al. (2010), data on advanced nursing was collected from 32 countries. The researchers noted a total of 13 advanced nursing titles and 22 countries providing formal advanced nursing education, with 11 of those identifying a master's degree as the most appropriate educational level. There was formal recognition of the NP-APN (nurse practitioner-advanced practice nurse) role in 23 countries, half of which had licensure maintenance or renewal requirements, including evidence-based continuing education and/or experience in clinical practice. Significantly, support for advanced nursing came from domestic nursing organizations (92%), individual nurses (70%) and governments (68%). The introduction of advanced nursing roles was opposed primarily by physicians and physician organizations (83% and 67%, respectively).

In the UK there is no doubt that many practitioners would like to see a new part of the register for advanced nurses. However, moves to regulate advanced nursing via the professional register in the 2000s unquestionably faltered, and formal statutory regulation is now regarded as at best unlikely, and at worst unworkable and financially prohibitive (CHRE 2008; Barton 2012). The current professional view is that the advanced nurse represents no greater risk to the public than the new registrant, and as such it is difficult to see what public protection benefit is to be gained from the considerable cost of a separate part of the nursing register. The prevailing wisdom is that the Code of Conduct (NMC 2015) offers fundamental public protection by offering guidance for nurses at all levels of practice. This view causes employers, educators and others concerns over practitioners who may be either 'conscious' or 'unconscious' incompetents (Longley et al. 2004). In contrast, there is a real-world lack of evidence that advanced nurses are failing in their duty of care in any significant number, while systematic reviews point to them enabling positive patient outcomes (Newhouse et al. 2011).

However, it is our contention in this text that the NMC's Code of Conduct may not alone be sufficient to manage a nursing career framework that seeks to encompass a transition from initial registration to advanced nursing, even within the clinical framework set out in the Agenda for Change (AfC). Although the advanced level of practice is associated with the higher AfC bands, there is no guarantee of a higher band or any national agreement on what roles should be assigned to which pay band. This adversely affects workforce planning, as well as succession planning. In short, the career pathway for the aspiring advanced practice nurse is not clear. Our general view, discussed in later chapters, is that well-structured and transferable mechanisms of employer-led governance and mandatory, appropriate master's-level education ensure fitness for practice (SGHS 2008; NLIAH 2010; DoH 2010). It is this framework that should form part of a national strategy that is sanctioned and guided at regulator and government level (SGHS 2008; NLIAH 2010; DoH 2010; Barton 2012).

We also need to consider the issue of structural and resource changes in the Health Service and the consequent need for service redesign. The UK Centre for Workforce Intelligence (Dunkley and Haider 2011) assessed the current and prospective workforce risks and opportunities for nursing and midwifery. They noted that the NHS is faced with the prospect of ongoing financial constraints and is simultaneously experiencing widespread organizational instability and change. They conclude that the resultant loss of experienced staff, and a potential reduction in recruitment, will have an impact across the health workforce, including nursing, medicine and the allied health professions.

Compounding that problem is the fact that innovative practice development (and any consequent improved patient care) is potentially constrained by dated organizational structures and cultures, characterized by rigid professional hierarchies, archaic working traditions and inefficient working practices (Ball and Cox 2004; Barton 2012). Indeed, the evidence continues to point to organizational models in the UK Health Service that hinder the effective use of advanced nurses (Barton and Mashlan 2011), and to the continuing existence of outdated, inflexible organizational structures (Ewens 2003). This will have a demoralizing impact on nurses and other health professionals, and thus underpins the pressing need to implement organizational structures and cultures that are new, that enable new ways of working and that facilitate new working roles (Woods 1999). Ewens (2003) sees the key responsibility for resolving problems of organizational structure and culture as lying with service nurse managers and organizational nurse executives, and it follows that this extends to managers of medicine and other health professions.

Norris and Melby (2006) observe that professional traditions were tested by the emergence of advanced nurses and their challenge to, and transgressions of, traditional professional boundaries between nursing and medicine. If new service models are to be effectively implemented, the organizational hurdles and areas of resistance to change need to be identified, pre-empted and resolved by service managers, and this before any innovation is stifled. Thus, what is clear is that any potential service improvement arising from the introduction of advanced nursing will not be possible unless senior management facilitates a culture that enables service innovation (Jones 2005; Barton et al. 2012).

However, despite the traditional resistance to change within health professions and organizations, the growing demand for new roles and service models can enable new opportunities. There is an urgent need for new ways of working in healthcare organizations, for strategic workforce planning and redesign, and for health managers and executives to respond to this. As we are all only too aware of the possible negative impact of austerity measures and resource restrictions, we must face those problems proactively. Anticipating changes to skill mix and skill deployment, strategically restructuring health organizations and managing new advanced practice ideas and roles will lead to improved efficiencies and better patient care (Dunkley and Haider 2011).

The Modernising Nursing Careers initiative (DoH 2006) sought to structure the nursing profession into the twenty-first century. With broad terms of reference, it considered all areas of the profession, from pre-registration education through to advanced nursing, and sought to ensure that the future nursing workforce is dependable, responsive and fit for purpose. It is notable that this in many ways mirrors what nursing and its leaders were striving for a century ago: the pursuit of a 'registered', assured and dependable front-line nursing workforce. Today we are engaged in a similarly complex and important development.

The most significant product of Modernising Nursing Careers in relation to advanced practice was the development of the Advanced Practice Toolkit (SGHS 2008). This lays out a foundation of four pillars of activity on which advanced nursing should be built: Clinical Practice, Research, Education and Management/Leadership. Although there are many variants to this model currently in use, it is becoming increasingly adopted throughout the UK as a set of first principles. In addition, the developers of the toolkit made two decisions that have enabled a more structured and professional debate on advanced nursing practice. First, they avoided the 'definition' trap. Definitions of advanced nursing abound, and reviewing them reveals certain core principles (clinical experience, expert knowledge, clinical history and diagnosis, complex decision making, leadership, evidence base). The point is that there are many entirely appropriate and accurate definitions of advanced practice, and as such it is somewhat fruitless to continue to seek the 'ultimate' definition.

Secondly, the developers avoided the competency trap. The RCN competency framework has served as a useful measure by which advanced nurse practitioners judge their knowledge, skill and competence. Internationally, the ICN definition of advanced practice nursing dating from 2002, and the subsequent competency framework published in 2008, also provide a common starting point that is widely acknowledged (ICN 2008). However, because competencies and competency frameworks are proliferating in all areas, reflecting the diversity of healthcare from critical care to community care, from child to adult, mental health and learning disability, any attempt to identify a definitive competency set for advanced nursing is doomed to failure. The stance of the toolkit is to promote practitioners' use of appropriate competencies to meet the needs and nuances of their role, and to articulate principles in the form of the pillars of practice. This is surely the way forward for advanced nurses and their employers.

Advanced nursing practice in context today

We have intentionally left to last what we believe to be the current status and foundations of advanced nursing practice in the UK. Although there have been considerable and positive developments in the last 25 years, it is still an unfinished story. Advanced nursing remains one of the least understood, yet most scrutinized and researched concepts in practice

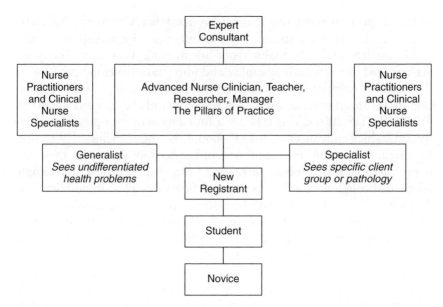

Figure 1.2 Novice to expert: specialists and generalists

development. It is varyingly described as a role or a level of practice, as encompassing both specialist and generalist features, and it ranges through clinical, managerial, educational and research areas. Figure 1.2 builds on Figure 1.1 to illustrate the notion that while commonly nurse practitioners have been associated with generalism and clinical nurse specialists with specialism, this need not be the case. Today nurse practitioners may specialize and clinical nurse specialists may deal with generalist case loads. It is more important that in future we embrace the continuum of advanced nursing and its diversity. The pillars of practice have moved advanced nursing beyond the purely clinical domain, and into the wider arena of the delivery of nursing.

Advanced nursing offers a significant opportunity to the UK Health Service at a time of severe austerity measures, resource restrictions and dramatic changes in health demography exemplified by an ageing population. That opportunity is founded on a long and complex history of professional development of advanced nursing, and can be contrasted with the widespread failure of health organizations and their managers to develop innovative services and new organizational models. It cannot be overstated that one of the major restraints has been the Health Service's failure to develop mechanisms of governance, and we have been held back by the notion that the only form of safe regulation is the statutory introduction of a new part of the register.

The Council for Regulatory Excellence (CHRE 2008: 6) made the following observations on the wider scope of regulatory options:

- **Registered health professionals** should only practise in areas in which they are competent to do so; they are responsible for the care that they provide to patients.
- **Employers** should have the appropriate support and performance management systems in place if they employ health professionals in extended roles.
- **Regulators** should ensure that their codes of conduct adequately reflect the requirement for health professionals to stay up to date and to operate safely within their areas of competence.
- **Regulators** should only pursue the option of creating a specialist list or annotation on the register when all other approaches have been exhausted.
- **The Secretary of State for Health and Ministers in the Devolved Administrations** should assess any application to change legislation in relation to specialist lists or annotations on a register solely against the risks posed to patient safety and public protection.
- **All parties** should demonstrate an active commitment to cooperating and sharing information to manage risks to patient safety and public protection.

Thus, it can be seen that the responsibility for governance and regulation falls on all (practitioners, managers, educators, regulators and government) and is not confined to any one individual or group (Marsden et al. 2003; Barton 2012). CHRE (2008) suggests six main regulatory principles, which should guide us all in our approach to the development, regulation and governance of advanced nursing services. These principles are proportionality, consistency, targeting, transparency, accountability, and checking for unintended consequences. Properly applied, these should enable advanced nursing practice innovations to be introduced with due consideration from all parties. Only then can we truly assure the public that proper and due process is in place to ensure the best care (Livesley et al. 2009).

Finally, advanced nursing has been strategically advocated as a cost-effective service redesign tool and resource that can overcome healthcare staff shortages and other problems facing the UK Health Service (DoH 1989, 2006, 2007). Our current understanding of what advanced nurses are, what could regulate their practice, the potential scope of their roles and what education is required for their preparation implies that advanced nurses are the cutting edge of nursing innovation.

Conclusion

It is now possible for us to visualize a hierarchy of skill and expertise in advanced nursing, in order to identify novice and expert advanced practitioners (Maylor 2005). We have a better understanding of the nature of generalist and specialist practice, and the intimate relationship between these concepts. With this developing body of evidence and emerging career framework, we can move forward with more confidence to tackle the constraints on the full and best use of this emergent new resource for health service provision.

By now we hope to have convinced you that the idea that advanced nursing may be captured by titles, definitions and competencies is simplistic. There is in reality a complex matrix of professional, cultural and organizational issues. That advanced nursing has the potential to improve patient care and enable efficient service delivery is supported by the developing evidence base. That its deployment is hampered by dated organizational and professional structures and traditions is also a fact.

Finally, we believe that the concept of and evidence base for advanced nursing are maturing and attaining wider acceptance. The responsibility for moving advanced nursing forward to benefit patient care and service delivery falls on all of us: the practitioners themselves, employers and managers, educators, the regulator and government. The historical struggle for formal registration of nurses is today being taken another step further as we strive to build a flexible career framework and a national strategy that are enabled by, and accommodate, the diversity and totality of advanced nursing.

References

AANPE (Association of Advanced Nursing Practice Educators) (2011) Literature Lists. http://www.aanpe.org/ANPTheLiteratureLists/tabid/1387/language/en-US/Default.aspx (accessed in July 2011).

Ball, C. and Cox, C. (2004) Part two: The core components of legitimate influence and the conditions that constrain or facilitate advanced nursing practice in adult critical care. *International Journal of Nursing Practice* 10: 10–20.

Barton, T.D. (2006) Nurse practitioners – or advanced clinical nurses? *British Journal of Nursing* 15(7): 370–376.

Barton, T.D. (2012) Comment: Embrace the opportunities that advanced practice offers. *Nursing Times* 108(24): 15.

Barton, T.D. and Mashlan, W. (2011) An advanced practitioner led service: The consequence of radical service redesign for health care managers and organisational infra-structure. *Journal of Nursing Management* 19(7): 943–949.

Barton, T.D., Thorne, R. and Hoptroff, M. (1999) The nurse practitioner: Redefining occupational boundaries? *International Journal of Nursing Studies* 36: 57–63.

Birnbach, N. (1985) The nurse registration movement in Great Britain. *Advances in Nursing Science* 7(2): 13–19.

Borsay, A. and Hunter, B. (2012) *Nursing and Midwifery in Britain since 1700.* Basingstoke: Palgrave Macmillan.

Campbell-Heider, N., Kleinpell, R.M. and Holzemer W.L. (1997) Commentary about Marchione and Garlands 'An emerging profession? The case of the nurse practitioner'. *Journal of Nursing Scholarship* 29(4): 338–339.

Carnwell, R. and Daly, W. (2003) Advanced nursing practitioners in primary care settings: An exploration of the developing roles. *Journal of Clinical Nursing* 12(5): 630.

Center for Health Workforce Studies (2004) *A Comparison of Changes in the Professional Practice of Nurse Practitioners, Physician Assistants, and Certified Nurse Midwives: 1992 and 2000.* Washington, DC: Bureau of Health Professions.

Council for Healthcare Regulatory Excellence (2008) *Advanced Practice: Report to the four UK Health Departments.* London: CHRE.

Department of Health (1989) *Working for Patients.* London: HMSO.

Department of Health (2004) *NHS Knowledge and Skills Framework (KSF).* London: HMSO.

Department of Health (2005) *Evaluation of Extended Formulary Independent Nurse Prescribing: Executive Summary.* London: HMSO.

Department of Health (2006) *Modernising Nursing Careers: Setting the Direction.* London: HMSO.

Department of Health (2007) *Trust, Assurance and Safety: The Regulation of Health Professional in the 21st Century.* London: HMSO.

Department of Health (2010) *Position Statement on Advanced Practice.* London: HMSO.

Dunkley, L. and Haider, S. (2011) *Nursing and Midwifery: Workforce Risks and Opportunities.* London: Centre for Workforce Intelligence.

Ewens, A. (2003) Changes in nursing identities: Supporting a successful transition. *Journal of Nursing Management* 11(4): 224–228.

Fenton, M.V. (1992) Education for the advanced practice of clinical nurse specialists. *Oncology Nursing Forum* 19(1): 16–20.

Fondiller, S.H. (1995) Loretta C. Ford: A modern Olympian, she lit a torch. *N & HC Perspectives on Community* 16(1): 6–11.

Ford, L. and Silver, H. (1967) Expanding the role of the nurse in child care. *Nursing Outlook* 15: 43–45.

Fulbrook, P. (1995) What is advanced practice? *Intensive and Critical Care Nursing* 11(1): 53.

Griffon, D.P. (1995) 'Crowning the edifice': Ethel Fenwick and state registration. *Nursing History Review* 3: 201–212.

Hamric, A.B. and Spross, J.A. (1989) History and overview of the CNS role. In A.B. Hamric and J.A. Spross (eds), *The Clinical Nurse Specialist in Theory and Practice*, 2nd edn. Philadelphia, PA: W.B. Saunders.

Helmstadter, C. (2007) Florence Nightingale's opposition to state registration of nurses. *Nursing History Review* 15: 155–168.

Hodnicki, D.R. (1998) Advanced practice nursing certification: Where do we go from here? *Advanced Practice Nursing* 4(3): 34–43.

Hodson, R. and Sullivan, T. (2001) *The Social Organization of Work*. Belmont, CA: Wadsworth/Thomson Learning.

Holliday, I. (1995) *The NHS Transformed*. Manchester: Baseline Books.

Hunt, J.A. (1999) A specialist nurse: An identified professional role or a personal agenda? *Journal of Advanced Nursing* 30(3): 704–712.

ICN (2008) Advanced Practice Nursing Network. Definitions and Characteristics of the Role. Accessed at http://international.aanp.org/Practice/APNRoles

Jones, M.L. (2005) Role development and effective practice in specialist and advanced practice roles in acute hospital settings: Systematic review and meta-synthesis. *Journal of Advanced Nursing* 49(2): 191–209.

Ketefian, S., Redman, R.W., Hanucharurnkul, S., Masterson, A. and Neves, E.P. (2001) The development of advanced practice roles: Implications in the international nursing community. *International Nursing Review* 48(3): 152–163.

Livesley, J., Waters, K. and Tarbuck, P. (2009) The management of advanced practitioner preparation: A work based challenge. *Journal of Nursing Management* 17: 584–593.

Longley, M., Magill, J. and Warner, M. (2004) *Innovation and Protection: A Framework for Post-registration Nursing*. Report for the Nursing and Midwifery Council Task and Finish Group. London: NMC.

Manton, J. (1971) *Sister Dora: The Life of Dorothy Pattison*. London: Methuen.

Marchione, J. and Garland, T.N. (1980) An emerging profession: The case of the nurse practitioner. *Journal of Nursing Scholarship* 12(2): 37–40.

Marsden, J., Dolan, B. and Holt, L. (2003) Nurse practitioner practice and deployment: Electronic mail Delphi study. *Journal of Advanced Nursing* 43(6): 595–605.

Maylor, M. (1997) Nurse practitioners: What difference does a title make? *Nursing Standard* 12(13–15): 54–55.

Maylor, M. (2005) Professional development: Differentiating between a consultant nurse and a clinical nurse specialist. *British Journal of Nursing* 14(8): 463–468.

McKenna, H., Keeney, S. and Bradley, M. (2003) Generic and specialist nursing roles in the community: An investigation of professional and lay views. *Health and Social Care in the Community* 11(6): 537–545.

Morgan, S. (2010) What are the differences in nurse practitioner training and scope of practice in the US and UK. *Nursing Times* 106(27): 21–24.

Newhouse, R.P., Stanik-Hutt, J., White, K.M. et al. (2011) Advanced practice nurse outcomes 1990–2008: A systematic review. *Nursing Economics* 29(5): 230–250.

NLIAH (National Leadership and Innovation Agency for Health Care) (2010) *All Wales Guidelines for Advanced Practice*. Llanharan: NLIAH.

Norris, T. and Melby, V. (2006) The acute care nurse practitioner: Challenging existing boundaries of emergency nurses in the United Kingdom. *Journal of Clinical Nursing* 15: 253–263.

Nursing and Midwifery Council (2004) *Code of Professional Conduct: Standards for Conduct, Performance and Ethics*. London: NMC.

Nursing and Midwifery Council (2015) *The Code: Professional Standards of Practice and Behaviour for Nurses and Midwives*. London: NMC. http://www.nmc-uk.org/Documents/NMC-Publications/revised-new-NMC-Code.pdf (accessed 1 March 2015).

Offredy, M. (2000) Advanced nursing practice: The case of nurse practitioners in three Australian states. *Journal of Advanced Nursing* 31(2): 274–281.

Pearson, A. and Peels, S. (2002) Advanced practice in nursing: International perspective. *International Journal of Nursing Practice* 8(2): S1–S4.

Peplau, H.E. (1965) Specialisation in professional nursing. *Nursing Science* 3(8): 268–287.

Ponto, J., Sabo, J., Fitzgerald, M. and Wilson, D. (2002) Operationalizing advanced practice registered nurse legislation: Perspectives from a clinical nurse specialist task force. *Clinical Nurse Specialist* 16(5): 263–269.

Pulcini, J., Jelic, M., Gul, R. and Loke, A.Y. (2010) An international survey on advanced practice nursing education, practice, and regulation. *Journal of Nursing Scholarship* 42(1): 31–39.

Read, S.M., Roberts-Davis, M., Gilbert, P. and Nolan M. (2000) Preparing Nurse Practitioners for the 21st Century. Executive Summary. Unpublished Review. Sheffield: School of Nursing and Midwifery, Sheffield University.

Royal College of Nursing (2008) *Advanced Nurse Practitioners: An RCN Guide to the Advanced Nurse Practitioner Role, Competencies and Programme Accreditation*. London: RCN.

Scottish Government Health Service (2008) *Supporting the Development of Advanced Nursing Practice – A Toolkit Approach.* Edinburgh: SGHS. http://www.advancedpractice.scot.nhs.uk/home.aspx (accessed April 2011).

Shaw, M.C. (1993) The discipline of nursing: Historical roots, current perspectives, future directions. *Journal of Advanced Nursing* 18: 1651–1656.

Spitzer, W.O. and Sackett, D.L. (1990) 25th anniversary of nurse practitioners: The Burlington randomised trial of the nurse practitioner. *Journal of the American Academy of Nurse Practitioners* 2(3): 93–99.

Stilwell, B. (1988) Patients' attitudes to a highly developed extended role: The nurse practitioner. *Recent Advances in Nursing* 21: 82–100.

Storr G. (1988) The clinical nurse specialist: From the outside looking in. *Journal of Advanced Nursing* 13: 265–272.

Styles, M.M. (1988) An international perspective: APN credentialing. *Advanced Practice Nursing* 4(3): 1–5.

UKCC (United Kingdom Central Council for Nursing, Midwifery and Health Visiting) 1990 *The Scope of Professional Practice.* London: UKCC (NMC).

UKCC (United Kingdom Central Council for Nursing, Midwifery and Health Visiting) 1997 *PREP – Specialist Practice: Consideration of Issues Relating to Embracing Nurse Practitioners and Clinical Nurse Specialists within the Specialist Practice Framework.* London: UKCC (NMC).

UKCC (United Kingdom Central Council for Nursing, Midwifery and Health Visiting) 1998 *Higher Level of Practice – Consultation Document.* London: UKCC (NMC).

Walby, S. and Greenwell, J. (1994) *Medicine and Nursing: Professions in a Changing Health Service.* London: Sage.

Waller, S. (1998) Higher level practice in nursing: A prerequisite for nurse consultants? *Hospital Medicine* 59(10): 816–818.

Woods, L.P. (1999) The contingent nature of advanced nursing practice. *Journal of Advanced Nursing* 30(1): 121–128.

Advanced nursing practice: The theoretical context and evidence base

Helen Rushforth

Chapter outline

- Introduction
- The origins of advanced nursing practice
- Advanced nurse practitioner regulation: International perspectives
- UK development of advanced nursing practice
- Regulation of the advanced nurse practitioner role in the UK
- Exploring the evidence base for advanced nursing practice
- The future direction of advanced nursing practice evidence
- Being able to use evidence effectively

Introduction

The focus of this chapter is the evidence base that underpins the concept of advanced nursing practice. While a comprehensive presentation of the vast evidence base is well beyond its scope, the aim is to provide an overview of some of the key features and findings as the evidence has evolved alongside the development of advanced nursing practice. However, in order to appreciate fully the nature of the evidence, it is necessary first to take a closer look at some of the underlying theoretical assumptions that underpin advanced practice itself. As noted in Chapter 1, the modern-day understanding of advanced practice is complex and lacking in a clear, consensus view or definition. Consequently, the somewhat elusive nature of advanced practice inevitably influences the evidence base, or perhaps more accurately the several evidence bases, underpinning it.

The origins of advanced nursing practice

There are different viewpoints about the origins of advanced nursing practice, but as Chapter 1 indicated, there are clear suggestions that it began with the development in the USA of specialist nursing roles in the late nineteenth and early twentieth centuries (Pulcini 2013). More formal recognition of the role emerged in the mid-twentieth-century 'nurse practitioner (NP) movement', with its origins in primary care and practice at the interface between nursing and medicine. Starting in the USA and Canada, role development extended over the next 20–30 years to the UK, Australia, New Zealand and the Republic of Ireland, as well as to parts of Africa and Asia where the term 'advanced practice nurse' is sometimes the preferred or regulated title.

More recent role development can be seen in a number of European countries, including Scandinavia, Belgium and the Netherlands (Sheer and Wong 2008; Pulcini et al. 2009). The parallel development of the clinical nurse specialist (CNS) role within the acute care setting is also important. This was initially clearly delineated from the NP role not only by its care setting, but also by its much clearer 'nursing' and 'educational' orientation (Daly and Carnwell 2003). However, as Dunn (1997) describes, by the mid-1990s the roles were becoming blurred as acute care NP roles started to develop. Despite this, the two roles have remained largely distinct, albeit with some overlap (Roberts-Davis and Read 2001; Pulcini et al. 2009).

In the USA, nurse practitioner and clinical nurse specialist sit alongside the nurse anaesthetist and the nurse midwife to form the four roles within the regulated title of 'advanced practice registered nurse' (APRN Consensus Working Group 2008). In the UK, as will be discussed shortly, advanced practice roles are far less distinct. It is thus perhaps not surprising that the evidence base surrounding advanced practice, particularly the UK-specific evidence, is also diverse and multifaceted.

Advanced nurse practitioner regulation: International perspectives

Consideration of the regulation of advanced nursing practice is central to consideration of its evidence base, because in many ways the evidence influences several aspects of regulation and the surrounding debate. Formal regulation of advanced practice, usually via the title of nurse practitioner or advanced practice nurse (advanced nurse practitioner in Ireland), is seen in many countries that use the title; Pulcini et al. (2009) describe 23 countries as having some form of formal role recognition.

However, such regulation is invariably complex, sometimes with a mixture of federal (country-wide) and state-specific control. For example, in the USA each state has its own regulation of the APRN role, some with and some without prescriptive authority, which invariably restricts the NP role to a significant degree in many states (Pearson 2012).

There is little merit in detailing such regulation in a text of this nature; policies change rapidly and the only way to gain up-to-date information at any given point is by consulting websites and policy documents from the relevant national boards and governing bodies. Within the USA, the annually published *Pearson Report* (Pearson 2012) offers an extremely valuable update on the current regulation of advanced practice roles state by state.

UK development of advanced nursing practice

The UK has a well-established history of advanced nursing practice, but no regulation for advanced practice roles, with the exception of a clear and separate regulatory process for non-medical prescribing. Indeed, overall the development of advanced practice in the UK has been somewhat piecemeal, as noted in Chapter 1. The emergence of the NP role since the mid-1980s has largely mirrored the emphasis on clinical assessment, diagnosis and treatment seen in the USA and Canada, with the earlier UK evidence base from that period similarly mirroring the US focus on the safety and effectiveness of NP roles when compared to the medical roles that they replaced. However, establishment of the NP title over the last 30 years has very much been at employer level, with the consequence that the underpinning evidence base has been much more inconsistently applied than in countries where regulation of roles and titles is more firmly established. The development of the CNS role in the UK has been similarly inconsistent. Manley (1997), as a precursor to developing her own evidence-based view of advanced practice, describes how from its UK inception the CNS role was less clearly defined than in the USA, and its educational and consultancy functions much less overt. This in turn may have led to the evidence base in respect of the CNS role, particularly in the UK, also being much more limited.

Other factors have also affected the development of clarity surrounding advanced nursing practice in the UK and its underpinning evidence base. One of these was the concurrent establishment in the 1980s of Nursing Development Units (Vaughan 1988) and the subsequent wide range of initiatives falling under the umbrella of nurse-led care. Another was the 1992 United Kingdom Central Council for Nursing Midwifery and Health Visiting (UKCC) publication of *The Scope of Professional*

Practice. This document liberated nurses to make decisions much more independently surrounding the expansion of their role, and to take on a large number of roles that were previously the domain of medicine. However, the parallel emergence of the overlapping concepts of expanded and advanced practice may well have contributed to confusion regarding to the distinction between the two. Consequently, the current UK picture is of a plethora of roles, titles and job descriptions related to CNS, NP and numerous other advanced nursing practice titles and roles, with a marked lack of consensus, variable levels of educational preparation and repeatedly failing attempts to achieve formal regulation.

Also relevant, and potentially adding to the current lack of clarity and consensus, was the UKCC's 1994 decision not to regulate or set educational standards for advanced practice. Instead, it offered a rather fluid and inclusive definition of advanced practice that arguably had more to do with the advancement of nursing itself than the practice role of particular individuals:

> Advanced practice is concerned with adjusting the boundaries for the development of future practice, pioneering and developing new roles responsive to changing needs, and with advancing clinical practice, research and education to enrich professional practice as a whole. (UKCC 1994: 8)

In contrast, though, the UKCC (1994) did somewhat confusingly set standards for specialist practice, but with a very different orientation to the CNS role. The resultant recordable qualification subsequently became aligned with specialist community public health nursing and district nursing, rather than with the role of the CNS.

In a similar vein, seminal work by Manley (1997) to develop an evidence-based model of advanced nursing practice challenged the notion of its being at the 'medical–nursing' interface. Manley drew on the CNS movement rather than the NP movement, building on the work of Hamric and Spross (1989), and developed the advanced nursing practice role to include elements of consultancy. In many ways what she describes is more a forerunner of the consultant nurse role that became more clearly established via *Making a Difference* (DoH 1999), thereby adding further complexity. Importantly, though, the consultant nurse (later consultant practitioner) role is probably more tightly controlled and more specific in its requirements than any other UK advanced practice role, apart from non-medical prescribing. The evidence base underpinning the added value of the consultant practitioner role is yet again somewhat limited, and at the time of writing the future of the role is far from certain.

Importantly, Manley (1997) also made links with the notion of expert practice as a key component of advanced nursing practice, echoing the seminal research of Benner (1984). Benner drew on parallels from the aviation industry to describe the development of nursing on a continuum from 'novice' to 'expert', via the intermediate steps of 'advanced beginner', 'competent' and 'proficient'. Thus, although Manley (1997) saw the role of advanced practitioner/consultant as very senior, its breadth and nursing centricity aligned advanced practice more closely with the notion of expertise and away from the NP interface with medicine. This broader perspective was further perpetuated by the development of the NMC 'Higher Level of Practice' pilot project (UKCC 1999; McGee 2009), which added yet another layer of confusion. This overly complex and unsatisfactory attempt at 'quasi advanced practice regulation' floundered before the pilot phase of the project was even complete.

Regulation of the advanced nurse practitioner role in the UK

As UK advanced nursing practice moved into the twenty-first century, the wealth of advanced practitioner roles and titles continued to develop, alongside repeated failure in respect of any developments towards regulation of the role. Importantly, however, 2005 saw an important change at the Nursing and Midwifery Council (NMC), with the formalization of proposals for nurse practitioner regulation, leading to widespread consultation. Interestingly, there were two key outcomes that potentially pulled in opposite directions in respect of the likelihood of successful regulation. The first was the definition of advanced/nurse practitioner, which started off pre-consultation rather broadly and inclusively as:

A registrant who has command of an expert knowledge base and clinical competence, is able to make complex clinical decisions using expert clinical judgement, is an essential member of an interdependent health care team and whose role is determined by the context in which s/he practices. (NMC 2005)

After consultation, it emerged much more precisely focused at the nursing/medical interface as:

Advanced nurse practitioners are highly experienced and educated members of the care team who are able to diagnose and treat your healthcare needs or refer you to an appropriate specialist if needed. (NMC 2006)

This latter definition, accompanied by a list of key roles linked to assessment, diagnosis and treatment, was seen by some as helpful in terms of setting standards, but left others feeling excluded. Key within this perhaps was a return to a clear recognition of the interface between advanced nursing practice and medicine, something that McGee (2009) argues has to be recognized as a key aspect of advanced nursing practice, but in the context of complementary rather than competitive roles.

The second important outcome of the consultation was in respect of the title. Respondents were given the option of seeking regulation of the title 'nurse practitioner (NP)' or 'advanced nurse practitioner (ANP)', and they chose the latter. The addition of the prefix 'advanced' to the NP role/title was actually far from helpful. Despite research attempting to establish the difference between ANP and NP (Ball 2005), arguably *all* NPs practise nursing at an advanced level, drawing also on certain aspects of medicine to fulfil their hybrid 'nursing medical role'. Thus, it may be that adding the word 'advanced' to NP allowed the distinction between an ANP and advanced nursing practice to become blurred; in many cases the two were used interchangeably, as evidenced in Mantzoukas and Watkinson's key 2006 international review of the generic features of advanced nursing practice. This in turn may have led to uncertainty regarding whether it was the precise ANP role – that is, the nurse working at the nursing/medical interface – or a more inclusive view of 'advanced nursing practice', akin to expert practice, that the NMC was seeking to regulate. Indeed, although the Republic of Ireland regulated the 'advanced nurse practitioner' title, most other countries with regulation regulate either the NP title or 'advanced practice nurse' (Pulcini et al. 2009).

The NMC consultation was only one factor contributing to the ongoing confusion surrounding titles. Another key adverse influence was the concurrent emergence of 'Agenda for Change' as the framework within which all NHS non-medical healthcare roles were described and salaried. Underpinned by the levels of practice outlined by Skills for Health (2007), those at band 7 were clearly designated as 'advanced practitioners' and those at band 8 as 'consultant practitioners', although it is unclear what evidence base underpinned this decision. Thus, rather than NPs and CNSs being a clearly defined subgroup of all the practitioners working at an advanced level, a much more inclusive view of advanced practice emerged, with everyone working at band 7 or above effectively becoming an 'advanced practitioner'.

Other factors have undoubtedly also played their part in the complexity of the UK definitions of advanced practice, as explored in Chapter 1. Whatever the contributory causes, the reality is that during the three-year period between 2006 and 2009 in which the government considered the case for regulation and ultimately sought the advice of the Council for Healthcare Regulatory Excellence (CHRE), the mandate for regulation was no longer seen as a priority. Thus, the CHRE's (2009, 2010) response in respect of advanced practice regulation (by this time inclusive of all healthcare professions, not only nursing) was that advanced practice was a natural evolution of the healthcare practitioner role; that is, congruent with Benner's notion of developing expertise. Thus, as described in Chapter 1, it saw advanced practice as adequately covered by the relevant professions' code of conduct or equivalent, and as not requiring regulation. This is unsurprising, since there is of course no logical requirement to regulate 'expertise' within a particular profession (Brook and Rushforth 2011).

Interestingly, though, the CHRE (2009) also suggested that, exceptionally, where the role of the practitioner was sufficiently different from that of the original profession in which the practitioner was registered, a case for regulation may exist. This key point *could* be applied to the NP role given its nursing/medical interface or hybrid status, provided that the NP role and that alone were put forward as requiring regulation. However, to date this point has received minimal recognition, and more recent attempts to advocate regulation made by the NMC (cited in Snow 2010) and supported by the former Labour Government (DoH 2010a) were stalled once again by changes both in government and in the senior leadership of the NMC. The underpinning financial crisis across the UK is another key factor, since regulation is inevitably costly. Consequently, it is the self-governance principles advocated by the Department of Health (2010b) in England, the National Leadership Agency for Health (2010) in Wales, NHS Education for Scotland (NES, 2012), the Royal College of Nursing (RCN, 2012) and the Department of Health (2011) 'Enabling Excellence' white paper that currently prevail. Interestingly, as Chapter 1 notes, the Department of Health (2011) cites a lack of evidence of risk as the key reason for not advocating advanced practice regulation.

The current UK health department's position thus endorses that of the CHRE (2009, 2010) that regulation of advanced practice is not required. This arguably leaves risks arising from the unregulated aspects of medical practice undertaken by the NP/ANP, for which he or she may or may not have been adequately educated and assessed as competent (Brook and Rushforth 2011). Yet this is an unsubstantiated view with which some will disagree, rather than one that can be backed by evidence. This position also leaves advanced nursing practice uncertain in respect of its identity. Increasingly, it seems that there is a dichotomy of viewpoints, where some see advanced practice as clearly positioned at the nursing/medical interface, but others view it much more inclusively as linked to the *advancing* of nursing practice, and as more congruent with expert practice (Por 2008; Brook and Rushforth 2011). In some countries this dichotomy is recognized but relatively unproblematic. For example, in Australia regulation of the narrower NP role is complemented by a more inclusive (but unregulated) conceptualization of advanced practice nursing (Gardner et al. 2007; Chang et al. 2011). However, in the UK the absence of regulation means that confusion regarding the nature of advanced practice is perpetuated, with a risk that a broader but much more diverse view will prevail. This in turn means that a lack of regulation *and* a lack of contemporary evidence could both pose a risk to public protection.

Exploring the evidence base for advanced nursing practice

The remainder of the chapter will explore much more systematically a number of the different subgroups of evidence that underpin advanced nursing practice, and also highlight gaps in the evidence base. Understanding the evolution of advanced practice and the atypicality of the UK position is important here, because the evidence base inevitably reflects the ethos in the country and at the time at which the research was undertaken. Thus, what is evident in the USA and Canada is a long history of a wealth of studies debating the safety and efficacy of the 'substitution' of doctors with nurses in a whole variety of NP roles, as well as a substantial literature exploring the interface between the NP and CNS roles, and that between the NP role and the quasi-medical role of the physician's assistant (PA). A smaller but similar literature is seen in other countries where the role is more clearly defined. Indeed, in the UK in the 1990s and early twenty-first century a similar literature also emerged, alongside an emergent literature focusing on the 'added value' arising from NP, CNS, nurse-led and other advanced nursing practice roles.

However, as the more recent UK evidence is scrutinized, the focus seems to change, congruent perhaps with the evolving and increasingly fluid definitions of advanced nursing practice. Consequently, although the 'added value' of advanced nursing roles continues to be explored, recent UK evidence seems to lack the explicit focus on safety, efficacy and role substitution inherent within earlier work, even though key studies made clear that more work in this domain needed to be done (Lattimer et al. 1998; Kinley et al. 2002; Horrocks et al. 2002; Laurant et al. 2004; Rushforth et al. 2006). Yet not only is there a gap in the current literature in respect of evidence of safety, there is also one in terms of evidence of risk – evidence essential if the case for regulation is to be made in the foreseeable future (DoH 2011). Nevertheless, as will become clear as a recurrent theme within this chapter, 'absence of evidence is not evidence of absence' (Altman and Bland 1995: 485).

Early evidence regarding safety and efficacy

Much of the early literature on advanced nursing practice, and almost certainly the greatest body of evidence, comes from the largely US- and Canadian-focused literature on the substitution of doctors by NPs in a variety of primary care, and more latterly secondary care, roles. A full review of this literature is beyond the scope of this chapter, but some perspective will be provided by noting that by the time Brown and Grimes (1993) wrote their review and meta-analysis on the topic, they could identify some 200 primary studies. Key early US research included the work of Silver and colleagues in paediatric primary care (Day et al. 1970; Duncan et al. 1971) and by Lewis and colleagues in the field of adult long-term condition care in outpatient settings (Lewis and Resnick 1967; Lewis et al. 1969). In the following 15–20 years dozens of similar studies emerged. What most of these had in common was a methodology involving a small number of nurses (sometimes just a single nurse) being compared with one or more junior doctors in their management of a particular patient population in a particular healthcare setting. Some studies were condition specific, while others included a range of conditions. Most put forward evidence of similar performance by nurses when compared with doctors in a variety of roles, with some also citing evidence of nursing superiority, especially in respect of patient satisfaction. Consequently, studies made repeated recommendations regarding the safety, efficacy and acceptability to patients of nurses replacing doctors in a variety of roles (Sox 1979; Brown and Grimes 1993; Richardson and Maynard 1995).

Despite their considerable quantity, such studies were repeatedly methodologically flawed. A key problem with some of the earlier studies (e.g. Duncan et al. 1971) was the 'historical control assumption'; that is, that if a doctor and nurse disagreed the doctor was always assumed to be right! Fortunately, this flaw was fairly quickly recognized and most studies subsequently offered some form of independent verification in the form of observation, retrospective audit, expert opinion or gold-standard comparison to determine which practitioner was correct in cases of disagreement. Many studies also included just one or two nurses, a methodological flaw that persists even in contemporary studies, inevitably leaving questions regarding the typicality or atypicality of the practitioner studied. While later studies do include a greater number of nurses, most are powered in respect of the number of patients included rather than the number of practitioners, and most feature fewer than ten nurses. Furthermore, many studies focus on health professionals whose training for their advanced practice roles has taken place on the same or similar courses; transferability of findings to all nurses must thus be undertaken with extreme caution.

Perhaps the least well-recognized flaw in most of this early work, and something key to all such research, was the repeated failure to power most of the studies adequately to include sufficient patients to allow meaningful comparison between those receiving care from nurses and those receiving care from physicians (Laurant et al. 2004; Rushforth et al. 2006). This risk is important in any quantitative research, but is far more important in research of this nature, because exceptionally such studies do not require nurses to be 'better than the doctors' in order to underpin safe or effective practice; what they are looking for is care of at least the same standard.

And herein lies the problem. Most randomized controlled studies are designed to look for a significant difference; that is, to establish whether a new drug or intervention is better than a previous one or a placebo. Consequently, since changing practice based on wrongly believing that a new drug or intervention is better than the previous one carries a high risk, statistical procedures and sample size calculations seek to keep the risk of finding a difference that did not really exist (often described as type one error) as low as possible – normally a minimum of 1 in 20. However, there also remains a possibility that a significant difference *did* exist but was not found, referred to as type two error. The clinical risk here is seen to be much lower, because the worst that can happen is that the benefits of a new treatment will be overlooked and the status quo maintained. Thus, to avoid impossibly large sample sizes being required, the risk of type two error is normally kept at around 1 in 5 (sometimes expressed as 80% power; Rushforth et al. 2006; Campbell et al. 2007).

However, these important factors need to be viewed very differently in the case of nurse/doctor substitution research. Because, unless unexpectedly nurses turn out to be better than doctors, the researcher essentially draws conclusions that the substitution of doctors with nurses is safe if the study does *not* find a significant difference. Yet, as noted above, the risk of this happening using standard methodology is 1 in 5, even if the sample size was sufficiently powered or 'big enough'. This is a far greater risk than any researcher would normally view as acceptable. Furthermore, if a study is underpowered – that is, it has fewer subjects – then the risk of *not* finding a significant difference is greater still. Nevertheless, numerous studies from this period (and regrettably also some more contemporary studies) repeatedly draw assumptions that a finding of 'no significant difference' means that it is safe for nurses to replace doctors in whatever domain of practice is being explored – an assumption that may be statistically and clinically unsafe. And this is despite seminal work by Dunnett and Gent (1977) highlighting both the problem and the solution.

The way to overcome this risk is by undertaking an explicit equivalence methodology, which is a study with a sample size far larger than a conventional significant difference trial, where methodologically the whole study is oriented towards the aim of determining whether the two things being studied are sufficiently similar for one to be substituted for the other (Jones et al. 1996; Rushforth et al. 2006; Campbell et al. 2007). The methodology is well established in clinical drug trials where a new drug is compared with an active comparator (another drug as opposed to a placebo), because the researcher wants to know if the new drug is similar in performance to the usual drug, rather than wanting to know whether it is better. Common reasons for doing this are on the grounds of the new drug having fewer side effects, for example, or lower cost. But for some reason, this well-established methodology took a very long time to be applied to NP research, with the consequence that numerous studies have been used to justify practice changes despite their conclusions being potentially unsafe.

Interestingly, within the time period during which much of this North American research was being conducted, one Canadian study (Spitzer at al. 1974) stands out above the rest for employing a rigorous methodology that few have followed until comparatively recently. Using a robust sample size of 1600 patients and an explicit equivalence methodology, the researchers demonstrated statistical similarity in the care given by NPs and physicians in primary care. Yet even here, the inclusion of just two NPs resulted in limited transferability of the study findings.

What is disappointing is that, apart from one further attempt to replicate the methodology (Chambers and West 1978), none of the subsequent considerable body of North American research during the latter half of the twentieth century replicated the rigour of this approach. Thus, although the 1990s saw an increased focus on acute care research, widening the potential transferability of the evidence base to acute care NPs and some CNSs, many of the earlier flaws are perpetuated. One exception to this is the work of Alba Mitchell-DiCenso, a pioneer of the evidence-based practice movement, whose work in the field of neonatal care maximized sample size and came as close to equivalence as was possible (Mitchell et al. 1991; Mitchell-DiCenso et al. 1996). This work contributed substantially to the evidence base indicating that neonatal nurse practitioners could replace junior doctors in neonatal intensive/high-dependency care.

UK evidence regarding safety and efficacy

Within the UK, the evidence exploring NP and other nurse-led roles in comparison with doctors emerged much later, reflecting the later development of the role itself. Nevertheless, early UK research replicated many of the earlier flaws seen in the North American evidence base. Some of the earliest work included that of Barbara Stilwell (Stilwell 1983, cited in Bowling and Stilwell 1988), who in a non-comparative chart review of 858 NP consultations in general practice concluded that around 45% of cases could have been managed solely by an NP. Subsequent studies ranged in scope but were fairly limited in number overall, with examples from this period including some of the earlier work in UK primary care (Salisbury and Tettersell 1988), rehabilitation care (Griffiths 1996), pre-operative assessment (Whitely et al. 1997) and early work in non-medical prescribing (Luker et al. 1998). All offer evidence of similar or superior nursing performance when compared with doctors. There is evidence of methodological developments compared with earlier North American evidence, but key problems include failure to use an explicit equivalence methodology. Other design flaws also emphasize the importance of reading such studies in full; for example, Whitely et al. (1997) assert the similarity of nurse-led pre-operative assessment compared with pre-registration house officers, but excluded nurses from undertaking the physical examination component of the assessment. It is also important to note that not all studies identified nurses as being similar or better than doctors. For example, James and Pyrgos (1989) compared determination of the need for X-ray between emergency nurse practitioners (ENPs) and registrars in a repeated measures design (i.e. both practitioners saw the same patients). Of the 332 adult and child cases included, they noted 40 cases of disagreement, of which 12 were determined by experts to be nursing errors of clinical significance. Lack of formal training of the nurses was felt to be a key factor in this finding.

During the 1990s, a number of large-scale, nationally funded UK studies were conducted, underpinned by the mandate at that time to reduce junior doctors' hours and workload (NHS Management Executive 1991). Particularly notable within these was the widely cited Greenhalgh report (Greenhalgh et al. 1994). This was a large-scale 'in-depth' study of practice in 24 hospital wards across the UK, which sought to identify roles that could safely be transferred from doctors to nurses. The researchers identified 35 distinct 'transferable' spheres of practice that a nurse could safely undertake. However, despite this list being widely reported in the NP and other literature, careful consideration of the full report reveals that the sole outcome measures used were 'number of attempts made' and 'length of wait', with the latter the only feasible outcome measure in many instances (e.g. patient history taking). This emphasizes the caution that must be used in accepting secondary citation, and the ease with which practitioners can be convinced that evidence to support practice is robust without this ever being so.

Another similarly funded study from the period is Touche Ross (1994), which considered 20 NP pilot roles, 16 of which were in primary care. The researchers again drew conclusions regarding the safety of nurses substituting for doctors, but again closer examination of the evidence reveals judgements about consultation appropriateness being made by retrospective review of audio tapes and case notes; thus physical examination skills and the safety of the judgements made compared with the patient presentations were left largely unexplored. Furthermore, 10% of nursing consultations reviewed by medical experts, and interestingly 18% of those reviewed by nursing experts, were felt to be unsatisfactory. Also from this period is the work of Coopers and Lybrand (1996), again often cited as positively demonstrating the benefits of NP roles in primary and ambulatory care, with their in-depth study of 10 primary and ambulatory care settings. Despite high levels of patient satisfaction being a key finding, patient compliance with medical prescriptions was found to be far higher than with nursing prescriptions (98% to 63%, respectively). Blind expert review also deemed 88% of medical referrals appropriate compared with 80% of NP referrals. Notably, lack of explicit inferential analysis is also a key flaw in a number of these studies.

Clearly, these and other similar studies from this period were conducted almost 20 years ago. Much has changed in respect of NP roles, NP education, medical education and the very nature of primary and secondary care. But what close scrutiny of these studies clearly demonstrates is that the evidence base on which the modern advanced practitioner (especially NP) role is founded is perhaps somewhat less robust than a more superficial reading of the evidence might suggest. What is therefore important is to consider the more contemporary evidence base carefully, and also to assess whether an ongoing evidence base for safe and effective advanced nursing practice can or should be maintained in the absence of funding for large-scale research.

Key developments in the UK evidence base

A marked turning point in the UK evidence base came with the key work of Lattimer et al. (1998), who conducted a robust large-scale equivalence study exploring the safety of nurse-led telephone triage of patients making out-of-hours contact with general practice. The study had a sample size of 14,492 calls, and demonstrated equivalence between nurse-led triage and traditional approaches to out-of-hours care, in a study that was effectively the forerunner to NHS Direct. It is however noteworthy that substantial funding from British Telecom was an essential component of this research.

Other studies pertaining to primary care from the same period employ more robust methodologies than earlier work, although none fully mirrors the rigour in Lattimer's work. Three studies from 2000 offer key evidence regarding the NP role in primary care (Venning et al. 2000; Shum et al. 2002; Kinnersley et al. 2000). All these studies were multi-centred, and included in excess of 1000 patients and larger numbers of NPs than earlier studies (e.g. 20 NPs in Venning et al.'s work). Overall, all three offered supporting evidence of the value and appropriateness of NP roles in general practice, with comparable patient outcomes. Venning et al. and Shum et al. both reported greater satisfaction with NP care when compared with GP care, although Kinnersley et al.'s findings were less clear in this respect. All the studies also reported NP consultations taking longer than GP consultations, a finding widely echoing observations in many earlier studies. However, higher referral rates and ordering more investigations were also a feature of NP care in Venning et al. and higher prescribing rates in Shum et al. Thus, while there is evidence in favour of NP care, there is also a need to recognize that this may have cost implications that are not wholly offset by the lower salaries paid to NPs compared with GPs. Importantly, cost differentials may be even more of a consideration in acute care, where more senior advanced practitioners (e.g. band 7 or 8a in 'Agenda for Change') may earn more than their junior medical counterparts. Findings such as longer consultations, more investigations and higher prescribing rates also suggest that nurses' inherent caution may have direct implications for patients, in terms of inconvenience and concern if not safety.

Methodologically, most advanced practitioner studies use real patients as subjects. An interestingly different approach to primary care research is seen in the work of Grant et al. (2002), exploring the quality of care delivery in the new NHS Walk-in Centres. Here, simulation with actors was used to explore 297 nurse vs GP consultations based on five standardized care scenarios, thus exceptionally facilitating a study where the sample size was focused on the number of practitioners involved rather than the number of patients. Notably, nurses scored better overall, but there was scenario variation, with GPs scoring better in the chest pain scenario. Also nurses were significantly better history takers, but there was a non-significant difference in favour of GPs demonstrating better physical examination skills; a difference that may have potentially been significant in a larger study.

Finally, providing some conclusions about much of the primary care evidence base are the key systematic review of Horrocks et al. (2002) and the Cochrane review by Laurant et al. (2004). Both acknowledge the considerable existing evidence base, which overall attests to the safety and appropriateness of nurse-led roles in primary care. Yet they also identify some caveats where nurses' performance may not be equal to or better than that of doctors, as well as the lack of methodological quality, as discussed above. Interestingly, these reviews also seem to have brought closure to the development of the evidence base in respect of primary care, as is often the case when a Cochrane review is published. Rashid (2010) found minimal new evidence when reviewing similar studies published in a five-year period following Laurant et al. (2004), and it will be interesting to see what new studies emerge in a planned 2015 update of the Laurant et al. Cochrane review.

Within acute care, the evidence base comparing nursing (usually NP roles) and medical roles is more limited. However, important studies have underpinned contemporary practice developments. Freij et al. (1996), Thurston and Field (1996) and Meek et al. (1998) all studied nursing roles in radiology. Freij et al. (1996) demonstrated comparable performance between senior house officers (SHOs) and NPs in ordering and interpreting 300 distal limb injuries, and Meek et al. (1998) demonstrated comparable performance between nurses and experienced SHOs, and superior performance when nurses were compared with novice SHOs. Thurlston and Field's (1996) retrospective survey of 1833 X-rays found a modest but significant difference between nurses and junior doctors, with nurses requesting 4% more X-rays and making 3.2% more referral errors. Inadequate training was identified as the main issue, a recurrent theme in studies where nursing performance is inferior. Importantly, once again none of these studies used an explicit equivalence methodology, although precise reporting of p values and confidence intervals does aid auditability.

Within emergency care, Sakr et al. (1999) conducted a large-scale study involving 1453 patients and care provided by two NPs compared with that provided by SHOs. Using expert verification of practitioner performance, no significant difference in clinically important errors between the two groups was reported (9.7% for nurses, 10.7% for SHOs); the errors that were noted mostly pertained to treatment decisions rather than history taking or examination. Although no explicit equivalence methodology is recorded, sample size and other safeguards to ensure comparability offer stronger external validity than other smaller studies from the same period based in emergency care (Tye et al.

1998; Byrne et al. 2000). Importantly, though, a recurring theme, as in much of the literature regarding advanced nursing practice, is evidence of increased patient satisfaction. Also interesting to note is a more recent study (Sandhu et al. 2009) that notes similarities and differences in communication patterns between different practitioner groups (including GPs, emergency department [ED] doctors and SHOs) compared with emergency nurse practitioners (ENPs). Patient satisfaction seems to be closely related to communication and relationship building. ENPs and GPs were both valued in respect of education and counselling, and ENPs rated highly in respect of information giving and support. These characteristics are probably key reasons for the recurrent evidence of high levels of satisfaction within nurse-led care. Interestingly, in contrast to earlier studies, Sandhu et al. (2009) showed no significant difference between the consultation times of nurses and doctors, with SHOs and ED practitioners both taking longer than nurses and GPs. As noted previously, any finding of 'no significant difference' must be viewed with caution. Nevertheless, if corroborated, this finding does perhaps offer some important insight into how nurses' consultation times decrease with greater experience, and also suggests that patient satisfaction is not necessarily attributable to nurses taking longer in their consultations.

In respect of neonatal care, there is an important evidence base attesting to the scope of practice of advanced neonatal nurse practitioners (ANNPs) and their potential to substitute for junior and middle-grade staff on the medical rota (Aubrey and Yoxall 2001; Lee et al. 2001; Leslie and Stephenson 2003). This evidence base again spans a number of years, although the relatively modest number of ANNPs again constrains the scale of the UK evidence to some extent. Well-conducted UK trials build on the earlier Canadian work of Mitchell-DiCenso and colleagues, and suggest that ANNPs can effectively substitute for both junior and middle-grade practitioners. However, Smith and Hall (2011) urge that a more integrated career path for ANNPs is required, and that recognition is needed of their finite number to ensure that they are utilized most effectively in future neonatal care delivery.

A key turning point in acute care research mirrors the quality of Lattimer's work in primary care with the 'Op check' study (Kinley et al. 2002). This multi-site study demonstrated comparable performance between NPs and pre-registration house officers in a large-scale non-inferiority randomized controlled trial (RCT), non-inferiority being a derivation of equivalence whereby the investigator seeks to ensure that the group of interest is 'no worse' than the comparison group, with equivalence or superiority both acceptable outcomes. However, only three NPs were involved, and one of these performed less well in the history-taking component than medical counterparts, which re-emphasizes the risks of only studying a small number of practitioners.

Rushforth et al. (2006) conducted a paediatric pre-operative assessment non-inferiority RCT in a single-site study that compared SHOs with eight ward-based nurses trained in history taking and physical examination, involving 595 children. The findings demonstrated overall non-inferiority in nursing assessment of abnormalities of potential perioperative significance, and non-inferiority when history taking was viewed in isolation. However, power was insufficient to demonstrate certainty in respect of non-inferiority in the physical examination component of the role. Nurses also identified significantly more 'false positives' than SHOs, with potential implications for over-investigation of some children; once again, nurses' inherent caution is a possible risk factor here, although this is something that is perhaps under-recognized in many studies and is seldom a primary outcome measure.

While there are other, smaller-scale acute care-focused studies from the same time period, as with primary care research there seems to be something of a change from the mid-2000s onwards in terms of the direction that advanced practice evidence has followed. As the more recent evidence, both UK and internationally, is scrutinized, it becomes apparent that a different orientation is emerging.

Contemporary evidence

Searching the evidence across the last ten years in relation to advanced practice reveals a number of different approaches, but largely there is a shift away from seeking to demonstrate comparative performance between doctors and nurses in relation to particular aspects of clinical practice. One factor in this might be a growing reluctance to think about nurses in advanced practice primarily in terms of medical 'substitution' and a companion desire to reinforce the secondary findings from many earlier studies regarding the 'added value' that nurses in advanced practice roles bring to the patient experience and the quality of care delivered. Certainly, in their key paper Bryant Lukosius et al. (2004) make a clear plea for this approach. There is also some suggestion of an emergent evidence base that is congruent with contemporary approaches to healthcare, where throughput, achieving targets and outcome measures are priority areas in respect of measuring the quality of service delivery.

That being said, it is also important to recognize that the new roles that nurses are being required to undertake, especially in relation to non-medical prescribing or the role of the community matron, are roles in which earlier evidence regarding safe care at the nursing–medical interface has limited transferability. Thus, the shift in the orientation of advanced practice research in recent years could leave practitioners in new roles at that interface especially vulnerable. Key here is the nursing role in non-medical prescribing, which will be discussed much more fully later in this text, so it is not explored in detail here. It is however interesting to note that the evidence base in this respect is smaller than might be imagined, with significant gaps and limited evidence pertaining to clinical outcomes (Bhanbhro et al. 2011). In respect of community matron development and case management, evidence is also limited despite the rapid initiation of this approach to community care (DoH 2005). The future of the role is currently far from certain, with anecdotal evidence suggesting that many trusts are reducing the number of community matrons/case managers in post, or replacing the role with other approaches to community care. It is possible that a lack of robust underpinning evidence for the role may be a key factor in its potential lack of sustainability, despite an anecdotal and common-sense view of its benefits, and several qualitative studies attesting to the patient satisfaction, care coordination and quality of life that the role offers (Brown et al. 2008; Chapman et al. 2009; Williams et al. 2010).

What thus emerges is a marked shift in methodological approach. Whereas in many traditional areas of enquiry qualitative evidence forms the theoretical basis for more focused quantitative enquiry, the current shift over the last ten years in relation to advanced practice seems to be away from the RCT and other forms of enquiry at the top of the evidence-based hierarchy, and towards more inductive modes or non-comparative research. The benefits and risks of this approach are an interesting area to debate.

For example, Ball and Cox (2003) offer a grounded theory study to explore the role of the advanced nurse practitioner in adult critical care nursing, suggesting that enhanced patient stay and improved patient outcome are the perceived benefits of advanced practice roles in critical care that merit further enquiry. The inductive approach to this study in some ways makes sense, because historically at this point critical care had only comparatively recently begun to establish the ways in which the advanced practitioner role might best be applied in this environment. However, a much more recent critical care study by Fleming and Carberry (2011) similarly uses a grounded theory methodology to explore the challenges of 25 experienced critical care nurses transitioning into an advanced practice role. The transition emerges from the study as a challenging one, with concerns regarding professional ability, potential conflict with traditional medical roles, and nurses having to re-establish their place within the clinical team being identified as some of the main difficulties. However, as the roles became established, so a unique ability to provide holistic care and integrate nursing and medical expertise emerged.

In Australia, an interesting series of papers by Gardner and colleagues (Gardner et al. 2007; Chang et al. 2011) has again focused on theory generation as the basis for implementing new nursing roles. They have differentiated the role of the 'advanced practice nurse (APN)', including those working as nurse specialists and consultant nurses, from the much more clearly defined role of the NP. Their work has then sought to define the attributes of the APN (which for them excludes NPs, although in other countries the NP is a subgroup under the APN umbrella, as earlier noted) and concludes that the best fit is an adaptation of the 'Strong Model of Advanced Practice' (Ackerman et al. 1996, cited in Gardner et al. 2007), which the team describe as the 'Modified Advanced Practice Role Delineation Tool' (Chang et al. 2011). They suggest that the key attributes of the APN include 'direct comprehensive care; support of systems; education; research; and publication/professional leadership'. Such findings echo the domains identified by contemporary UK reports on advanced practice (DoH 2010b; NLIAH 2010).

Policy drivers and the need to demonstrate a quantifiable impact on practice are also clearly influencing contemporary evidence, with a move towards service evaluation approaches. For example, a multi-professional study on the impact of advanced practice roles on service delivery and patient care was conducted by Acton Shapiro/University of York (2009) on behalf of NHS North West. This regional study, focusing in particular on the Greater Manchester area, looked at the impact of advanced practice role developments by collating achievements, as well as factors thought to have positively or negatively affected the impact. Benefits were felt to include improved access to health services, reduced/more appropriate admissions, reduced waiting times and better teamworking/interprofessional working. Barriers appeared to include financial constraints after initial pump priming and lack of role clarity, with nurses in particular being pulled back into more traditional nursing roles. Studies such as this provided valuable insights into the impact of such roles, which are clearly congruent with the current health service agenda. However, it is important to recognize that service evaluation of this nature, while pragmatic and cost effective, does make it much more difficult to isolate variables. It is thus difficult to be confident that the perceived benefits are attributable to the advanced practitioner roles rather than to other factors.

It is also interesting to note a recent acute medicine-focused study also based in Manchester (Williamson et al. 2012), this time taking an ethnographic perspective to exploring the role of ward-based advanced

NPs in acute medicine. The study used participant observation and interview to conduct an in-depth exploration of the practice of five such NPs, with the key emerging finding being that NPs were a 'lynchpin', holding a pivotal role facilitating nursing and medical practice. Perceived enhancements to the patient journey, clinical communication and holistic care are clearly desirable outcomes for contemporary practice. These findings interestingly echo Fleming and Carberry's (2011) findings in critical care cited above, and also earlier work by Lloyd Jones (2005).

The future direction of advanced nursing practice evidence

What therefore emerges from considering exemplars of research exploring contemporary approaches to advanced nursing practice is an evidence base that has a clear focus on the 'added value' that advanced nursing practice roles can offer, but lacks clear irrefutable evidence to support the impact of those roles on service delivery. This is surely one of the key challenges for the short-term future of advanced nurse practitioner research as it debates the optimal approaches to the future evidence base.

Furthermore, there is no doubt that safety continues to be a prime consideration, especially as reports of suboptimal care continue to dominate the media. Yet there is little in contemporary evidence to verify that new roles undertaken by advanced practice nurses rather than doctors are safe. Spitzer et al. (1978: 163) argue that new nursing initiatives of this nature should be 'subject to the same rigorous scrutiny as any major new clinical method or new drug', and in respect of public protection this is difficult to argue against. Yet as Lattimer et al. (1998) point out, there is a tradition within UK nursing of putting new roles into place and *then* evaluating them, an observation that has clearly continued to hold true in recent years if initiatives such as the community matron and non-medical prescribing roles are considered.

It can of course be argued, as DoH (2011) clearly notes, that evidence of risk attributable to advanced nursing practice roles is minimal, and anecdotal evidence suggests that the NMC sees very few 'fitness for practice' cases linked to advanced practice roles. Perhaps nurses' inherent 'over caution', evidenced in a number of studies, is also their safeguard. However, arguably healthcare needs to be based on much more robust evidence than assumptions arising from an absence of evidence of risk. Furthermore, threaded throughout the evidence cited in this chapter are recurrent suggestions (often under-emphasized in the study write-up) of instances where new nursing roles may compromise rather than maintain or enhance care. Such observations are vital in a climate in which the patient's right to receive the same standard of care irrespective of who delivers it is the key legal principle on which safe care is judged (Dimond 2005). Yet finding meaningful ways of researching risk or suboptimal practice is far from easy; the queue of those willing to volunteer to have their practice scrutinized in this way is likely to be very short indeed.

Consequently, focusing advanced practice research on contemporary notions of 'impact' may well be the most productive way forward. One of the factors that could help in realizing this goal is a much more coordinated and collaborative approach to generating such evidence, a plea clearly made by Bryant Lukosius et al. (2004) but one that has, as yet, received limited recognition. These authors also note the dominance of the clinical aspect of the advanced practitioner role in research, with other facets having received limited attention. Another closely related key aspect of advanced practice that requires research is the impact of current UK policies around self-regulation, in terms of the ongoing diversity of job titles and role descriptions, and its consequences for care delivery. However, the irony may be that the very principles of self-regulation also militate against any coordinated attempts at large-scale research. So it is regrettably likely that it will take a major adverse incident in relation to an advanced nursing role to provide the catalyst for such an approach.

A final point is the observation in a number of studies that suboptimal care by nurses is potentially attributable to limited educational preparation. Thus, the other key challenge in respect of future evidence is perhaps to seek to quantify the impact of educational preparation on the successful articulation of advanced practice roles, so that optimal evidence-based approaches to education can be followed. Currently, though, despite a profession that advocates the importance of evidence-based practice, healthcare is remarkably limited in its provision of evidence-based education. Some helpful contemporary evidence does exist, such as work by Barton (2006), but collectively the evidence base regarding optimal advanced practitioner preparation is limited in both quantity and scope. However, if master's-level education for all who practise nursing at an advanced level is to become mandatory rather than guidance (DoH 2010b), then evidence of the efficacy of such educational endeavours is arguably key.

Being able to use evidence effectively

Finally, a very important point to note in respect of advanced nursing practice and evidence: there would seem to be a persuasive argument that all who practise in advanced practice roles should be able to apply evidence critically and insightfully to their practice. The guidance that those practising nursing at an advanced level should hold or be working towards a master's degree is key here (DoH 2010b), as is the recent move to an all-graduate nursing profession (NMC 2010). Scrutiny of curricula for master's degrees suggests that learning to read and apply evidence insightfully are invariably key requirements of such programmes. However, the challenge of securing funding and time for master's-level education, together with the lack of regulation and mandatory educational requirements for advanced practice in the UK, means that there are many practising advanced-level nursing in the UK whose education in respect of research and evidence-based practice is somewhat limited.

Where practitioners are able to access education at master's level, the opportunities to engage critically with the evidence base underpinning their practice are considerable. Moves away from the traditional requirement to undertake a piece of empirical research within a master's degree are arguably particularly helpful here, with most advanced practitioner students now able to undertake much more useful and transferable projects including systematic/evidence-based reviews, audits, service evaluations and preparation of business cases with appropriate evidence. The overarching goal should surely be that no advanced practice student leaves a programme of study without being fully prepared to read any piece of evidence critically, and with it being second nature to take no piece of evidence at face value. It will take many more years and some considerable cultural shifts to ensure that all who practise at an advanced level have the benefits of such educational preparation, and work in an environment in which these skills can be fully utilized. The move to ensuring that this happens has considerable potential to influence not only the efficacy of advanced nursing practice roles, but also, via much clearer practitioner advocacy, the evidence base underpinning advanced nursing practice itself.

References

Acton Shapiro/University of York (2009) *Rome Wasn't Built in a Day: The Impact of Advanced Practitioners on Service Delivery and Patient Care in Greater Manchester.* York: Acton Shapiro.

Altman, D. and Bland, J.M. (1995) Absence of evidence is not evidence of absence. *British Medical Journal* 311: 485.

APRN Consensus Working Group (2008) Consensus Model for APRN Regulation: Licensure, Certification, Accreditation and Education.

https://www.ncsbn.org/Consensus_Model_for_APRN_Regulation_July_2008.pdf (accessed 18 February 2015).

Aubrey, W.R. and Yoxall, C.W. (2001) Evaluation of the role of the neonatal nurse practitioner in resuscitation of preterm infants at birth. *Archives of Disease in Childhood Foetal Neonatal Edition* 85: F96–F99.

Ball, C. and Cox, C. (2003). Part one: Restoring patients to health – outcomes and indicators of advanced practice nursing in adult critical care. *International Journal of Nursing Practice* 9: 356–367.

Ball, J. (2005) Maxi Nurses: Advanced and Specialist Nursing Roles: Results of a Survey of RCN Members in Advanced and Specialist Nursing Roles. London: Employment Research Limited for the RCN.

Barton, D. (2006) Nurse practitioners – or advanced clinical nurses? *British Journal of Nursing* 15(7): 370–376.

Benner, P. (1984). *From Novice to Expert: Excellence and Power in Clinical Nursing Practice.* Menlo Park, CA: Addison-Wesley.

Bhanbhro, S., Drennan, V., Grant, R. and Harris, R. (2011) Assessing the contribution of prescribing in primary care by nurses and professionals allied to medicine: A systematic review of the literature. *BMC Health Services Research* 11: 330. http://www.biomedcentral.com/1472-6963/11/330 (accessed 18 February 2015).

Bowling, A. and Stilwell, B. (1998) *The Nurse in Family Practice.* London: Scutari.

Brook, S. and Rushforth, H. (2011) Why is the regulation of advanced practice essential? *British Journal of Nursing* 20(16): 996–1000.

Brown, K., Stainer, K., Stewart, J., Clacy, R. and Parker, S. (2008) Older people with long term conditions. Their views on the community matron service: A qualitative study. *Quality in Primary Care* 16: 409–417.

Brown, S. and Grimes, D. (1993) *Nurse Practitioners and Certified Nurse Midwives: A Meta-Analysis of Studies on Nurses in Primary Care Roles.* Washington, DC: American Nurses Publishing.

Bryant Lukosius, D., DiCenso, A., Browne, G. and Pinelli, J. (2004) Advanced practice nursing roles: Development, implementation and evaluation. *Journal of Advanced Nursing* 48(5): 519–529.

Byrne, G., Richardson, M. and Brunsdon, J. (2000) Patient satisfaction with emergency nurse practitioners in A and E. *Journal of Clinical Nursing* 8: 83–93.

Campbell, M., Machin, D. and Walters, S. (2007) *Medical Statistics: A Textbook for the Health Sciences.* Oxford: Wiley-Blackwell.

Chambers, L. and West, A. (1978) The St. John's randomised trial of the family practice nurse: Health outcomes of patients. *International Journal of Epidemiology* 7(2): 153–161.

Chang, A., Gardner, G., Duffield, C. and Ramis, M.-A. (2011) Advanced practice nursing role development: Factor analysis for a modified role delineation tool. *Journal of Advanced Nursing* 68(6): 1369–1379.

Chapman, L., Smith, A., Williams, A. and Oliver, D. (2009) Community matrons: Primary care professional views and experiences. *Journal of Advanced Nursing* 65(8): 1617–1625.

Coopers and Lybrand (1996) *Nurse Practitioner Evaluation Project, Final Report.* London: National Health Service Management Executive.

Council for Healthcare Regulatory Excellence (2009) *Advanced Practice: Report for the Four UK Health Departments.* London: CHRE.

Council for Healthcare Regulatory Excellence (2010) *Right Touch Regulation.* London: CHRE.

Daly, W. and Carnwell, R. (2003) Nursing roles and levels of practice: A framework for differentiating between elementary, specialist and advanced nursing practice. *Journal of Clinical Nursing* 12: 158–167.

Day, L., Egli, R. and Silver, H. (1970) Acceptance of pediatric nurse practitioners: Parent's opinion of combined care by a pediatrician and a pediatric nurse practitioner in a private practice. *American Journal of Diseases in Childhood* 119: 204–208.

Department of Health (1999) *Making a Difference: Strengthening the Nursing, Midwifery and Health Visiting Contribution to Health and Healthcare.* London: HMSO.

Department of Health (2005) *Care Management Competences Framework for the Care of Older People with Long Term Conditions.* London, DoH.

Department of Health (2010a) *Front Line Care: Report by the Prime Minister's Commission on the Future of Nursing and Midwifery in England.* London: DoH.

Department of Health (2010b) *Advanced Level Nursing: A Position Statement.* London: DoH.

Department of Health (2011) *Enabling Excellence: Autonomy and Accountability for Health and Social Care Staff.* London: DoH.

Dimond, B. (2005). *Legal Aspects of Nursing,* 4th edn. Harlow: Pearson Education.

Duncan, B., Smith, A. and Silver, M. (1971) Comparison of the physical assessment of children by pediatric nurse practitioners and pediatricians. *American Journal of Public Health* 61(6): 1170–1176.

Dunn, L. (1997) A literature review of advanced clinical nursing practice in the United States. *Journal of Advanced Nursing* 25: 814–819.

Dunnett, C. and Gent, M. (1977) Significance testing to establish equivalence between treatments, with special reference to data in the form of 2x2 tables. *Biometrics* 33(4): 593–602.

Fleming, E. and Carberry, M. (2011) Steering a course towards advanced nurse practitioner: A critical care perspective. *Nursing in Critical Care* 16(2): 67–76.

Friej, R.M., Duffy, T., Hackett, D., Cunningham, D. and Fothergill, J. (1996) Radiographic interpretation by NPs in a minor injuries unit. *Journal of Accident and Emergency Medicine* 13: 41–43.

Gardner, G., Chang, A. and Duffield, C. (2007) Making nursing work: Breaking through the role confusion of advanced practice nursing. *Journal of Advanced Nursing* 57(4): 382–391.

Grant, C., Nicholas, R., Moore, L. and Salisbury, C. (2002) An observational study comparing quality of care in walk-in centres with general practice and NHS Direct using standardised patients. *British Medical Journal* 324(7353): 1556–1566.

Greenhalgh, C., Roberts, J. and Hill, I. (1994) *The Interface between Junior Doctors and Nurses: A Research Study for the Department of Health.* Macclesfield: Greenhalgh and Co.

Griffiths, P. (1996) Clinical led outcomes for nurse-led inpatient care. *Nursing Times* 92(9): 40–43.

Hamric, A. and Spross, J. (eds) *The Clinical Nurse Specialist in Theory and Practice.* Philadelphia, PA: W.B. Saunders.

Horrocks, S., Anderson, E. and Salisbury, C. (2002) Systematic review of whether nurse practitioners working in primary care can provide equivalent care to doctors. *British Medical Journal* 324: 819–823.

James, M. and Pyrgos, N. (1989) Nurse practitioners in the Accident and Emergency department. *Archives of Emergency Medicine* 6: 241–246.

Jones, B., Jarvis, P., Lewis, J. and Ebbutt, A. (1996) Trials to assess equivalence: The importance of rigorous methods. *British Medical Journal* 313: 36–39.

Kinley, H., Czoski-Murray, C., George, S. et al. (2002) Effectiveness of appropriately trained nurses in pre-operative assessment: Randomised controlled equivalence/non-inferiority trial. *British Medical Journal* 325: 1323–1327.

Kinnersley, P., Parry, K., Clement, J. et al. (2000) Randomised controlled rrial of nurse practitioner versus general practitioner care for patients requesting same day consultations in primary care. *British Medical Journal* 320: 1043–1044.

Lattimer, V., George, S., Thompson, F. et al. (1998) Safety and effectiveness of nurse telephone consultation in out of hours primary care: Randomised controlled trial. *British Medical Journal* 317: 1054–1059.

Laurant, M., Reeves, D., Hermens, R., Braspenning, J. and Sibbald, R. (2004). Substitution of doctors by nurses in primary care. *The Cochrane Database of Systematic Reviews,* Issue 4, Art No: CD001271.pub2. DOI:10.1002/ 14651858. (Edited with no change to conclusions 2009.)

Lee, T.W., Skelton, R.E. and Skene, C. (2001). Routine neonatal examination: Effectiveness of trainee paediatrician compared with nurse practitioners. *Archives of Disease in Childhood Foetal Neonatal Edition* 85: F100–F104.

Leslie, A. and Stephenson, T. (2003). Neonatal transfers by advanced neonatal nurse practitioners and paediatric registrars. *Archives of Disease in Childhood Foetal Neonatal Edition* 88: F509–F512.

Lewis, C. and Resnik, B. (1967) Nurse clinics and progressive ambulatory patient care. *New England Journal of Medicine* 277: 1236–1241.

Lewis, C., Resnik, B., Schmidt, G. and Waxman, D. (1969) Activities, events and outcomes in ambulatory patient care. *New England Journal of Medicine* 280(12): 645–649.

Lloyd Jones, M. (2005) Role development and effective practice in specialist and advanced practice roles in acute hospital settings: Systematic review. *Journal of Advanced Nursing* 49(2): 191–209.

Luker, K., Austin, L., Hogg, C., Ferguson, B. and Smith, K. (1998) Nurse–patient relationships: The context of nurse prescribing. *Journal of Advanced Nursing* 28(2): 235–242.

Manley, K. (1997) A conceptual framework for advanced practice: An action research project operatiionalising an advanced nurse practitioner/consultant nurse role. *Journal of Clinical Nursing* 6: 179–190.

Mantzoukas, S. and Watkinson, S. (2006) Review of advanced nursing practice: The international literature and developing the generic features. *Journal of Clinical Nursing* 16: 28–37.

McGee, P. (2009) *Advanced Nursing Practice in Nursing and the Allied Health Professions.* Oxford: Wiley-Blackwell.

Meek, S., Kendall, J., Porter, J. and Freij, R. (1998) Can accident and emergency nurse practitioners interpret radiographs? A multicentre study. *Journal of Accident and Emergency Medicine* 15: 105–107.

Mitchell, A., Watts, J., Whyte, R. et al. (1991) Evaluation of graduating neonatal nurse practitioners. *Pediatrics* 88(4): 789–794.

Mitchell-DiCenso, A., Guyatt, G., Marrin, M. et al. (1996) A controlled study of nurse practitioners in neonatal intensive care. *Pediatrics* 98: 1143–1148.

National Health Service Management Executive (1991) *Junior Doctors: The New Deal.* London: NHSME.

National Leadership and Innovation Agency for Health (2010) *Framework for Advanced Nursing, Midwifery and Allied Health Professional Practice in Wales.* Llanharan: NLIAH.

NHS Education for Scotland (2012) Advanced Nursing Practice Toolkit. http://www.advancedpractice.scot.nhs.uk/ (accessed 18 February 2015).

Nursing and Midwifery Council (2005) *The Proposed Framework for the Standard of Post Registration Nursing.* London: NMC.

Nursing and Midwifery Council (2006) *Report on NMC Consultation on a Proposed Framework for the Standard for Post Registration Nursing.* London: NMC.

Nursing and Midwifery Council (2010) *Standards for Pre-Registration Nursing Education.* London: NMC.

Pearson, J. (2012) *The Pearson Report: A National Overview of Nurse Practitioner Legislation and Healthcare Issues.* Cranbury, NJ: NP Communications.

Por, J. (2008) A critical engagement with the concept of advanced nursing practice. *Journal of Nursing Management* 16: 84–90.

Pulcini, J. (2013) Advanced practice nursing: Beyond the basics. In S. DeNisco and A. Barker (eds), *Advanced Practice Nursing*, 2nd edn. Burlington, VT: Jones and Bartlett Learning.

Pulcini, J., Jelic, M., Gul, R. and Loke, A. (2009) An international survey on advanced practice nursing education, practice and regulation. *Journal of Nursing Scholarship* 42(1): 31–39.

Rashid, C. (2010) Benefits and limitations of nurses taking on aspects of the clinical role of doctors in primary care: Integrative literature review. *Journal of Advanced Nursing* 66(8): 1658–1670.

Richardson, G. and Maynard, A. (1995) Fewer Doctors? More Nurses? A Review of the Knowledge Base of Doctor-Nurse Substitution. Discussion Paper 135. York: Centre for Health Economics, University of York.

Roberts-Davis, M. and Read, S. (2001). Clinical role clarification: Using the Delphi method to establish similarities and differences between clinical nurse practitioners and clinical nurse specialists. *Journal of Clinical Nursing* 10: 33–43.

Royal College of Nursing (2012) *Advanced Nurse Practitioners: An RCN Guide to Advanced Nursing Practice, Advanced Nurse Practitioners and Programme Accreditation.* London: RCN.

Rushforth, H., Burge, D., Mullee, M. et al. (2006) Nurse-led pre operative assessment: An equivalence study. *Paediatric Nursing* 18(3): 23–29.

Sakr, M., Angus, J. and Perrin, J. (1999) Care of minor injuries by emergency nurse practitioners or junior doctors: A randomised controlled trial. *Lancet* 354: 1321–1326.

Salisbury, C. and Tettersell, M. (1988) Comparison of the work of a nurse practitioner with that of a general practitioner. *Journal of the Royal College of General Practitioners* 38: 314–316.

Sandhu, H., Dale, J., Stellard, N., Crouch, R. and Glucksman, E. (2009) Emergency nurse practitioners and doctors consulting with patients in an emergency department: A comparison of communiation skills and satisfaction. *Emergency Medicine Journal* 26: 400–404.

Sheer, B. and Wong, F. (2008) The development of advanced nursing practice globally. *Journal of Nursing Scholarship* 40(3): 204–2011.

Shum, C., Humphreys, A., Wheeler, D., Cochrane, M.A. and Clement, S. (2002) Nurse management of patients with minor illnesses in general practice:

Multicentre, randomised controlled trial. *British Medical Journal* 320: 1038–1043.

Skills for Health (2007) *Key Elements of Career Framework*. London, Skills for Health.

Smith, S. and Hall, M. (2011) Advanced neonatal nurse practitioners in the workforce: A review of the evidence to date. *Archives of Disease in Childhood Foetal and Neonatal Edition* 96: F151–F155.

Snow, T. (2010) New head of NMC prepares to end impasse on advanced practice. *Nursing Standard* 2(24): 21.

Sox, H.C. (1979) Quality of patient care by nurse practitioners and physicians assistants: A ten year perspective. *Annals of Internal Medicine* 91: 459–468.

Spitzer, W. (1978) Pediatric nurse practitioners. *New England Journal of Medicine* 298(3): 163–164.

Spitzer, W., Sackett, D.,Sibley, J. et al. (1974) The Burlington randomised trial of the nurse practitioner. *New England Journal of Medicine* 290: 251–256.

Thurston, J. and Field, S. (1996) Should accident and emergency nurses request radiographs? Results of a multicentre evaluation. *Journal of Accident and Emergency Medicine* 13: 86–89.

Touche Ross and Co. (1994) *Evaluation of Nurse Practitioner Pilot Projects, Summary Report*. London: NHSE, South Thames.

Tye, C., Ross, F. and Kerry, S.M. (1998) Emergency nurse practitioner services in major Accident and Emergency departments: A United Kingdon postal survey. *Journal of Accident and Emergency Medicine* 15: 31–34.

UKCC (1992) *The Scope of Professional Practice*. London: United Kingdom Central Council for Nursing, Midwifery and Health Visiting.

UKCC (1994) *The Future of Professional Practice: The Council's Standards for Education and Practice Following Registration*. London: UKCC.

UKCC (1999) *A Higher Level of Practice: Report of the Consultation on the UKCC's Proposals for a Revised Regulatory Framework for Post-Registration Clinical Practice*. London: UKCC.

Vaughan, B. (1988) The story of NDUs – how nursing, midwifery and health visiting nursing development unit programme began. *Journal of Research in Nursing* 3(4): 272–274.

Venning, P., Durie, A., Roland, M., Roberts, C. and Leese, B. (2000) RCT comparing the effectiveness of GPs and NPs in primary care. *British Medical Journal* 320: 1048–1053.

Whitely, M., Wilmott, K. and Galland, R. (1997) A specialist nurse can replace pre-registration house officers in surgical pre-admission clinic. *Annals of the Royal College of Surgeons of England* 79: 257–260.

Williams, V., Smith. A., Chapman, L. and Oliver, D. (2010) Community matrons: An explanatory study of patients' views and experiences. *Journal of Advanced Nursing* 67(1): 86–93.

Williamson, S., Twelvetree, T., Thompson, J. and Beaver, K. (2012) An ethnographic study exploring the role of ward-based advanced nurse practitioners in an acute medical setting. *Journal of Advanced Nursing* 68(7): 1579–1588.

Advanced nursing practice: Education for competence

Lynne Gaskell, Susan Beaton and Lillian Neville

Chapter outline

- Introduction
- Governance
- Key characteristics and competencies
- Collaboration between higher education and the health service
- The business case
- Triangulation of assessment
- Clinical skills logs
- Individual learning pathway
- Portfolio development
- Direct observation
- Work-based learning
- Methods of assessing competencies
- Work-based assessors
- Work-based case studies
- Service evaluation of advanced practitioner roles
- Conclusion

Introduction

This chapter will focus on aspects of education that are relevant to developing the competencies of advanced practice. While it is acknowledged that on a global level there is no consensus on a definition of advanced practice, nor how it should be governed, there are some important commonalities. As authors, we have drawn on our wide experience of facilitating learning on advanced practitioner programmes and offer examples of assessment strategies that have been used both to develop and to test competence in relation to advanced practice. Examples of the experience of clinical assessors are included that highlight the value of work-based learning in this important field of practice. For the purpose of this chapter all aspects are related to advanced nurse practitioners (ANPs), although they may apply to other professionals employed or training in an advanced practice role.

Governance

Advanced nurse practitioners must meet the professional standards and requirements mandated by their location's regulatory body. All ANPs are personally accountable for their actions and must be able to justify their decisions using appropriate evidence. They are professionally accountable to their regulator, as well as having a contractual accountability to their employer, and they are accountable in law for their actions (Shannon 2012: 7). It is inherent in ANP roles that new responsibilities are taken on and therefore there is a need for organizations to ensure that robust governance arrangements, surrounding all types and levels of practice, are in place prior to their establishment. This is necessary in order to allow ANP roles to function fully. New professional support arrangements, which recognize the nature of the role and the responsibilities involved, will be required and existing professional support mechanisms may not be sufficient. This approach offers the most effective means of controlling risks to service user safety from an individual professional's practice and provides a proportionate response. Good governance regarding role development and implementation must, therefore, be based on consistent expectations of the level of practice required to deliver the service. This is best achieved through benchmarking such posts against nationally agreed standards and processes.

Concern about 'new' roles is both prudent and understandable. It has been argued that risks to service user safety arise when professionals take on roles and responsibilities for which they lack competence or where they practise without adequate safeguards. However, work by the Council for Healthcare Regulatory Excellence (CHRE 2009) has emphasized that the activities that professionals undertake at advanced-level practice do not lie beyond the scope of existing regulation, unless the nature of their practice changes to such a significant extent that their scope of practice is fundamentally different from that at initial registration. It is proposed that advanced-level practice reflects a set of responsibilities, competencies and capabilities that act as an indicator of a particular stage on the career development ladder, and that such practitioners are always accountable to their regulatory body whatever the level or context of practice (NLIAH 2010: 34).

ANPs are practising in a number of countries, including the USA, Canada, Australia, New Zealand and the UK. The International Council of Nurses (ICN; Affara, 2005) states within its Standards for ANP Education that 'Advanced Practice has its foundations in educational institutions that are recognised by accrediting/approving bodies of the specific nation or international community' (2005: 5). Master's-level education is recommended, with curricula being specific to each country and its healthcare system.

The core competencies for advanced nursing practice roles that the ICN has developed reflect the international value of the nursing profession. The ICN suggests that academic programmes preparing ANPs should adhere to the following four guidelines:

- Provide students with the opportunity to gain knowledge, experience and the necessary skills to function competently in the role of the ANP.
- Prepare the nurse to practise in the national context.
- Staff programmes with qualified faculty and have them accredited by the authorized national body.
- Ensure that programmes facilitate lifelong learning and the maintenance of competency.

In the UK, current government policy is to reduce regulation. The Nursing Midwifery Council (NMC), as the regulatory body along with the Health and Care Professions Council (HCPC), has no plans to implement a separate professional register for ANPs. Although the Prime Minister's Commission on the Future of Nursing and Midwifery (2010) recommended that the NMC 'must regulate ANP practice, ensuring that they are recorded as such on the register and have the required competencies', this is no longer either government or professional policy.

The concept of advanced practice in the UK is at a pivotal point in its development, with position papers regarding the role from the governments of England, Wales and Scotland (Scottish Government 2010; NHS Wales 2010). What is agreed, however, is that all clinicians working at an advanced level are expected to demonstrate expertise in a core set of competencies. Governance of qualified ANPs is the responsibility of the individual professional (within the bounds of their current registration) and their employers (through job descriptions and local governance arrangements).

The Australian Nursing and Midwifery Council (ANMC) has developed standards against which ANPs practising in Australia are assessed in order to obtain and retain their licence to practise. Universities in Australia also use the standards when developing curricula and to assess student performance (ANF 2005).

Canadian provincial registering nursing organizations have identified clinical expertise as one of the fundamental criteria of ANP practice (Donnelly 2003). In Canada regulation is the responsibility of the province in which the ANP is practising. In some provinces formal ANP education can be either at baccalaureate or master's level. However, those who have graduated from a master's-level programme are not required to undergo the Detailed Competency Assessment Process before taking the registration exams (written and objective structured clinical examination, OSCE).

The minimum education required to become an ANP in the USA is a graduate degree (AANP 2007). After completing their MSc, NP students in the USA must pass the licensing exam in their specialty before they can begin to practise (APRNJDG 2008). It may be argued that the public can be confident that students who pass the exam have demonstrated a standard level of knowledge and reasoning skills, regardless of the university in which they trained. After passing the exam, individuals are licensed as ANP registered nurses and can legally use the 'nurse practitioner' title. Falsely identifying oneself as an ANP in the USA is a criminal act and carries penalties that can include fines or a jail term (Board of Registered Nursing 2009).

In the UK, where ANPs are not licensed or have their own registration with the NMC, there is not even agreement on what the name of the role should be. It was recognized, however, that introducing the ANP role had the potential to enhance the existing capacity and capability of the workforce, helping to deliver service improvements (Swift 2009) and, more recently, to help deliver the NHS's Quality, Innovation, Productivity and Prevention (QIPP) agenda (Neville and Swift 2012). Guidance has been provided by the RCN Advanced Practitioner competencies (RCN 2008), NHS Scotland's Advanced Nurse Practitioner toolkit (Scottish Government 2010), NHS Wales's Advanced Practitioner Framework (2010) and in a position statement on Advanced Level Nursing (DoH, 2010). However, most of this guidance encompasses only one profession and does not take account of ANP roles outside of nursing; only the Welsh document covers nursing and allied health professionals.

Thus, in the UK it seems likely that for the foreseeable future, governance will remain the concern of individual ANPs and their employers. Consequently, it is incumbent on individual ANPs to document evidence of the impact of their role, while universities need to ensure that ANP students are equipped with the relevant knowledge and skills to engage in this process post-qualification (Neville and Swift 2012). For example, providing opportunities to engage in auditing practice and service evaluations and development should be an integral part of the assessment process. ANPs also need to develop skills in selecting and recording good-quality evidence within a professional portfolio. This is strongly advocated by the Royal College of Nursing (2012).

Key characteristics and competencies

This book emphasizes throughout that advanced practice may be conceptualized in many ways. It may be viewed philosophically, ethically, as a concept, as a level of practice and expertise, as a career pathway, or indeed as a role with competencies. To meet the needs of our discussion in this chapter, we will focus at this point on 'role' and 'competencies'.

Key characteristics to be achieved in order to undertake the role of an advanced nurse practitioner have been defined within the concordat for advanced practice (NHS Northwest 2009). That agreement includes the following:

- Definitions of advanced nurse practice.
- Common characteristics of the advanced practitioner role.
- The agreed level of education and development required for this role.
- Guidance about the current level for the post.
- An outline of the differences between a number of cadres of practitioners.

The role is described as multi-professional and clinical in focus, functioning at level 7 of the Career Framework for Health (Skills for Health 2006).

For England, the Department of Health in its 2010 position paper identified four themes under which all competencies should be benchmarked:

- Clinical/direct care or practice.
- Leadership and collaborative practice.
- Improving the quality and developing the practice.
- The development of self and others.

The expectation is that nurses working at advanced levels will have achieved these competencies following a structured academic and clinical curriculum at master's level.

Master's degree preparation is used widely for ANPs, as advocated by the ICN (2008). A majority of countries participating in a recent study reported that the importance of appropriate educational opportunities is key in the development of ANP roles (Delamaire and Lafortune 2010). Master's-level preparation serves as a professionalizing strategy that legitimizes the achievement of graduates. The award enhances the credibility of ANPs in the eyes of the public, employers and colleagues, particularly medical staff (Gerrish et al. 2003). There is broad agreement that the development of master's degree programmes needs to be innovative in order to meet the clinical, leadership, research and autonomous requirements of ANPs in response to changes in technology, demographics, politics, consumer knowledge, litigation and the demands of an efficient and effective health service (Ham 2003; Callaghan 2008; Richardson and Cunliffe 2003).

ANPs need to be assessed against established competencies to determine their cost and clinical effectiveness within a modern NHS. Demonstrating improvements in patient and service outcomes has been deemed essential, since service costs may not be significantly different between ANPs and their medical peers (Venning et al. 2000; Kleinpell and Gawlinski 2005; Bryant-Lukosius and DiCenso 2004).

Collaboration between higher education and the health service

Collaboration between students, employers and higher education institutions can enable both managers and students to unravel the network of factors affecting advanced nursing practice in health and social care. Additionally, collaborative working can help to create opportunities to facilitate and audit change (Livesley et al. 2009).

Commissioning flexible, collaborative and service-led educational programmes can assist in ensuring that change is sustainable and produce practitioners who are fit for practice, purpose and award. Inherent within the concept of ANP is the assumption that the goal is to improve the patient's experience in a cost-effective and efficient manner (Callaghan 2008; Por 2008). The need for the role and the context of the service should be clearly articulated through a service redesign specification, a job description and a person specification to ensure a sustainable and economically viable workforce and service provision (Acton Shapiro 2009).

The business case

As we stated at the beginning of this chapter, we aim here to use our experience of facilitating education and advanced nursing practice competence. To that end, we now specifically draw on a business case in which we have participated, a collaboration between the NHS in North West England and a higher education institute (HEI).

As part of the changes to the NHS brought about by the Health and Social Care Act 2012, Primary Care Trusts (PCTs) and Strategic Health Authorities (SHAs) ceased to exist on 31 March 2013. Their responsibilities were taken over by Clinical Commissioning Groups and the NHS Trust Development Authority. At the time, Northwest NHS produced a good practice guide and checklist for the introduction of new roles. Based on the NHS National Practitioner Programme, the guide offers a framework of nine points, each with an aide-mémoire to ensure that all relevant factors have been considered:

- Advanced nurse practitioner role description.
- Service needs analysis.
- Education, training and development.
- The new AP role.
- The learning environment.
- Management and assessment roles, arrangements, accountability and supervision.
- Communication.
- Safety and effectiveness.
- Costs and sustainability of the service.

The framework is used in the development of a business case to support the introduction of any new trainee ANPs. All parties sign a partnership agreement that details the roles, responsibilities and expectations of managers, mentors, assessors, higher education institutes and Northwest NHS. A collaborative process assists each partner to clarify their unique contribution to the training of ANPs, and facilitates an evidence-based framework for the implementation of advanced nursing practice, with recognition of the importance of environmental factors and an organizational infrastructure for new roles (Rutherford et al. 2005; Bryant-Lukosius and DiCenso 2004).

Advanced nursing practice is contingent on context; it is not a homogeneous role, since heterogeneity is a key feature (Mantsoukas and Watkinson 2006; Abbott 2007). The continued developments in health and social care have resulted in the need for ANPs to take greater responsibility, autonomy and accountability for developing service provision. In an interpretive, qualitative examination of ANP roles, Gardner et al. (2007) found that ANPs' roles included different aspects of management, education, clinical service and consultancy, and that some ANP roles spanned several specialty environments. ANPs described their advanced skill in direct clinical care as the ability to respond quickly to the demands of clinical practice in a changing and demanding age, taking a lead in service improvements and meeting the requirements laid out in the knowledge and skills framework, providing opportunities for their future career advancement. Interprofessional collaboration and networking to promote the ANP role are essential to demonstrate the significance and role of ANPs in providing care, reducing healthcare costs and developing innovative models of care as appropriate (Brooten et al. 2012). Therefore, while the core of advanced nursing practice should be constant (Nursing and Midwifery Council 2008; ICN 2008), bespoke elements of the role, such as surgical interventions and specialized investigations and treatments, will be contingent on the needs of the patients to whom the service is being delivered (Acton Shapiro 2009; Scottish Government 2010).

Interviews for the trainee ANP position are completed with representatives from the HEI, service managers and workplace assessors present. It is important that each potential candidate is assessed on clinical and academic suitability for the programme. The interview may involve questions and discussions on a number of unseen clinical cases and/or scenarios involving risk, interdisciplinary teamworking and legal/ethical decision making. Alternatively, the students give formal presentations of how they will develop their role within the department to affect the service and improve patient care. The interview tasks allow the interview panel to differentiate students who are prepared and have vision regarding their trainee ANP role and clinical reasoning skills.

In addition, clear communication between stakeholders and strong partnerships between employers and the HEI can ensure that the individual ANP's progress is monitored from the beginning of the programme. Finally, organizational readiness and collaboration with the education providers are fundamental to ensure that the full potential of ANPs is realized.

The university programme

The University of Salford MSc Advanced Practice Programme is monitored by an advisory board that meets two to three times annually. The board consists of health service commissioners, employers, advanced

Table 3.1 Modular programme overview

	Semester 1	Semester 2	Semester 3	Credits
Year 1	Principles Advanced Practice (30)		Contextualising Advanced Practice (30)	60
Portfolio	Individual Learning Pathway	Tripartite Agreement Core and Bespoke Skills	Organisational Pathway Analysis	30
Year 2	Research Methods (30)	Advanced Practitioner Competence (30) Clinical Reasoning (30)		90

nursing practice students and academic staff. Within these meetings key decisions regarding programme developments and assessments are made that take into account stakeholders' needs.

The programme runs over 45 weeks a year and advanced practice students are allowed two days each week for training. Often one day is university based and the second day is used to develop clinical competency/experience/mentorship and engage in work-based assessments. The modular programme (see Table 3.1) consists of core elements including life sciences, clinical assessment diagnosis and project management, as well as evidence-based practice and leadership, and has a strong focus on work-based learning.

Formative assessment and development of competencies

Students are encouraged to be actively engaged with every stage of the assessment, in order that they truly understand the requirements of the process and the criteria and standards being applied to facilitate deeper learning, as advocated by Rust et al. (2005). Explicit within the timetable are revision sessions, as well as opportunities for verbal feedback from lecturers and peers. Students rate timely, specific and detailed feedback as very important in developing and improving their skills by identifying weaknesses and providing positive reinforcement for the enhancement of skill development (Aliner 2003; HEA 2009). Explicit learning outcomes for modules and assessments are provided at the beginning of the module and within it.

Discussion around assessment guidelines, marking criteria, active engagement in tutorials, group discussion and feedback is actively encouraged. Creating and negotiating individual criteria are encouraged during formative teaching and assessment sessions. Feedback is seen as a dialogue rather than a monologue and is given both individually and as a group session, as advocated by Angelo (2008). The interaction of being self-directed and using assessments formatively has been shown to promote greater educational achievement (Brown et al. 2007). Explicit links between assessment strategies from module to module are used to consolidate and contextualize learning.

Triangulation of assessment

Strategies can be designed to evaluate clinical skills development; clinical reasoning; problem solving and testing the underpinning clinical science in addition to research; and communication and teamworking skills. Through exploring clinical themed objective structured clinical examinations (OSCE), multiple choice questions (MCQ), written assignments, vivas, written examinations and practice-assessed clinical cases and skills, it can be argued that this approach to educational competency assessment provides depth and breadth as well as triangulation to the assessment process.

Objective structured clinical examination or assessment (OSCE/OSCA)

The OSCE is defined as a circuit of assessment stations where an examiner assesses a range of practical clinical skills using a previously determined objective marking scheme (Selby 1995). The OSCE tests the student's communication skills, underlying anatomical/pathological knowledge and ability to perform a systematic patient assessment within a given timeframe. It evaluates practical skills and communication, which are dependent on each other for cooperation and concordance (Pfeil 2001; Aliner 2003). This form of examination is used in the earlier part of the master's-level programme, where the student has received taught theoretical content and has already had the opportunity to engage in supervised practice within their employing organization, as advocated by Ward and Barrett (2005) and Roberts and Fenton (2012). In terms of validity, OSCE stations involve model patients briefed on their role, assessors marking against specific criteria and moderators working across stations to ensure parity of assessment. It can also be classed as best practice to involve external clinical assessors and verifiers in this assessment to ensure its validity.

OSCEs are variable and in some cases they can assess skills such as insertion of vascular lines, airway intubation, communication skills and aspects of specific clinical examination. To ensure parity, each OSCE station is structured into five sections and assessors give a verbal instruction to commence that aspect of the exam. Moderators rotate between stations to ensure parity of prompting, clarity of questions and awarding of marks. Utilizing the same assessors for individual stations and having a consistent pool of assessors within the module teams improves the overall reliability of the assessment process (O'Neill and McCall 1996).

Biological systems may be used to structure the OSCE, most commonly the six core systems of respiratory, cardiovascular, abdominal, musculoskeletal, neurological and mental health. Students are required to pass each component on a grade, which is an award of 2 out of 4. No compensation is allowed between sections of any particular OSCE. Referral on any station would necessitate the student not passing the module overall and hence needing to be reassessed on that particular station during the resit period.

The design and assessment criteria for OSCE examinations vary from on HEI to another, but our experience shows us that the core principles that HEIs use are consistent and equitable. Students' criticisms of OSCEs have included the fact that (depending on how the stations are designed) they represent only a 'snapshot' rather than a whole examination, and that they are commonly conducted on 'healthy patients' (actors). However, a section linking life sciences, pathology and clinical skills and rationale for procedures can test clinical reasoning. Furthermore, increasing the number of OSCE scenarios ensures assessment on a breadth of knowledge and skills, which can easily and flexibly be aligned with the curriculum and enables students to be flexible, adaptable employees in a rapidly changing health arena.

There is insufficient evidence to show whether OSCE assessments can measure competence, despite the process being embedded in the assessment of students across the health professions, postgraduate medical education and ANP programmes. Two studies did demonstrate an improvement in performance after OSCE, however (Mason et al. 2005; Baez 2005).

Reported benefits of OSCEs include enhancement of skills acquisition through a hands-on approach, the opportunity for students to practise skills in a safe and controlled environment and the opportunity to combine both teaching and assessment. Furthermore, OSCEs have been identified as a satisfactory way of assessing communication, clinical skills, knowledge and intention by a number of authors (Short et al. 2009; Rennie and Main 2006; Aliner 2006).

However, OSCEs have been reported in some studies to be costly to run and time consuming (Aliner 2003; Mason et al. 2005). A

number of studies reported the OSCE setting to be stressful or intimidating for participants – although none of these compared the level
of stress to other forms of formal examination (Chabeli 2001;
Franklin 2005). Time constraints at each station can also limit the
ability for reflection. Inconsistencies between assessors and actors
have been reported as a source of frustration and inconsistency for
those being examined.

Viva voce examinations

The viva voce involves extended pieces of work such as patient assessment and management/poster presentations, which may be partly
assessed by an oral examination. In these situations, the viva voce is a
useful tool to assist in authenticating that the work is that of the student
and allows a flexible method of discussing and reviewing aspects of the
student's work in detail.

Carrochio and Burke (2010) advocate that various assessments are
needed to test the integration of competencies across the whole educational and clinical continuum. The viva can be identified as a link to
connect competencies to the real world of practice. One of the key
competencies pertaining to clinical practice involves the presentation of
the findings from the patient assessment to the clinical assessor. To be
able to perform this efficiently, the student needs to have knowledge of
the signs and symptoms of illness, undertake an examination of the
patient, formulate a management plan and communicate this to their
assessor.

The viva aims to measure clinical competence in an authentic manner
and to demonstrate clinical reasoning and professional communication
skills (Ryding and Murphy 1999). It offers the opportunity to test both
clinical and academic knowledge and skills that are closely aligned to
daily clinical practice. The viva should be based on a real case that has
been verified by the student assessor and enhanced to fit the programme
requirements. Both Ryder and Murphy (1999) and Cobourne (2010)
have demonstrated that the viva is a viable and reliable approach to
assessing clinical reasoning.

Poster presentation

This assessment allows students to demonstrate an understanding of
physiology at postgraduate level by relating pathophysiology and pharmacology to an individual patient or patient group. The student presents their knowledge to the two examiners and is then questioned on the
content of their poster. This assessment format allows the student to

demonstrate in-depth knowledge, but may increase stress in students who struggle with some of the concepts of 'hard science'.

Multiple choice question examinations (MCQs)

MCQ examinations allow assessment of students' knowledge in specific educational contexts, such as factual science subjects. They are valuable in the assessment of anatomy and physiology in the taught content of the advanced practice programme curriculum. The major parameter that MCQs assess is factual knowledge, but with careful attention to question formulation it has been argued that critical thinking and different cognitive categories such as comprehension, application and analysis can also be tested (Morrison and Free 2001).

MCQs are used to test the breadth rather than the depth of knowledge. They have the advantage of greater differentiation of ability by of the minimal writing involved, which permits the assessment of a larger body of knowledge; the ability to cover a higher number of subjects; encouragement of background reading; elimination of communication skills as a discriminator; lack of disadvantage for those with poor written skills; and not penalizing a candidate with poor grammar, handwriting or articulation. Disadvantages include not permitting construction and presentation of an argument; failure to assess novel ideas and innovative thinking; and not assessing the best answer or risk, especially in professional exams.

Written examinations

In our advanced practice MSc, students research around complex cases and sit a two-hour examination on the assessment, differential diagnosis and management of these. The cases may include patient groups that are not from within their own area of practice, such as paediatrics, elderly or palliative care. They may have psychological or serious pathologies and involve a broad multi-disciplinary team, integrating anatomy, physiology, pharmokinetics, imaging, medical and surgical management and health promotion issues. Written examinations provide evidence of authenticity, which guarantees that the student's work is their own and guards against the potential for plagiarism. Students have the opportunity to discuss evidence-based clinical examination, investigations, differential diagnosis and a management plan with evidence of clinical reasoning and contemporary guidelines/QIPP agenda where appropriate. Risk, ethical, legal, psychosocial and holistic aspects of care can also be considered.

Clinical skills logs

Given the wide range of clinical specialties from which students are drawn, along with considerable variance in their experience and skills, they are required to achieve competency in a number of core skills, including the six core systems of musculoskeletal, neurological, cardio-vascular, respiratory, abdominal and mental health. Students are expected to have the opportunity to practise and develop these skills through the taught university sessions and workshops, and skills acquisition progresses from the opportunity to observe through to practising regularly with and without supervision. Gaskell and Beaton (2010) suggest that teaching and assessing levels of competency in the core systems requires a pool of experienced, clinical assessors competent in teaching and assessing across the range of specialties. Skills are system specific and include observation, palpation, auscultation and special tests appropriate to the system. While the optional or bespoke skills that ANPs identify become extremely important, the exact focus for their work as an ANP determines the extent and level to which these skills are needed (Bryant-Lukosius and DiCenso 2004).

Individual learning pathway

In our MSc, trainee ANPs negotiate an individual learning pathway (ILP) based on the ANP competencies and the specific needs of the service. This may encompass both core and bespoke knowledge and skills and is agreed by the manager, student and clinical supervisor. Evidence of achievement is collected in a portfolio, which is formally assessed. On completion, the student will not only have the necessary knowledge and skills to undertake the role, but will also be able to identify, measure and record the impact of their role.

One possible organizing framework for the ILP and the portfolio is that developed by the Faculty of Emergency Nursing (www.fen.uk.com), described as the 'Elements of Advanced Practice'. This includes 51 sub-elements of ANP grouped into four themes:

- Knowledge
- Intervention
- Patient/client management
- Development of themselves and others

The milestones in the ILP provide a developmental roadmap for the individual student's competencies and sub-elements. They are behavioural

Table 3.2 Example of one sub-element personalized by an AP student in their ILP

THE ELEMENTS OF ADVANCED PRACTICE

ELEMENT 1: KNOWLEDGE

Code & subject	Personalised Competency Statements	Method of achievement (generating evidence) – Resources: taught, independent, clinical	Skills required for role & possible timescales
1.1 Anatomy & Physiology	Apply extensive knowledge of anatomy, physiology and psychology to differentiate a wide range of patient presentations with complex care needs, to determine the appropriate diagnosis **Aims:** Increase knowledge of: Respiratory system Cardiovascular system Neurological system Kidney function Liver function Gastro-intestinal system Metabolic and endocrine system Musculoskeletal system Biochemistry Haematology Oncology Apply greater knowledge of critical care pathophysiology	**Taught:** First two modules **Independent learning:** Personal study, extensive reading of pathophysiology text books and on-line Tortora resources **Clinical:** Learning from mentors and assessors. Working in critical care areas. Clinical workshops arranged by LF **Resources:** Oncology CNS	Building a portfolio of skills Build upon existing knowledge and skills Formal assessment – clinical and academic **Time frame:** Currently identify myself as Advanced beginner Aim to be competent by 2 years Proficient in 3 years Expert in 3 to 5 years

descriptions of the progression of knowledge, skills and attitudes that define each of the sub-competencies' domains. They serve to inform learners of where they are and the knowledge, skills and attitudes they require to progress to the next level(s). Evidence of achievement is contained within a portfolio.

Professional activities represent the core clinical activities of an ANP, appropriately scaled to level of experience. Performing these four core elements requires the ANP to integrate the competencies and sub-elements. Since the milestones map directly to the sub-elements, they help to pinpoint at what level in the developmental progression a student is performing and to address any specific sub-elements that may be a barrier to graduation. Specific milestones must be reached for competence and a pass mark to be achieved. Additionally, the local context and tripartite agreement between the student, assessor and learning facilitator are important in prioritizing which additional competencies and sub-competencies are highlighted.

Portfolio development

Portfolios are evidence of the development of knowledge and skills, are patient focused and should evaluate clinical outcomes/services in line with government incentives, as advocated by Oermann and Floyd (2002) and Wilkinson et al. (2002). Sargent (2003) suggests that APs should evaluate their role against core ANP competencies and include a practitioner enquiry/service review to evaluate the impact on patient care. Quality indicators should include the reduction of waiting times, better outcomes, reduced length of stay, inappropriate referrals and reduced overall costs (Furlong and Smith 2005; Richardson and Cunliffe 2003; McCormack 2009).

A report commissioned by the Carnegie Foundation (Cooke et al. 2010) to review medical education and make recommendations outlines four goals that are key to the development of the portfolio concept:

- Standardization of learning outcomes and individualization of the learning process.
- Integration of formal knowledge and the individual clinical experience.
- Development of enquiry and innovation.
- Focus on professional identity.

A portfolio has been described as 'a collection of materials chosen by an individual to provide evidence of skills, knowledge, attitudes and achievements that reflect the current development and activity of that individual' (Byrne et al. 2007: 24). It relies on a level of self-regulation, writing and critical reflection on the part of the individual being assessed. While studies report the use of portfolios both as a personal development tool and an assessment tool, there is currently insufficient evidence to show whether they can measure competence (McCready 2006). However, they do provide an opportunity for individuals to document evidence of learning outcomes and processes, personal and professional development and areas for further development (Endacott et al. 2004).

Portfolios may be used in a variety of ways. There is a continuum from a collection of superficial evidence to a deep and meaningful array of evidence that is well signposted and earns its place in the individual's portfolio. However, all the evidence included must be authentic, sufficient, relevant and current. At its best, a portfolio should demonstrate the sum of an individual's worth as a practitioner. In the context of advanced practice preparation, this should be the culmination of the student's journey from commencing the programme to qualification as an ANP.

On our master's degree, as with many others, there is a specific module at the end of the programme that is assessed by the final version of the portfolio. This has been supported by employers, education commissioners, students and academic staff, as it demonstrates evidence of competence and the impact of the trainee ANP role. At the end of this module, students will be able to demonstrate evidence of:

- Critical engagement with everyday practice through reflection and action.
- Collaborative and ongoing evaluation of practice through audit and service development.
- Advancement of knowledge and skills through clinical cases and skills.
- New knowledge about the transformation of self through reflexivity with reference to the individual learning pathway.
- An ability to select appropriate, high-quality evidence.

Portfolio processes

Signposting the evidence

A list of evidence should be accompanied by a grid or matrix that demonstrates how the evidence relates to the organizing framework. Each piece of evidence must earn its place and must therefore be meaningful to the student in relation to their specific ANP role. As there is no opportunity to defend the portfolio verbally, the student needs to narrate the evidence carefully, making it clear to the reader why it is included and what they wish the reader to understand by its presence.

Triangulation of evidence

This requires the student to present three pieces of diverse evidence against a particular sub-element of advanced practice to add weight to the portfolio. For example, a clinical case, a reflection and a testimonial can be combined to show the student's competence from different angles. It is important that triangulation is only used when there is strong evidence against the sub-element. Over-use of triangulation can be meaningless and dilutes the overall strength of the portfolio.

Breadth of evidence

Students should demonstrate a wide variety of sources and avoid over-reliance on one particular type of evidence, for example clinical cases.

Depth of evidence

The quality of evidence should be at a high level, commensurate with advanced practice and master's degree level. Students should provide an evaluation of activities such as teaching and give some commentary regarding learning points and future development.

Types of evidence for inclusion in the portfolio

Reflection

Reflection is a core concept in nurse education at both pre- and post-registration levels. It assists nurses to maintain and improve their practice by identifying strengths and areas that may need to be further developed and gives them conscious control over their practice (Cowan et al. 2007). However, some ANP students do not initially demonstrate the ability to reflect on learning using an appropriate model. They often rely on a model that they used as pre-registration students, which may not be the most appropriate for reflection at a higher level of study. Using a variety of reflective models demonstrates the student's ability to select the most appropriate model for the specific experience.

Reflective writing, risk assessment and change management

These are key to the student's development in a variety of ANP competencies. Such evidence may be generated as a result of a critical incident or an extract from a reflective journal. Some questions to prompt the discussion could include:

- Was the process influenced by professional or national guidelines, tools or frameworks?
- Did it result in a change in practice/change in the patient's or client's management?
- Was there any resistance, and if so from whom?
- How did you or could you have dealt with it?
- What professional knowledge, skills and personal attributes do you have or do you think that you need to develop in order to manage the change?
- What theoretical underpinnings have you drawn on to make your decisions?

Audit

Audits of new or existing services are frequently included in AP students' portfolios. They may be used to evaluate specific clinical interventions on validated outcomes, including waiting times, patient satisfaction, review of critical incidents and functional outcomes. McCormack (2009) suggests that ANPs are best placed for this role since they are engaged with everyday practice, evaluation of practice through audit and research enquiry. Students may also decide to include audits of their own practice to demonstrate competence in specific areas. For example, it may be possible to audit a sample of case notes and compare the final and differential diagnoses with the notes at a later stage in the patient's journey. It is likely that the student can then deduce the accuracy of diagnosis and the relevance of investigations ordered. On reflection, there may be specific learning points and areas for future development.

Garbett and McCormack (2002) suggest that practitioners who are committed to continuous, rigorous processes of change reflecting the perspectives of service users and providers can transform the culture and context of care.

Other types of evidence

There is a plethora of potential evidence that can be used from the ANP student's everyday practice. The following list serves as an example of types of evidence that have been used and signposted effectively:

- Research critiques
- Literature reviews
- Critical incident analysis
- Documentation produced, e.g. policy, patient pathways, guidelines along with minutes of meetings
- Published work
- Testimonials
- Programme-generated work
- Teaching materials
- Certificates accompanied by evaluation of learning in relation to the AP role

Students can disseminate their portfolios to managers and commissioners of services. It is imperative that ANPs can showcase their work and network with peers to improve and standardize practice with best evidence. Gaskell and Beaton (2010) suggest that the portfolio should provide evidence of teamwork, open communication and collaborative working, all of which are crucial to productivity and enable other members to take risks and grow professionally while striving for a common purpose.

Direct observation

Direct observation has been proposed as a useful tool for prior learning assessment. There is currently little evidence to determine the effectiveness of direct observation as a method for assessing competence, however. Potential issues include the need for assessors to be familiar with the clinical and practical setting of the assessment and the impact of direct observation on the reliability of results.

Brown (2002), in a survey of 150 clinical mentors in university settings in the UK, identified that, while 80% felt that consistent supervision was given in a supportive environment, 30% considered that areas of practice that require evaluation are not identified on a regular basis. The survey highlighted the importance of nurses involved in direct observation having a good understanding of the role and expectations of the individual being assessed, as well as an understanding of the range of learning opportunities available outside the limitations of the assessment. Issues highlighted for consideration in relation to direct observation included the need for accuracy and consistency of assessment, awareness of the range of variables that can influence practice in the clinical setting and the role of personal characteristics.

Cowan et al. (2005) identified a number of factors that may bias assessment observation: the process of socialization; familiarity; the assessor favouring or disfavouring the person being assessed; the nervousness of the person being assessed; resource deficiencies with which an external assessor is unfamiliar; workplace assessors who are not sufficiently involved in practice to know what constitutes acceptable competence; educators who are not sufficiently involved in practice to know what constitutes acceptable competence; and the fact that successful performance on one day is no guarantee of it on another. However, many of these issues can be overcome with extensive preparation and support of assessors and the use of consultant physicians and experienced ANPs to assess the competencies in practice. Carrying out the assessments over a period of time will also facilitate the reliability of the testing, as will the use of more than one assessor.

Work-based learning

The challenge facing academic institutions and employers is how to enmesh clinical competencies while achieving the academic requirements of a programme. One approach involves the integration of work-based learning (WBL) as a philosophy of knowledge and skill development underpinned by a triangulation approach to assessment. This can include university-assessed skills and knowledge and patient-based assessment by practising physicians within the NHS. Integrating work-based and university assessments facilitates the internalization of learning through repeating skills within different contexts, and it also forms links between the workplace and university. Because the ANP programme is competency based, the competencies are strengthened by specialist supervision and collaboration, as advocated by Furlong and Smith (2005).

Both HEI and Health Trust assessment sites must be clear about the purpose of each assessment, which needs to be carefully designed against the competencies to be assessed, the learning objectives of each module and the demands of the employing and/or statutory bodies. A clear standard is defined, below which any ANP would not be judged 'fit to practise'. This raises a challenge for all involved in the education and assessment of ANPs. Assessment must involve formative learning opportunities to support the final summative competency achievement.

At the MSc Advanced Practice programme at the University of Salford, students are assessed on clinical competence, communication, knowledge, technical skills, clinical reasoning, academic writing, research and reflection in daily practice. A core philosophy of the assessment process was to develop interprofessional, lifelong learners incorporating role extension, role expansion and role development (Daly and Carnwell 2003). Self-directed learning and self-reflection are promoted to produce practitioners who may subsequently drive institutional change (Epstein and Hundert 2002). The ILP and WBL ensure that the student's work and intended ANP role remain at the centre of their learning. Analysis of each student's knowledge and skill deficits alongside an analysis of the organization's readiness to support them as qualified ANPs is instrumental to ensuring that organizations are ready to support practitioners in new roles.

Methods of assessing competencies

ANPs' provision of safe and effective care to their client group requires a professional with advanced problem-solving skills, sound underpinning knowledge and accurate and proficient clinical skills. To ensure that graduates of ANP programmes are competent to fulfil their role and job description, competency assessment tools that measure performance must be reliable and validated. However, even the most widely used competency scales, including Bloom's Taxonomic Scales (Bloom et al. 1956), the Dreyfus Model for Skill Acquisition (Dreyfus and Dreyfus 1980) and Benner's from Novice to Expert model (Benner 2000), have not been adequately tested for reliability and validity and therefore one cannot be cited as superior. By developing these tools from a sound theoretical and evidence base, competence can be achieved.

Competencies are defined as the foundation for safe and quality patient care (Kubin and Fogg 2010; Pearson 2002). The challenge facing education providers is to devise assessment strategies that, while demonstrating the acquisition of clinical skills, also accommodate critical thinking and problem solving. Ultimately, to ensure validity and veracity, any assessment contained within the programme needs to be more than a checklist.

The standards for competency outcomes were constructed following a functional analysis of different occupational roles in relation to ANP, which were then translated into clinical competencies and outcomes to be assessed. In relation to ANP, clinical competencies were based on Association of Emergency Nurses guidelines. These competencies are assessed in the clinical setting, where the assessor makes judgements on each trainee's achievements (Leu 2002). To ensure a more comprehensive approach to competency development and the wide range of clinical settings in which the ANP would be working, the functional analysis of one role was problematic and therefore required a critical analysis of

> ### Box 3.1 Using more than one assessor
>
> Sally is an orthopaedic trainee advanced nurse practitioner and has identified through her ILP that she needs to develop her skills in respiratory assessment. However, she works in an acute orthopaedic setting and her identified clinical assessor does not routinely assess respiratory function. Armed with her clinical skills learning log, Sally arranges a placement with a respiratory physician, who uses the CSL respiratory competencies as a formative development tool. During this process, any deficits in skills and/or knowledge can be identified and actioned. One initial area requiring improvement may be the development of correct percussion technique or the ability to distinguish between crackles and wheezes. While the student may be able to perform the competencies, the underpinning knowledge relating to the presenting pathology is lacking and requires further practice and skill development to achieve summative level competence.

junior doctor training and the assessment of clinical competence. Such an assessment cannot be broken down into individual tasks. It involves the complex interplay between the application of underpinning knowledge and clinical reasoning that leads to successful achievement of academic and clinical outcomes via a competency approach. Use of a number of examiners adds to the validity and reliability of the assessment of competence (Wass et al. 2001), as illustrated in Box 3.1.

Competency levels 0–4

The University of Salford devised five levels of competence within its Taxonomy of Achievement, scoring from 0–4:

- 0 denotes unsafe practice.
- 1 denotes inexperienced practice.
- 2 denotes competent under supervision.
- 3 denotes proficient practice and ability to work autonomously.
- 4 denotes expert practice.

Students are expected to achieve a minimum of level 2 by the end of Year 1 and a minimum of level 3 by the end of the programme.

Looking at the scenario in Box 3.1, Sally would have scored 0–1: she was working in an area of unfamiliar practice; she had little theoretical knowledge but was able to observe relevant practice; she was able to practise under the close supervision of her assessor while gaining confidence and competence in a new skill.

The competencies, grade descriptors and taxonomy were developed by a team approach that utilized and reviewed curriculum and assessment strategies from undergraduate medical education (Livesley et al. 2009). In an attempt to ensure validity, they were also reviewed by medical practitioners involved in curriculum development. As the role of the ANP is developed to undertake some of the roles presently carried out by junior doctors, similar competencies are required. These standards for the assessment framework are what separates ANPs from other healthcare professionals, resulting in a valuable resource for employers (Pearson et al. 2002).

Assessors use the approved marking criteria to assess student skill and knowledge through a 15-minute presentation followed by 15 minutes of questioning. This shows that students can present a comprehensive history and physical examination and defend their actions on management. It is also a useful tool to measure student progression in terms of documentation, differential diagnosing and investigations, measuring cognitive reasoning ability and transfer of concepts between different patient groups. This connects the competencies to 'real-world' and 'real-time' practice.

A potential 'bridge', described in a seminal article by Ten Cate and Scheele (2007), is the identification of 'entrustable professional activities' (EPAs). EPAs are simply the routine, professional-life activities of physicians based on their specialty and sub-specialty (Carraccio and Burke 2010). For example, an EPA for an orthopaedic ANP may be to 'serve as the primary admitting orthopedic surgeon for previously well adults suffering from common acute problems that may require surgery'. In order to perform this professional activity, the ANP must have knowledge of the signs and symptoms of these illnesses; perform a physical examination to elicit confirmatory findings; search for outcomes/tests associated with specific therapeutic interventions; communicate with the patient and the family about the management plan; and act as a liaison to the consultant surgeon who may see this patient in follow-up.

Distinguishing between different levels of competence has been demonstrated to be problematic when assessing clinical skills (Girot 2000; Gardner et al. 2007). It is inappropriate to focus merely on the technical procedure component of advanced practice, since the finished product will not involve the necessary intellectual development and knowledge to underpin the clinical decision making. Relying on purely competency-based education is adopting a reductionist approach and will inhibit the ANP's development (Goldsmith 1999). However, the ANP has to be able to function in complex clinical situations that require interaction between specific skills and advanced clinical decision making. Watson et al. (2002) argue that measuring the performance of a master's-level ANP poses challenges that can be best addressed by assessing practice through competency-based standards. Indeed, Hase and Kenyon (2000) argue that ANPs need to demonstrate capability as well as competence. 'Capability' suggests that the AP is able to fulfil the requirements and expectations of an advanced level of practice. Educational achievement combined with students who are employed and capable of functioning in AP trainee roles that require them to practise at advanced level develops individual capability.

Work-based assessors

Assessors receive a formal induction into the programme, assessment criteria and grading criteria to improve the reliability and validity of the assessment process, along with deadlines and schedules of cases, as outlined by Gaskell and Beaton (2010). They are given time to discuss the documentation, marking criteria and type of feedback. Assessors new to the post may also review previous anonymous scripts as good examples. The assessor is marking the student's ability to perform competently under supervision in the early stages, but demonstrating increasing ability to apply theoretical concepts to clinical practice. Thus, the role of the assessor is to promote more than just clinical skill competence, including the development of clinical reasoning skills.

Assessors are consultants, both medical and nursing, registrars or advanced nurse practitioners with at least three years of experience. Committed assessors may also be honorary and regular lecturers and are involved in university-based assessments. Nikolou-Walker and Garnett (2004) suggest that this improves the reliability and validity of all programme assessments and develops closer partnerships between the NHS employer and the university.

Bespoke learning agreements and ILPs encourage and develop specialized knowledge and skills pertinent to the ANP's area of practice. This is best achieved by agreement between the student, learning facilitator, consultant assessor and line manager (Gaskell and Beaton 2010). It also places the needs of the student and the service first, as advocated by Nikolou-Walker and Garnett (2004).

Assessors are offered moderation from the university whereby learning facilitators can review the process and give feedback. This ensures parity between assessors and the NHS employer and improves the validity and reliability of the marks awarded. Students can complete formative cases during the early part of the assessment to develop their skills and to be given specific action points to develop their own learning. Assessors are advised to do this along with action points.

Students are expected to complete cases on patients with increasingly complex care needs and should incorporate the majority of different systems within the first modules. This may be facilitated by having an experienced group of assessors and collaborative working with mentors. Work-based cases include observation and discussion of history taking and consultation, clinical examination and assessment and effective communication. Students are expected to demonstrate clinical decision-making skills and to implement and critically evaluate investigations and interventions. An underpinning of theoretical knowledge, multi-disciplinary team collaboration, patient referrals and discharge, legal, ethical and professional issues and appropriate documentation should be demonstrated and/or discussed.

Formative assessments performed early within the module allow students to gauge their own strengths and weaknesses. Students award themselves a score against all the defined criteria and assessors give them appropriate and specific action points. The formative case-based assessments are used to demonstrate the progression of marks awarded between Year 1 and Year 2 and are used as reflective practice by students. They are included within the 40 portfolio cases for submission.

Work-based case studies

To illustrate competence in clinical reasoning and client management further, a series of work-based assessed clinical cases is a valuable tool. In our programme, in order to complete the MSc the ANP students need to complete 40 work-based cases, of which 15 are marked summatively by the work-based assessor. These assess the integration of knowledge and skills, context of care, information management, teamwork, health systems and patient–physician relationships, which are more appropriately assessed within the workplace. Summative workplace assessments are assessed on real patients in real-life situations, incorporate the perspectives of consultants, peers and patients, use investigations as part of routine differential diagnosis and incorporate measures that predict clinical outcomes.

In addition to assessments of clinical skills, new formats that assess clinical reasoning, expert judgement, management of ambiguity, professionalism, time management, individual learning strategies and teamwork encourage specialism and flexibility while maintaining adequate reliability and validity. Institutional support, reflection and mentoring accompanying the development of assessment programmes are paramount to this dimension.

Boxes 3.2 and 3.3 are commentaries from two experienced consultant work-based assessors of ANP students in clinical practice.

Box 3.2 Commentary from Consultant Nurse, Medical Assessment Unit

It is imperative that the assessor has a working knowledge of the university programme content, expectations of you as a mentor/assessor and outcomes expected from student placement. Establishing links with programme leaders and key staff within the HEIs is a must and it is beneficial for assessors to have a peer assessment when assessing students for quality assurance purposes.

Clarity about the role you adopt as a mentor/assessor allows you to teach, observe and monitor students allowing them to develop at a rate they are comfortable with, depending on the range of knowledge, skills and attitudinal behaviours already adopted from their previous clinical and professional experience. For these reasons, formative and summative assessments need to be individualized and organized to capture the advancement in clinical skills.

A combination of assessments are used such as work-based summative assessments, direct observational practices, clinical examinations and history taking. Assessors are well placed to link in evidence-based practice and current thinking to inform the student of how this influences their developing practice, but that cannot be exclusively defined or assessed through the core competencies alone.

Throughout the assessment process, it is vital for a mentor to raise their own awareness of the elements against which they are making an assessment. Not simply knowledge and skills are being assessed but an appropriate professional attitude to the situation to achieve all outcome measures that are patient centred and support patient safety and quality of care. Unfortunately, there are some students who do not achieve the level of competency required. It is of value to follow an agreed process that enables mentors to escalate the concern to the HEI and, with their assistance and joint ownership, devise an action plan with the student to allow development and support to occur. If the structure and processes are transparent and robust, then all students can aspire to achieve their goals with the necessary reassurance that there is a master plan.

Box 3.3 Commentary from Associate Specialist in Emergency Medicine

Taking a history, remembering what questions to ask, examining a patient, documenting and presenting your findings logically are all skills that take years to refine. These are some of the skills mentors and medical assessors pass on to the student ANP. APs already have good communication skills, experience of talking and interacting with patients and their relatives, and have an awareness of other professionals' roles and abilities that needs to be retained.

Mentoring involves allowing the students to develop new clinical skills, history taking, examination techniques, diagnostic abilities and therapeutic management techniques while not losing the skills they already possess.

In the first year the students develop their history-taking abilities (a full system review seems to be a common stumbling block). They practise examination techniques, developing cardiovascular, respiratory, abdominal, musculoskeletal and neurological examination. Setting up an examination workshop with healthy volunteers in these early stages is very useful to the students. They need to be encouraged to consider differential diagnoses at all stages of the clinical encounter, and to justify the use of appropriate investigations. Interpreting results and formulating management plans should be developing by the end of the first year.

The mentor/assessor role is to ask questions of the students and encourage them to research the answers themselves. Pointing the student in the right direction, showing them where and how to look for an answer, is preferable to delivering a result; there is also a need to check findings and outcomes and ensure patient safety. Clinical examination techniques need to be refined, correct findings reinforced and missed findings demonstrated.

In the second year the process is refinement. The students' examinations should be becoming more fluent. Use of the skills templates is a handy way to analyse and focus on areas for development. Students should be comfortable presenting patients to other professionals and referring where appropriate. They should be formulating management plans confidently and be capable of autonomous practice within their usual field of practice. Students should be encouraged to work with other professionals and to know when and how to seek senior or expert advice.

Inevitably this whole process takes time, but it can often be incorporated into the usual clinical environments. Students can be encouraged to see new patients while you carry on clinical duties, and then present them to you and findings/results checked between your own clinical encounters. However, some time needs to be set aside for focused discussions or tutorial meetings. A half hour or hour can offer the opportunity to assess progress and develop short-term learning aims.

While this may sound onerous, there are enormous benefits in being a mentor. Teaching patient examination means you critique your own skills and improve your techniques. Discussing clinical cases, reviewing evidence and critiquing inevitably have an effect on your own clinical knowledge. Discussions have often provided me with the opportunity to be updated by the latest evidence, and have improved my own knowledge. In short, mentoring will improve your own development, knowledge and abilities as well as giving you pride in observing the development of a fellow clinical colleague.

Service evaluation of AP roles

As part of its evaluation strategy, NHS England North is using a range of different methods to demonstrate the difference that skill mix changes such as the ANP role make to services and the patient experience. Sources of evidence include formal longitudinal studies, case studies of practitioner-led services and individual roles, local business cases and audit results, award nominations, conference posters and presentations. An early longitudinal study by Acton Shapiro (2009) to evaluate the ANP role in Greater Manchester, focused on the first two cohorts of students, reported difficulties in monitoring the effects of posts and collecting concrete data. It suggested that ANP roles were fulfilling some of the original aims and gave some examples from across local NHS organizations where ANP roles had improved access to services and reduced waiting times. Its broad conclusion was that 'ANP roles are having a positive impact on patient care and service delivery in their Trusts' (Acton Shapiro 2009: 6).

Across North West England case studies have been used to provide evidence of the impact of individual ANPs in specific service areas. This is consistent with a wide range of evaluations of advanced practice roles that provide evidence of improving access to services and reducing waiting times, particularly in relation to individual practitioners in unique roles (Neville and Swift 2012). Some examples are given in this section in relation to improving the quality of care and productivity (all from Neville and Swift 2012).

Improving quality of care

- Clinical outcomes of an ANP-led neonatal transfer team. Timings and physiological measurements on arrival at the receiving unit are closely matched for babies transferred by ANPs and babies transferred by doctors.
- Within an ANP-led children's walk-in centre, children with minor illness/injury have been assessed and treated since 2006, improving access to services and providing care closer to home.
- The introduction of ANPs within a Rapid Assessment Unit has had a positive impact on the achievement of European working time directive compliance. The ANP is able to do some aspects of work from the junior medical staff's very demanding workload. This can help to maximize access to expert opinion and diagnosis, as well as provide holistic care, which increases patient satisfaction.

Improving productivity

- ENT services are now meeting a five-week target for new referrals, whereas prior to the ANP role average waiting time to see the consultant was over 10 weeks. Clients can now attend the ANP-led clinic within 2–3 weeks.
- An ANP-led community DVT service was found to have treated on average 115 patients per year with medium/high-risk DVTs (positive D Dimer results). The average length of stay was 5 bed days per patient. These avoided admissions save approximately 575 bed days per year, which equates to a cost saving of £115,000.
- An ANP in pharmacy has had success in simplifying regimens, optimizing therapy and reducing the side effects and overall costs of prescribed medicines.

Conclusion

A range of issues emerging from the education and competency debate have been discussed in this chapter. The development of competencies for advanced practice and the challenges that this presents are widely acknowledged. The examples of assessment methods and strategies provided here should be helpful to readers who wish to develop their repertoire further in relation to advanced practice.

The focus of this chapter has been on trainee advanced nurse practitioners. Chapter 13 will offer insights into maintaining and developing competence beyond qualification as an advanced practitioner.

Reflective questions

1 To what extent do you consider that registration or formal regulation of advanced practice affords protection to practitioners, employers, the public and the profession?
2 Discuss with colleagues the extent to which there should be collaboration between stakeholders in relation to assuring the quality of advanced practice education.
3 In what ways do you think formative assessment should be used to enhance the development of advanced practice competencies?
4 On consideration of the various assessment strategies proposed in this chapter, which do you think should be given the most weight and for what reasons?
5 Which of the assessment strategies do you consider would be preferred by students, employers and clinical mentors?

References

Abbott, S. (2007) Leadership across boundaries: A qualitative study of the nurse consultant role in English primary care. *Journal of Nursing Management* 15: 703–710.

Acton Shapiro (2008) *Evaluating the Implementation and Impact of AP across Greater Manchester: Progress and Challenges.* Consultancy and Research Report. York: Department of Health Sciences, University of York.

Acton Shapiro (2009) *Rome Wasn't Built in a Day – The Impact of Advanced Practitioners on Service Delivery and Patient Care in Greater Manchester. Final Report.* Commissioned by NHS North West. York: University of York.

Advanced Practice Registered Nurse Joint Dialogue Group (2008) *Consensus Model for APRN Regulation: Licensure, Accreditation, Certification & Education.* Chicago, IL: APRNJDG.

Affara, F.A. (2005) *Standards for ANP Education.* Geneva: International Council of Nurses.

Aliner, G. (2003) Nursing students' and lecturers' perspectives of objective structured clinical examination incorporating simulation. *Nurse Education Today* 23(6): 419–426.

American Academy of Nurse Practitioners (2007) *Scope of Practice for Nurse Practitioners.* Washington, DC: AANP.

Angelo, R. (2008) Distance learning in higher education: A programme approach to planning, design, instruction, evaluation and accreditation. *The Internet and Higher Education* 12(4): 179–180.

Australian Nursing Federation (2005) *Competency Standards for the Advanced Registered Nurse.* Rozelle: Amanda Adrian & Associates.

Baez, A. (2005) Development of an objective structured clinical examination (OSCE) for practicing substance abuse intervention competencies: An application in social work education. *Journal of Social Work Practice in the Addictions* 5(3): 3–20.

Benner, P. (2000) *From Novice to Expert.* Englewood Cliffs, NJ: Prentice Hall Health.

Bloom, B.S., Engelhart, M.D., Furst, E.J., Hill, W.H. and Krathwohl, D.R. (1956) *Taxonomy of Educational Objectives, Handbook I: The Cognitive Domain.* New York: David McKay.

Board of Registered Nursing (2009) *Business and Professions Code.* Sacramento, CA: Board of Registered Nursing. http://www.rn.ca.gov/regulations/bpc.shtml#2701 (accessed 1 March 2015).

Brooten, D., Youngblut, J., Haanan J. and Guido-Sanz, F. (2012) The impact of interprofessional collaboration on the effectiveness, significance, and future of advanced practice registered nurses. *Nursing Clinics North America* 47(2): 283–294.

Brown, N. (2002) What are the criteria that mentors use to make judgements on the clinical performance of student mental health nurses? An exploratory study of the formal written communication at the end of clinical nursing practice modules. *Journal of Psychiatric and Mental Health Nursing* 7: 407–416.

Brown, G.T.L. and Hirschfield, G.H.F. (2007) Student's Conceptions of Assessment and Mathematics: Self Regulation Raises Achievement. *Australian Journal of Educational and Developmental Psychology* 7: 63–74.

Bryant-Lukosius, D. and DiCenso, A. (2004) A framework for the introduction and evaluation of advanced practice nurse roles. *Journal of Advanced Nursing* 48: 530–540.

Byrne, M., Delarose, T., King, C.A. et al. (2007) Continued professional competence and portfolios. *Journal of Trauma Nursing* 14(1): 24–31.

Callaghan, L. (2008) Advanced nursing practice: An idea whose time has come. *Journal of Clinical Nursing* 17: 205–213.

Carraccio, C. and Burke, A. (2010). Beyond competencies and milestones: Adding meaning through context. *Journal of Graduate Medical Education* 2(3): 419–422.

Chabeli, M.M. (2001) Nurse educators' perceptions of OSCE as a clinical evaluation method. *Curatonis* March: 84–91.

Cobourne, M.T. (2010) What's wrong with the traditional viva as a method of assessment in orthodontic education? *Journal of Orthodontics* 37(2): 128–133.

Cooke, M., Irby, D. and O'Brien, B. (2010) *Educating Physicians: A Call for Reform of Medical School and Residency.* San Francisco, CA: Jossey-Bass.

Council for Healthcare Regulatory Excellence (2009) Performance review of health professional regulatory bodies 2008/2009. Providing improvement in regulation. Annual Report and Accounts. Volume 2. London: CHRE.

Cowan, D.T., Norman, I.J. and Coopamah, V.P. (2005) A project to establish a skills competency matrix for EU nurses. *British Journal of Nursing* 14(11): 613–617.

Cowan, D.T., Wilson-Barnett, J. and Norman, I.J. (2007) A European survey of general nurses' self assessment of competence. *Nurse Education Today* 27: 452–458.

Daly, W. and Carnwell, R. (2003) Nursing roles and levels of practice: A framework for differentiating between elementary, specialist and advanced nursing practice. *Journal of Clinical Nursing* 12: 158–167.

Delamaire, M.-L. and Lafortune, G. (2010) Nurses in advanced roles: A Description and evaluation of experiences in 12 developed countries. OECD Health Working Paper No. 54. Paris: OECD.

Department of Health (2010) *Advanced Level Nursing: A Position Statement.* London: DoH.

Donnelly, G. (2003) Clinical expertise in advanced practice nursing: A Canadian perspective. *Nurse Education Today* 23(3): 168–173.

Dreyfus, Stuart E. and Dreyfus, Hubert L. (1980) *A Five-Stage Model of the Mental Activities Involved in Directed Skill Acquisition*. Washington, DC: Storming Media.

EdCaN (n.d.) Assessment fact sheet: Performance assessment using competency assessment tools. National Education Framework for Cancer Nursing. http://www.edcan.org/pdf/EdCanFactSheetCAT.pdf (accessed 18 February 2015).

Endacott, R., Gray, M.A., Jasper, M.A. et al. (2004) Using portfolios in the assessment of learning and competence: The impact of four models. *Nurse Education in Practice* 4: 250–257.

Epstein, M. and Hundert, M. (2002) Defining and assessing professional competence. *Journal of the American Medical Association* 287(2): 226–235.

Evans, A. (2008) Competency Assessment in Nursing. A summary of literature published since 2000. EdCaN, http://www.edcan.org/pdf/EdCancompetenciesliteraturereviewFINAL.pdf (accessed 19 February 2015).

Franklin, P. (2005) OSCEs as a means of assessment for the practice of nurse prescribing. *Nurse Prescribing* 3(1): 14–23.

Furlong, E. and Smith, R. (2005). Advanced nursing practice: Policy,education and and role development. *Journal of Clinical Nursing* 14: 1059–1066.

Gallagher, L. (1992) Positive reinforcement in clinical teaching. *Nurse Educator* 17(4): 35–36.

Garbett, R. and McCormack, B. (2002) A concept analysis of practice development. *Nursing Times Research* 7(2): 87–100.

Gardner, G., Chang, A. and Duffield, C. (2007). Making nursing work: Breaking through the role confusion of advanced practice nursing. *Journal of Advanced Nursing* 57(4): 382–391.

Gaskell, L. and Beaton, S. (2010) Inter-professional work based learning within an MSc in Advanced Practice: Lessons from one UK higher education programme. *Nurse Education in Practice* 10(5): 274–278.

Gerrish, K., McManus, M. and Ashworth, P. (2003) Creating what sort of professional? Masters level nurse education as a professional strategy. *Nursing Enquiry* 10(2): 103–112.

Girot, E.A. (2000) Graduate nurses: Critical thinkers, or better decision makers? *Journal of Advanced Nursing* 31(2): 288–297.

Goldsmith, S. (1999) Beyond competencies in Australian Nursing. *Australian Electronic Journal of Nursing Education* 5: 1.

Ham, C. (2003) Improving the performance of health services: The role of clinical leadership. *The Lancet* 61: 1978–1980.

Hanson, C.M. and Hamric, A.B. (2003) Educating advanced practice nurses for practice reality. *Journal of Professional Nursing* 19(5): 262–268.

Hase, S. and Kenyon, C. (2000) From andragogy to heutagogy. *UltiBASE*, December.

Higher Education Academy (2009) *Postgraduate Taught Experience Survey* (PTES). Heslington: HEA. https://www.heacademy.ac.uk/node/4198 (accessed 18 February 2015).

International Council of Nurses (2005) *Standards and Core Competencies for Advanced Practice Nursing.* Taipei: INP/APNN.

International Council of Nurses (2008) Definition and characteristics of the role. http://international.aanp.org/Practice/APNRoles (accessed 18 February 2015).

Khattab, A.D. and Rawlings, B. (2001) Assessing nurse practitioner students using a modified objective structured clinical examination (OSCE). *Nurse Education Today* 21: 541–550.

Kleinpell, R. and Gawlinski, A. (2005) Assessing outcomes in advanced practice nursing practice: The use of quality indicators and evidence based practice. *AACN Clinical Issues* 16: 43–57.

Kubin, L. and Fogg, N. (2010) Back to basics boot camp: An innovative approach to competency assessment. *Journal of Pediatric Nursing* 25(1): 28–32.

Leu, Wai-Ching (2002) Competency based medical training: Review. British Medical Journal 352: 7366.

Laurant, M., Harmsen, M., Faber M. et al. (2010) *Revision of Professional Roles and Quality Improvement: A Review of the Evidence.* London: The Health Foundation, London.

Livesley, J., Waters, K. and Tarbuck, P. (2009) The management of advanced practitioner preparation: A work-based challenge. *Journal of Nursing Management* 17: 584–593.

Major, D. (2005) OSCEs – seven years on the bandwagon: The process of an objective structured clinical evaluation programme. *Nurse Education Today* 25: 442–454.

Mantzoukas, S. and Watkinson, S. (2006) Review of the advanced nurse practitioner: The international literature and developing the generic features. *Journal of Clinical Nursing* 16: 28–37.

Mason, S., Fletcher, A., McCormick, S., Perrin, J. and Rigby, A. (2005) Developing assessment of emergency nurse practitioner competence: A pilot study. *Journal of Advanced Nursing* 50(4): 425–432.

McCormack, B. (2009) Practitioner research. In S. Hardy, A. Titchen, B.G. McCormack and K. Manley (eds) *Revealing Nursing Expertise through Practitioner Inquiry.* Oxford: Wiley-Blackwell.

McCready, T. (2006) Portfolios and the assessment of competence in nursing: A literature review. *International Journal of Nursing Studies* 44: 143–151.

Morgan, S. (2010) What are the differences in nurse practitioner training and scope of practice in the US and UK? *Nursing Times* 106: 27.

Morrison, S. and Free, K.W. (2001) Writing multiple-choice test items that promote and measure critical thinking. *Journal of Nursing Education* 40(1): 17–24.

National Leadership and Innovation Agency for Healthcare (2010) *Framework of Advanced Nursing, Midwifery and Allied Health Professional Practice in Wales.* Llanharan: NLIAH.

Neville, L. and Swift, J. (2012) Measuring the impact of advanced practice: A practical approach. *Journal of Nursing Management* 20(3): 382–389.

NHS Confederation (2010) *Dealing with the Downturn: Using the Evidence.* London: NHS Confederation.

NHS Improvement (2011) QIPP and NHS reform. http://www.nhsiq.nhs.uk/ (accessed 1 March 2015).

NHS Northwest (2009) http://www.nwwmhub.nhs.uk/media/34081/nwest-concordat-final-2009-2-.pdf (accessed 1 March 2015).

NHS Wales (2010) Framework for Advanced Nursing, Midwifery and Allied Health Professional Practice in Wales. Llanharan: NLIAH. http://www.wales.nhs.uk/sitesplus/documents/829/NLIAH%20Advanced%20Practice%20Framework.pdf (accessed 18 February 2015).

Nikolou-Walker, E. and Garnett, J. (2004) Work-based learning. A new imperative: Developing reflective practice in professional life. *Reflective Practice* 5(3): 297–312.

Oermann, M. and Floyd, J. (2002) Outcomes research: An essential component of the advanced practice nurse role. *Clinical Nurse Specialist* 16(3): 140–144.

O'Neill, A. and McCall, J. (1996) Objectively assessing nursing practices: A curricular development. *Nurse Education Today* 16: 121–126.

Pearson, A. (2002) The 'competent' nurse. *International Journal of Nursing Practice* 8(5): 233–234.

Pearson, A., FitzGerald, M. and Walsh, K. (2002) Nurses' views on competency indicators for Australian nursing. *Collegian* 9(1): 36–40.

Pfeil, M. (2001) Re-introducing skills teaching to nurse education: An action research project. *Nurse Education Today* 21: 616–623.

Por, J. (2008) A critical engagement with the concept of advancing nursing practice. *Journal of Nursing Management* 16: 84–90.

Prime Minister's Commission on the Future of Nursing and Midwifery Care in England (2010) *Front Line Care.* London: HMSO.

Rennie, A.M. and Main, M. (2006) Student midwives' views of the objective structured clinical examination. *British Journal of Midwifery* 14(10): 602–606.

Richardson, A. and Cunliffe, L. (2003) New horizons: The motives, diversity and future of nurse led care. *Journal of Nursing Management* 11: 80–84.

Roberts, J. and Fenton, G. (2012) Assessing success. *Nursing Standard* 24(35): 64.

Royal College of Nursing (2008) *Advanced Nurse Practitioners: An RCN Guide to the Advanced Nurse Practitioner Role, Competencies and Programme Accreditation.* London: RCN.

Royal College of Nursing (2012) *Advanced Nurse Practitioners: An RCN Guide to the Advanced Nurse Practitioner Role, Competences and Programme Accreditation.* http://www.rcn.org.uk/__data/assets/pdf_file/0003/146478/003207.pdf (accessed 1 March 2015).

Rust, C., O'Donavan, B. and Price, M. (2005) A social constructivist assessment process: How the research literature shows us this could be the best practice. *Assessment and Evaluation in Higher Education* 30(3): 231–240.

Rutherford, J., Leigh, J., Monk, J. and Murray, C. (2005) Creating an organizational infrastructure to develop and support new nursing roles – a framework for debate. *Journal of Nursing Management* 13: 97–105.

Ryding, H.A. and Murphy, H.J. (1999) Employing oral examinations (viva voce) in assessing dental students' clinical reasoning skills. *Journal of Dental Education* 63(9): 682–687.

Sargent, J. (2003) A proposal to develop a national framework for assistant and advanced practitioners. Workforce Development Confederation Standing Conference, August.

Scottish Government (2010) Advanced Nursing Practice Roles: Guidance for NHS Boards. http://www.advancedpractice.scot.nhs.uk/media/614/sg-advanced-practice-guidance-mar10.pdf (accessed 18 February 2015).

Selby, C. (1995) How to do it: Set up and run an objectives structured clinical exam. *British Medical Journal* 310: 1187.

Shannon, M. (2012) Strategic Framework for the Development of Clinical Advanced Practice Roles in NHS Lanarkshire. NHS Lanarkshire. http://www.lanpdc.scot.nhs.uk/Resources/Lists/Publications/Attachments/69/Framework%20for%20Development%20of%20Clinical%20AP%20Roles.pdf (accessed 18 February 2015).

Short, M.W., Jorgensen, J.E., Edwards, J.A., Blankenship, R.B. and Roth, M.D. Assessing intern core competencies with an objective structured clinical examination. *Journal of Graduate Medical Education* 1(1): 30–36.

Skills for Health (2006) The Career Framework for Health. London: Skills for Health.

Swift, J. (2009) Advanced practitioners. *HSJ Online* 24 August. http://www.hsj.co.uk/resource-centre/your-ideas-and-suggestions/advanced-practitioners/5004160.article (accessed 18 February 2015).

Ten Cate, O. and Scheele, F. (2007) Competency-based postgraduate training: Can we bridge the gap between theory and clinical practice? *Journal of the Association of American Medical Colleges* 82(6): 542–547.

Venning, P., Drury, A., Roland, M., Roberts, C. and Leese, B. (2000) Randomized controlled trial to compare the cost effectiveness of general practitioners and nurse practitioners in primary care. *British Medical Journal* 320: 1048–1053.

Ward, H. and Barratt, J. (2005) Assessment of nurse practitioner advanced clinical practice skills: Using the objective structured clinical examination (OSCE). *Primary Health Care* 15: 37–41.

Watson, G.B. and Glaser, E.M. (2002) *Watson-Glaser Critical Thinking Appraisal UK*. London: Psychological Corporation.

Wilkinson, T.J., Challis, M., Hobma, S.O. et al. (2002) The use of portfolios for assessment of the competence and performance of doctors in practice. *Medical Education* 36(10): 918–924.

CHAPTER 4

Advanced nursing practice: The strategic, cultural and organizational challenges

Fiona Paul, Mark Cooper, Mike Sabin and Margaret Smith

Chapter outline

- Introduction
- Concept exploration
- Challenges
- Analysis and discussion
- Conclusion: Lessons learnt and future challenges

Introduction

In this chapter we explore the service demand for nurse practitioner and advanced nurse practitioner roles, and where and why this demand originated. We examine how and why, in the UK healthcare system, a simple idea evolved rapidly into many different variants and possibilities, and the challenges this has caused strategic planners. We explore nursing practice beyond initial registration and some of the intra- and interprofessional tensions and challenges that have arisen nationally and internationally. We discuss how the 'Modernising Nursing Careers' initiative was pivotal in drawing together and establishing consensus around what advanced nursing practice is within the UK context, effectively splitting nurse practitioner practice into different levels. The evidence base and recommendations for advanced nursing practice are also reviewed. Finally, we explore some of the strategic, cultural and organizational challenges that lie ahead.

Nursing roles are evolving globally to fill the needs of primary and secondary healthcare. Within the UK the significant drivers for the

Box 4.1 Terminology

Different terminology is used across the literature and within practice settings to describe various roles beyond initial registration, including nurse practitioners and clinical nurse specialists. In this chapter we discuss how advanced nursing practice has been defined in the UK as a specific *level of practice*; in fact, it is one of several levels beyond initial registration (Scottish Government 2010; NHS Wales 2010; Department of Health 2010).

In some countries, nurse practitioner roles that have evolved to be at *advanced practice level* are increasingly being referred to as advanced nurse practitioner roles. Although sections of the literature appear to use the terms nurse practitioner and advanced nurse practitioner interchangeably, it could be argued that while some nurse practitioner roles have evolved to *advanced practitioner level*, others have not.

In this chapter, the term nurse practitioner will be used to describe a collection of roles beyond initial registration, whereas advanced nurse practitioner will be used to describe the sub-set of nurse practitioner roles that are at advanced practitioner level.

Additionally, from an international perspective, the terms advanced nursing practice and/or advanced practice nursing may be used interchangeably to encompass nursing practice beyond initial registration. In the USA, for example, advanced practice nursing is used to describe nurse practitioners who practise in a range of specialties and settings and who are practising at an advanced level (Kleinpell 2009). Whereas in other countries advanced nursing practice is often used to describe all nursing practice at advanced practitioner level or above (e.g. consultant level), in this chapter we will restrict ourselves to using it to describe nursing practice at advanced practitioner level, as described in the Career Framework for Health (Skills for Health 2006).

development of nursing practice have included relative reductions in medical staffing through the reduction in junior doctors' hours because of the New Deal and the European Working Time Directive; changes in training for junior doctors resulting from *Modernising Medical Careers*; changes in patient demographics and expectations; increased specialization; and the modernization of the health service.

The idea of a nurse who had further formal medical training and could fulfil what had historically been viewed as a medical role or at least part of a medical role was first mooted in the USA in the mid-1960s. Early randomized controlled trials comparing these new nurse practitioners with medical staff found no difference in the quality of care provided by nurse practitioners or doctors (Sackett et al. 1974; Spitzer et al. 1974; Chambers and West 1978; Hoekelman 1975; Burnip et al. 1976). From these early beginnings the idea of the nurse practitioner began to evolve into what we now understand as advanced-level nursing practice.

Concept exploration

In considering the spread of the concept, it is useful to consider advanced practice as a 'meme' – an idea (or even a style or behaviour) that has spread from one person to another through writing and speech. Dawkins (1976) argued that memes are analogous to genes, being subject to variation, mutation, competition and inheritance as they spread and evolve. He defined the meme as a unit of cultural transmission and gave examples of melodies, fashions and learned skills as examples of cultural items that can be copied. As people often refine, modify and combine memes with other memes to create new memes, they change and evolve over time.

Considering the early concept of the nurse practitioner in this way can help us make sense of how the idea has evolved into the advanced nurse practitioner and the concept of advanced-level practice. It can also explain why the role is so variable both within countries such as the UK and across different geographical, socio-political and healthcare system contexts.

Conditions

There are three conditions required for evolution to occur:

- 'Heredity or replication, or the capacity to create copies of elements;
- Variation, or the introduction of new change to existing elements;
- Differential "fitness", or the opportunity for one element to be more or less suited to the environment than another.' (Dawkins 1976)

Provided that it is shared, an idea has the capacity to be replicated. The notion of a nurse practitioner within various specialties has been shared through numerous papers in international professional journals (Carnwell and Daly 2003; Sheer and Wong 2008; Por 2008; Brooten et al. 2012), conference proceedings (Gilfedder et al. 2010), popular culture and television (e.g. *Scrubs*, *Casualty*, *Holby City* and community channels such as Nurse TV), the internet through websites and blogs, and textbooks (to name a few). Nurse practitioner roles have been more directly replicated through training on specific courses, initially on in-house hospital study days and latterly on university courses.

As with genetics, along with replication comes 'variation' or 'mutation'. Such variation can occur easily through individuals and groups making improvements to the idea, or indeed through miscommunication or misunderstanding, and these mutations of the meme become adopted and replicated in turn. Some variations may be more successful than others in a particular context (cultural or organizational) and may prosper and become the dominant and accepted perspective, while others may fail to prosper or have success only in a particular niche.

Such variation in role definition can be increased by reducing regulatory barriers, such as the withdrawal of the 1977 UK guidance on certification for extended roles (Department of Health 1992) and positive policy developments (e.g. the publication of the 'Scope of Professional Practice' by the then regulatory body for nursing and midwifery in the UK, the United Kingdom Central Council for Nursing and Midwifery, in 1992 (UKCC 1992) and 'Dispelling the Myths' (DoH 2003) in 2003. Alternatively, variation can be reduced by setting clear standards for NP practice, education and governance (e.g. Australian, New Zealand and Irish arrangements for NP practice).

Niche variation can occur through trying to 'fit' an NP role into specific service gaps. Gaps in service have arisen for many different reasons, including actual or relative shortages of medical staff, increasing patient numbers, changing models of service delivery, targets for service, financial considerations, changing patient aspirations, changes to patient demographics, and developments in medicine and healthcare delivery. These 'gaps' are unlikely to be exactly 'nurse practitioner' shaped, so the NP 'idea' may be stretched, moulded and reshaped to fill specific gaps. This additional variation is more likely to happen in countries where the NP idea is more fluid.

Differential 'fitness' of the concept relates to the notion that certain ideas may be more hardy or adept at surviving than others. The NP idea is more likely to survive in localities where there is a clear service gap that the NP can bridge. Conditions also have to be habitable, for example the role has to be accepted by peers and other professional colleagues, patients have to be comfortable and happy being treated by NPs, and workable referral and support arrangements need to be in place, along with education and organizational readiness to support practitioners in their new roles (Livesley et al. 2009). Additionally, NPs have to have access and authority to request and interpret appropriate investigations, there must be no legal impediments to practice, and appropriate financial systems need to be in place to fund the role and organizational commitment for succession planning (Currie and Grundy 2011). NPs also have to survive competition for the role. Gaps in the healthcare system that have appeared and given rise to the opportunity for NPs may change and contract. If the gap was partly created by the reduction in junior doctors' hours, then increasing the number of medical school places may put pressure on NPs' roles when the number of trainee doctors increases. Other professional groups may feel that they are also suitably equipped to fill the gaps. For example, in the UK physiotherapists, paramedics and radiographers are undertaking similar roles to some nurse practitioners (Mason et al. 2003; Hoskins 2011). New professional groups have also emerged, most notably the physician's assistant (DoH 2006a).

Roles may also be more likely to survive within specialties and localities where there is high-quality evidence of positive impact on patient outcomes and system processes. This is particularly evident in the USA, where a number of studies have identified positive outcomes in relation to NPs and ANPs across various specialties (Kleinpell 2009). European studies have shown similar positive outcomes, although a review of studies showed that these have mainly been undertaken in primary care and minor ailment clinics (Elsom et al. 2005). Many of the studies evaluating NP/ANP roles have tended to focus on qualitative outcomes such as patient satisfaction, although other evidence is emerging relating to clinical outcomes. Thompson and Meskell (2012) identified that the emergency nurse practitioners (ENPs) who participated in their study had equivalent or better skills than some of their medical colleagues, including radiology diagnostic skills, increased awareness of pain management practices and a greater impact on waiting times.

Roles that can demonstrate improvements in the quality of healthcare and reductions in cost will have the best chances of survival. Indeed, cost reductions are frequently highlighted as one of the key reasons for either replacing doctors with ANPs or setting up ANP services (Sheer and Wong 2008; Norton 2012). However, there is limited available evidence of the impact of advanced nursing practice on cost due to variations in how this has been evaluated in studies. For example, a systematic review of 16 studies that examined a range of outcomes for patients who had been managed by either a doctor or an ANP in primary care found minimal differences relating to cost, because of the complexities involved. While ANPs may save medical salary costs, this may be offset by them ordering more investigations and making additional patient referrals to other services (Laurant et al. 2004).

When evaluating cost effectiveness, it is also important to consider whether the focus of the ANP role was to substitute for a doctor, or to supplement a service through quality enhancement. For example, studies do not take into account longer-term savings such as a reduction in complications experienced by patients that might result from an improvement in the quality of care provided by an ANP (Delamaire and Lafortune 2010).

The factors influencing development

External factors

Various policies and legislative changes within the UK have either explicitly supported the development of the nurse practitioner role or have helped ensure a conducive environment for the role to flourish.

As attitudes have changed, it has become unacceptable for most people (including junior doctors) to work more than 48 hours a week in Europe. Government policy in the early 1990s (NHS Management Executive 1992), followed by the later implementation of the European Working Time Directive (Council Directive 93/104/EC 1993), placed legally binding maximum working hours on junior doctors. NHS organizations were financially penalized if medical staff rotas were not compliant. The 'New Deal' and the Working Time Directive effectively created gaps in medical staffing rotas, as there were now insufficient numbers of medical staff to fill them. The punitive costs to the NHS for non-compliant rotas gave an extra push to NHS organizations identifying creative solutions to fill these growing gaps.

Changes to specialist training for medical practitioners (DoH 2004a) and new contracts for general practitioners and hospital consultants (DoH 2004b) only increased the pressures on NHS organizations to find new ways of organizing and delivering services. One of the agreements in the new GP contract allowed GPs to 'opt out' of providing out-of-hours services. This meant that the responsibility fell to health authorities and health boards to provide replacement services.

While the number of medical school places had increased and new medical schools had opened, there were still too few doctors to fill all the existing medical rotas. Add to this an increasingly elderly population who are surviving into older age, often with multiple and complex health problems, as well as rising patient expectations and advances in medical care, that means that many more conditions are treatable and, therefore, that the demand on the Health Service is set to continue to increase.

Withdrawal of the 1977 guidance on certification for extended roles by the Department of Health (DoH 1992), publication of *The Scope of Professional Practice* (UKCC 1992) and changes to the law to permit non-medical prescribing (Medicinal Products: Prescription by Nurses Act 1992) both removed barriers to nurse practitioner practice and at the same time supported the expansion of the nurse's role.

The urgent need to find new ways of working to cover medical rotas and out-of-hours care caused by all of these different factors meant that intra- and interprofessional opposition to the development of nurse practitioner roles had limited impact.

Aspirations and tensions: Internal factors

A central issue in the development of advanced nursing practice has been the tension between two approaches that have emerged since the idea of an advanced nurse practitioner was first introduced. This tension is frequently highlighted within the international literature (Coombs et al. 2007). One relates to advancing the nursing profession by enhancing nurses' capabilities and practice and the quality of holistic nursing care. This may be described as a professionally focused/ professionallyaspirant/role enhancement approach. The other relates to meeting a service need or filling a gap such as some of the external factors discussed previously, which may involve role substitution. This may be described as an operationally focused/service-driven/role redesign approach.

It is important to consider, however, that these approaches may overlap and this has possibly led to some of the tensions and challenges within advanced nursing practice. For example, differences in titles internationally have led to confusion over the roles, scope of practice and professional boundaries of advanced practice nurses (Por 2008; Duffield et al. 2009). Elsom et al. (2005) highlight that advanced practice nursing roles and titles do not automatically entitle one to advanced status. Role boundaries have also created challenges within advanced nursing practice, not only from medical colleagues, but also nursing leaders and colleagues (Hinchliff and Rogers 2008). Therefore, it is recommended that ANPs continue to maintain their professional identity and focus on the nursing nature of advanced practice roles (Lowe et al. 2012). From a professionally focused/professionally aspirant/role enhancement perspective, this has been shown to some extent in studies that have compared medical practitioners with ANPs, for example those identifying that ANPs utilize their nursing expertise to provide more holistic care (Laurant et al. 2004). However, further research is needed, and this should focus more on ANPs' nursing contributions as opposed to comparing them with medical practitioners (Hinchliff and Rogers 2008).

Elsom et al. (2005: 182) state: 'Advanced nursing practice requires critical reflection on the nature of nursing practice and the beliefs, judgements and values that underpin it.' Therefore, advanced nursing practice should expand and offer new possibilities for holistic patient care (Nieminen et al. 2011). Additionally, it must be recognized as relating to developing nursing skills, relevant for a particular context, along with further education in a specific area of practice (Elsom et al. 2005).

There is no doubt that the purpose of advanced nursing practice is to deliver high-quality, evidence-based care that improves patient outcomes. This is achievable through leadership, legitimate influence, expertise and education (Coombs et al. 2007). However, this is dependent on the acceptance and formal recognition of advanced nursing roles. Despite the growing evidence of the effectiveness of such roles, resistance exists from various perspectives within healthcare internationally (Duffield et al. 2009).

From an operationally focused and service-driven perspective, there is a need for all healthcare professional disciplines (including nursing) to adopt aspects of advanced-level practice, such as clinical skills provision, management, leadership and professional roles, and this will inevitably lead to blurring of professional boundaries in order to provide better care to expanding populations (Asbridge 2012). Yet blurring of professional boundaries is frequently cited as a barrier to nurses working at an advanced level, because they have adopted some of the skills that were once traditionally conducted by medical practitioners, such as prescribing and physical examination (Whitaker 2006). These skills are increasingly required to be undertaken by other professions to assess patients rapidly and prevent delays in commencing treatment (West 2006; National Prescribing Centre 2010). However, criticisms have been raised about practitioners undertaking such skills without formal medical education (Wiseman 2007).

The structure, level and content of education for practitioners working in advanced practice roles have been contentious issues. In the UK, for example, this has been partly due to a lack of guidance on standards of education, supervision and assessment (Brook and Rushforth 2011). Concerns have also been raised internationally about education and preparation for ANP roles in addition to issues around regulation, which add to the challenges associated with advanced nursing practice. Some countries begin with the role and then develop the title, scope and regulation, while other countries begin with regulation and then progress with education and development of the role (Sheer and Wong 2008).

Brook and Rushforth (2011) argue that regulation is imperative, since nurses may be appointed as ANPs without adequate educational preparation in advance of taking on a role that requires high levels of decision making. Gerrish et al. (2011) found that less than one third of ANPs had a master's degree, which is frequently recommended as a core level of education for ANPs. Nevertheless, robust education programmes are in place in many areas, and specifically within courses such as non-medical prescribing (NMC 2006; National Prescribing Centre 2010). There are also robust monitoring and governance procedures relating to non-medical prescribing in many healthcare organizations (NPC 2010).

Role substitution, especially of medical roles, is frequently highlighted as a challenge within advanced nursing practice. In some areas, physicians and/or their professional organizations resist the use of APNs or restrict full use of their knowledge and skills, fearing competition with and invasion of the physician role (Brooten et al. 2012). Although the evolution of healthcare globally has allowed opportunities for disciplines, particularly nursing, to develop and advance their practice, this will inevitably blur professional boundaries and challenge traditionally held beliefs and values (Coombs et al. 2007). Nurses working in new advanced roles have indicated a need for support, trust and mutual respect from colleagues in their own discipline as well as others, especially medical colleagues (Nieminen et al. 2011; Kilpatrick et al. 2012). Support from colleagues is important due to the additional responsibilities involved in ANP roles. While some ANPs, particularly student or new ANPs, may embrace the responsibility and autonomy offered within an ANP–patient relationship, they may also perceive the additional responsibility as onerous or daunting (Nieminen et al. 2011). Cox (2012) adds that for nurses going through the transition from a basic professional role to an advanced practice professional role, it is essential that they continue to contribute to effective teamwork among other disciplines.

A key message from within the literature in relation to advanced-level nurses is that while they may take on various components of another profession's role, such as physical examination and prescribing, it is important that they retain their traditional nursing values and strengths to enhance patient care and to promote and facilitate evidence-based nursing practice with their colleagues (Byrne et al. 2000; Elsom et al. 2005; Nieminen et al. 2011; Gerrish et al. 2011; Norton 2012). Por (2008) adds that nurses have always expanded their practice to meet the needs of patients and clients within an evolving healthcare system; however, advanced nursing practice is not only related to an expansion of practice, but is also an expansion of clinical expertise, knowledge and research to further the scope of nursing practice.

It could be argued that the rise of professionalism within nursing in the 1980s reflected both an emerging confidence in the educational and research base for nursing practice, and a zeitgeist that was moving away from established health professions and embracing a more person-centred caring model.

Interestingly, while one strand of the subsequent developments supported the emergence of an advanced form of nursing practice where nurses moved into a medical substitution role, a parallel strand saw the characterization of advanced practice as a 'nursing plus' model, where the nursing element of the role remained broadly the same, but the range of skills (technical and non-technical) was expanded to meet a particular clinical, operational or patient/client need.

This mutation of the meme and plurality of development has played out against a rapidly developing socio-political context, and it is clear that there are now many advanced nursing practices in existence. Whether we see this as a problem or an opportunity is much more than merely a philosophical question for the profession, and requires us to consider issues of education, workforce planning, governance and professional identity.

It is important to consider whether advanced practice is an entity in itself, definable as a level of practice characterized by particular behaviours, skills and attributes and applicable across professions. Or is advanced practice in nursing only understandable as advanced nursing practice – one of many stages or levels of specifically nursing practice?

It could be argued that if nursing practice is in any way unique to the profession, whether in terms of specific actions or attitudes or in the way in which practice is collectively embodied, then any advanced nursing must be a level or stage of the development of that nursing practice only; a 'higher form' of nursing. However, if advanced practice is instead principally a level of clinical functioning, autonomy and decision making attainable by, and identifiable across, both nursing and other health professions, then the language with which we describe it, the way in which we support its development and the way in which we plan and enact its use will be fundamentally different.

We also need to consider whether the emergence of advanced practice in nursing was, and is, driven by a focus on improving patient/client outcomes and whether such enhancement of practice could be achieved through higher forms of nursing practice that were not previously available to clients; or whether this movement was more about sustainability of service delivery in the face of increasing demand or diminishing capacity, with new or different practitioner groups delivering the same care outcomes in more efficient ways.

Certainly, the professionalism agenda in the UK saw the development of advanced practice in nursing as an emancipatory and liberating force for nurses and a nursing profession that had hitherto been politically, socially and clinically or operationally subservient to other professional groups. However, it was also clear that the areas where most development was occurring were those where traditional delivery models were proving to be unsustainable (out-of-hours provision and Hospital at Night) and where there was a desire for nurses to be ushered into gaps left by reorganization in other professional groups, legislative change and/or fiscally driven service redesign.

Whether driven by enhancement or sustainability, the key test for advanced nursing practice has to be based on evidence that such an approach is in the patients' or clients' best interests. Subsequently, more robust research is required into the effectiveness of advanced nursing roles, as this is essential for future, evidence-based practice (Gardner et al. 2007). This is likely to be achieved by the careful and deliberate selection of clinical, educational, organizational and patient/family outcomes that truly measure ANPs' contribution to care (Brooten et al. 2012). As well as measuring the benefits to care, there is also a need to consider other important outcomes such as adverse events and resource utilization.

Changing patient demographics

An emergent area for expanding practice is long-term/chronic illness management, as a result of advances in medicine and the increasingly ageing population. In England, for example, the Department of Health (2005) estimates that 17.5 million people are living with a long-term health condition, and this figure will continue to increase, particularly for those over the age of 65. Consequently, complex and diversified services have been required (Asbridge 2012), providing opportunities for nurses to advance their skills and knowledge and for new nursing roles to fill the gaps in service that arise. However, studies have indicated that it is not always clear how service needs are identified in relation to advanced practice roles, therefore robust service needs analysis mechanisms are required in advance that reflect the region or country concerned (Chang et al. 2010; Zahran et al. 2012). It has also been suggested that decisions about new nursing roles and services should involve key stakeholders from the outset, otherwise these may be met with scepticism, particularly where there is blurring of professional boundaries (Iliffe et al. 2011). The management of long-term conditions and chronic disease is a global challenge and approximately two-thirds of emergency hospital admissions are related to chronic illnesses (DoH 2005). Consequently, nurse-led case management of these conditions has been recommended as a system that streamlines care and reduces hospital admissions. In England, community matrons undertake this, but an evaluation has indicated that some GPs may have negative perceptions of this role due to how it was implemented, which may have affected previously good working relationships with GPs and community nurses (Iliffe et al. 2011). These perceptions may change over time once the role becomes accepted, but research is required in this area.

Factors such as skill mix, succession planning and the long-term funding of services also need to be clarified before nurses undertake extensive education and training to prepare for advanced practice roles. Some nurses who have embarked on preparation for advanced practice may be unable to apply their new skills and knowledge if a service is discontinued, or if advanced-level nursing posts are unavailable (Currie and Grundy 2011).

Evidence shows that nurses working in advanced practice roles provide equivalent standards of care and management to physicians for patients in primary care (Laurant et al. 2004). Many of these patients have long-term conditions such as asthma, diabetes and coronary heart disease, and some of the key benefits for patients highlighted in systematic reviews are improvements in nurse-led consultations, including longer consultations, increased patient satisfaction and compliance, and higher rates of investigations (Brown and Grimes 1995; Horrocks et al. 2002). A systematic review revealed that care and management in the short term in primary care were comparable between doctors and ANPs, with a few similar improvements noted in some studies in favour of nurse-led consultations. However, the reviewers mentioned that increased patient satisfaction did not necessarily mean that patients preferred to be seen by a nurse, as patient preferences were found to be variable depending on the reason for the consultation (Laurant et al. 2004).

Examples of ANP roles

To illustrate the breadth of advanced nursing practice and its key drivers, examples of two different roles, one in primary and the other in secondary care within the UK, will now be presented and discussed.

The emergency nurse practitioner (ENP) role developed organically. Increasing waiting time in Emergency Departments, coupled with the idea that senior nurses could see and treat many of the minor injuries that attend them, encouraged many to experiment with utilizing nurse practitioners. Several hospitals opened up their in-house courses to emergency nurses from other departments and soon ENPs were being trained all over the country. Initially their scope of practice was quite limited, depending on the training hospital and then subsequently modified by the department in which the ENP went to work. However, as ENPs have proved that they are safe and effective (Sakr et al. 1999; Cooper et al. 2002), and as services have had to change for a variety of other reasons, including the unsustainability of smaller departments (often caused by other services like intensive care being moved off certain sites), nurse practitioner-led Minor Injury Units have been set up to meet the public's demand to retain as many services as possible as locally as possible (see Box 4.2).

Box 4.2 The emergency nurse practitioner

The first formal emergency nurse practitioner role in the UK can be traced back to a three-month trial of a nurse-led minor injuries service at Oldchurch Hospital in Essex in 1986 (Ramsden 1986; Head 1988; Morris et al. 1989). However, nurses have been treating patients in many of the smaller A&E Departments unofficially for many years, using their clinical judgement whether to consult the doctor, send the patient to a major A&E Department or treat the patient themselves, and therefore functioning in essence as nurse practitioners (Jones et al. 1986). The reason the service was introduced at Oldchurch related to increased numbers of complaints received by the local Health Authority concerning waiting times and a suggestion by the local Community Health Council that 'some form of "vetting" process should be carried out, say by a nurse practitioner' (Head 1988; Morris et al. 1989).

Over the next few years the idea that nurse practitioners in A&E could contribute to reducing waiting times and increasing patient satisfaction created considerable interest (Yates 1987; Walsh 1989; Booth 1992; Burgess 1992; Burgoyne 1992; Woolwich 1992). By 1991, 40% of all A&E Departments (major, minor and specialist) in England and Wales were reported to have nurses working in nurse practitioner roles, although the vast majority (34%) were considered to be 'unofficial' schemes and only 6% (n=27) were 'official' schemes (Read et al. 1992). Official schemes were classified in this survey, as were those where the title 'nurse practitioner' was used to denote nurses working in this role.

The idea continued to spread, fuelled by rising numbers of people seeking medical attention in A&E Departments every year and the fact that medical staff were being overstretched (National Audit Office 1992). 1992 was a pivotal year for nursing role development in the UK. Hurdles to nurses practising in extended roles were being removed and supportive policies put in place. Numerous articles and papers in the professional literature extolled the benefits of ENP services (for example, Marsden 2003; Jennings et al. 2008; Walsh 2001) and more and more departments began to set up services (see Figure 4.1).

A number of hospitals set up their own in-house ENP courses, which initially taught their own staff and then accepted nurses from other departments. This helped cross-fertilize the role into many new departments. In these early days the role of the ENP was locally defined by each department, usually through drafting written 'protocols' (Cooper et al. 1998). Many departments shared protocols and through nurses travelling to other hospitals to undertake training, a core scope of practice began to take shape. Subsequently major changes have been made to the way in which many A&E services are delivered, with larger and more centralized Emergency Departments with round-the-clock senior medical or consultant staffing replacing one or more smaller A&E Departments. Minor Injury Units, which are often nurse led, have been opened in communities when A&E Departments have closed.

Emergency nurse practitioners are now firmly embedded in most Emergency Departments as well as solely staffing many Minor Injury Units and NHS Walk-in Centres. As the role has evolved over nearly 30 years in many different settings, it is not surprising that different levels of practice have emerged, and variations in pay, scope of practice and title (Fotheringham et al. 2011).

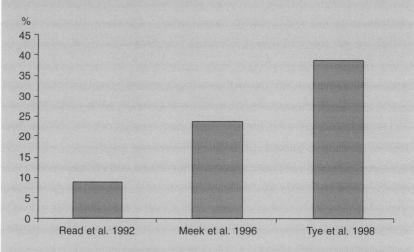

Figure 4.1 Growth of 'official' ENP services in major A&E Departments in England and Wales during the 1990s

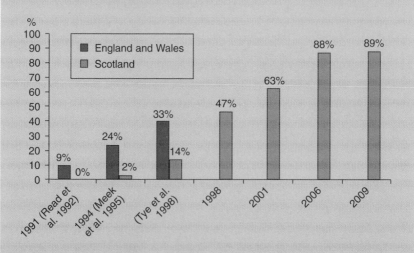

Figure 4.2 Growth of ENP services in England and Wales, and Scotland, between 1991 and 2009

The Hospital at Night nurse practitioner, on the other hand, is a good example of a role being planned, albeit quickly, to meet a specific service need. Changes to junior doctors' training in the mid-2000s, and punitive pay awards to junior doctors if they had to work excessive hours through rotas that were non-compliant with the Working Time Directive, caused hospitals throughout the UK to revise the way in which they provided medical cover overnight. The old system, where each individual specialty provided cover for its area only, was unsustainable. A new approach, a Hospital at Night (HaN) team, was first piloted by the NHS Modernisation Agency in England. Hospitals across the UK were quick to implement their own schemes to solve staffing problems and save money, and almost all saw nurse practitioners as having a pivotal role on these HaN teams. Alongside locally led hospital-level and SHA/NHS Board-level developments, the NHS Modernisation Agency in England and NHS Education for Scotland invested in developing the framework for Hospital at Night education and the training of nurse practitioners. A considerable amount of collaborative working went on to develop a nurse practitioner role to help fill places on these new teams (see Box 4.3).

Box 4.3 The Hospital at Night nurse practitioner

While the ENP role has evolved over the last three decades, a more recently developed role within acute hospital care in the UK is the Hospital at Night (HaN) nurse practitioner. This role emerged in 2003 with the inception of Hospital at Night teams, which were set up to deliver care out of hours as a result of the European Working Time Directive (Modernisation Agency 2004). The concept of HaN relates to a multi-disciplinary team approach to care overnight, coordinated by an advanced nurse practitioner. It was devised to ensure safe, prioritized and coordinated care and management of patients, utilizing a range of expertise within the team, and to enhance the support and education of all staff (DoH 2005). In most hospitals there are three levels of HaN nurse practitioners (bands 6, 7 and 8). Many of these practitioners have undertaken master's-level study, whereas others have received 'in-house' education. Their role involves coordinating the team overnight, exercising higher levels of decision making and competently performing skills that were traditionally the domain of medical staff, such as physical examination, history taking and prescribing (Gooding 2004; Whitaker 2006).

As the HaN service is fairly new, literature and research are minimal, especially in relation to advanced practice nursing roles within it. A few evaluations of this service have indicated positive trends in outcomes for patients, such as reductions in hospital stay and reduced mortality rates

(Parish 2007; Beckett et al. 2009). Positive perceptions have also been highlighted regarding the support and education provided by the HaN team for ward medical and nursing staff overnight (DoH 2005). Nevertheless, HaN nurse practitioner roles may not be fully accepted due to the challenges of professional working boundaries (Whitaker 2006) and issues around the bleep-filtering role of the HaN nurse practitioner, who is the first point of contact when a ward nurse is seeking advice or assistance from a medical practitioner (Clark and Paul 2012). Issues around bleep filtering were also highlighted in the Department of Health (2005) report. Previously ward nurses contacted a doctor directly and so they questioned why they could no longer do this. This indicated that they possibly lacked awareness or knowledge of the benefits of bleep filtering, such as minimizing interruptions to medical staff when they are engaged in the care of acutely ill patients. Despite the benefits of the multi-disciplinary HaN team approach for patients and ward staff, some medical and nursing staff may lack awareness of other key aspects of the HaN nurse practitioner role, for instance patient assessment, and may assume that it is mainly related to undertaking tasks such as cannulation and venepuncture. Therefore it is recommended that education on new nursing roles is incorporated into undergraduate healthcare curricula and staff induction sessions (Clark and Paul 2012).

Challenges

The evolution of the nurse practitioner role in the UK, whether slow as seen in the ENP role or rapid as in the HaN NP role, has ensured that there is wide variation in almost every aspect, from titles to scope of practice, educational preparation to salary. This variation, while it ensures that the role is highly adaptable, makes it difficult for strategic planners, educationalists, managers and practitioners to know exactly what a nurse practitioner can do.

This challenge also exists internationally, as there is wide variation between countries in terms of educational standards, regulation, titles, reimbursement, prescribing privileges and, fundamentally, no clearly identified scope and standards of practice (ICN 2002). In specific countries, including the USA, Canada, New Zealand, Australia and Ireland, regulation has been introduced and there is greater clarity around the role. However, in Canada and the USA there can be variation in educational standards, prescribing privileges and reimbursement arrangements, and even in titles between different internal jurisdictions (Donald et al. 2010; Goolsby 2011).

By 2006, there were hundreds if not thousands of nurses working in a wide range of nurse practitioner-type roles in the UK. Evidence from randomized controlled trials demonstrated that nurse practitioners were safe and effective (Sakr et al. 1999; Cooper et al. 2002; Horrocks et al. 2002) and this in turn helped support the development of further roles. In fact, from 1992 there had been a mushrooming of new roles (Read et al. 1999), facilitated by supportive policies and legislation.

To complicate matters, the meme mutated again and the term 'advanced practice' began to appear in the professional literature in the late 1980s and was widely embraced during the 1990s. In the eyes of many people the term became synonymous with nurse practitioner practice, but to others advanced practice in nursing could be applied to other nursing roles and not necessarily those that were clinical.

There were debates over whether nurse practitioners were nurses who had 'extended' practice into the territory of other professions (usually medicine), or had 'expanded' nursing practice to take in practice usually associated with other professions. There were others who argued that nurse practitioners had in fact left nursing and were forming a new profession. There were also debates about 'specialist' and 'advanced' practice and which could be considered the higher level.

Greater clarity around roles and terminology was urgently required. The RCN Nurse Practitioner Forum, along with groups such as the Association of Advanced Nurse Practitioner Educators (AANPE), argued that nurse practitioner practice should become regulated. In 2005, following a national consultation, the Nursing and Midwifery Council agreed and proposed that Advanced Nurse Practitioner should become a registered title. However, changes in legislation would be required, which would take time. Approval was sought from the UK Privy Council.

While regulation was being explored, it was becoming imperative for both practitioners and strategic planners that there was greater clarity around advanced practice and the whole nurse practitioner role in the UK.

Defining advanced nursing practice

While advanced nursing practice (ANP) seems to act as an umbrella term, defining it has been difficult because of the many variations in how nursing roles have developed and evolved according to the specific area/specialty and the resources available (Por 2008). There are also examples of formal and informal developments of expanded practice, which may add to the lack of clarity and consistency in relation to advanced nursing practice (Elsom et al. 2005). Consequently, it is becoming increasingly important to clarify the term 'advanced nursing practice' and also to differentiate between the various titles and roles that practitioners have adopted. This is important for nurses, healthcare professionals and patients, not only to ensure consistency and standards for benchmarking purposes, but also to provide evidence of efficiency, cost effectiveness and improved patient outcomes (Lowe et al. 2012).

While several countries have highlighted the need for national approaches to advanced practice, an international approach may be more relevant in today's evolving healthcare services, since perspectives are similar globally (Lowe et al. 2012). This need for clarity has been re-emphasized in countries where new nursing roles have been recently introduced (Nieminen et al. 2011; Zahran et al. 2012). Studies have highlighted the importance of achieving a consensual understanding among educationalists, employers and professional bodies about not only what advanced nursing practice is, but also its purpose, so that a common framework can be identified (Gardner et al. 2007; Chang et al. 2010; Nieminen et al. 2011; Zahran et al. 2012).

A criticism of much of the literature that has focused on defining advanced nursing practice has been the debate around what advanced practice nurses should be doing, as opposed to defining the concept itself (Zahran et al. 2012). This is compounded by the considerable variability in ANP roles, titles and responsibilities (Chang et al. 2010; Gerrish et al. 2011). In the UK, the Advanced Nursing Practice Toolkit (NHS Education for Scotland 2012) was developed, drawing on existing work from organizations such as the International Council of Nurses (ICN), RCN, NMC and Career Framework for Health, and this has significantly helped to achieve consensus on the concept, not only within nursing but within other healthcare professions (Eddy 2008; Brook and Rushforth 2011). The key message from this work indicates that advanced practice is a *level of practice* rather than a role or a title, representing a key shift in the meme.

Modernising Nursing Careers and advanced practice development

In the UK in 2006, *Modernising Nursing Careers* (MNC) set out an agenda for the review and revision of the profession, supported by the Chief Nursing Officers of the four UK countries (DoH 2006b; Scottish Government 2006). To some extent, this echoed the aspiration of the professionalism agenda from 20 years before and sought to advocate for nursing as both enabler and change agent. The original document reflected confidence in the growing contribution of nursing to healthcare, as well as a recognition that some existing professional structures were outdated and may be limiting further enhancement of that contribution.

The MNC Coalition, hosted by DoH England, drew together senior representatives from each of the four countries, the Council of Deans of Health, the NMC, professional organizations and NHS employers and commissioners. Importantly, and perhaps for the first time, the coalition also recognized the issue of devolved government and sought to support professional consensus in responding to potential divergence in health need and in strategic/operational models for delivery of healthcare. One key area within the MNC action plan was advanced nursing practice. NHS Scotland took forward this work on behalf of the coalition and the resulting Advanced Nursing Practice Toolkit, which was developed in 2007 (NHS Education for Scotland 2012), sought to bring together previously published work regarding definitions of advanced practice (ICN 2002; NMC 2005; Skills for Health 2006; RCN 2008; see also Box 4.4), the Career Framework for Health (Figure 4.3), competencies, education and governance into a consensus model.

Box 4.4 Definitions of advanced practice

International Council of Nurses
A Nurse Practitioner/Advanced Practice Nurse is a registered nurse who has acquired the expert knowledge base, complex decision-making skills and clinical competencies for expanded practice, the characteristics of which are shaped by the context and/or country in which s/he is credentialed to practice. A master's degree is recommended for entry level. (ICN 2002)

NHS Career Framework. Advanced Practitioners – Level 7
Experienced clinical professionals who have developed their skills and theoretical knowledge to a very high standard. They are empowered to make high-level clinical decisions and will often have their own caseload. Non-clinical staff at Level 7 will typically be managing a number of service areas. (Skills for Health 2006)

Nursing and Midwifery Council
Advanced nurse practitioners are highly experienced and educated members of the care team who are able to diagnose and treat your healthcare needs or refer you to an appropriate specialist if needed. Advanced nurse practitioners are highly skilled nurses who can:

- take a comprehensive patient history
- carry out physical examinations
- use their expert knowledge and clinical judgment to identify the potential diagnosis
- refer patients for investigations where appropriate
- make a final diagnosis

- decide on and carry out treatment, including the prescribing of medicines, or refer patients to an appropriate specialist
- use their extensive practice experience to plan and provide skilled and competent care to meet patient's health and social care needs, involving other members of the health care team as appropriate
- ensure the provision of continuity of care including follow-up visits
- assess and evaluate, with patients, the effectiveness of the treatment and care provided and make changes as needed
- work independently, although often as part of a health care team
- provide leadership
- make sure that each patient's treatment and care is based on best practice (NMC 2005)

Royal College of Nursing
An advanced nurse practitioner is: *A registered nurse who has undertaken a specific course of study at least first degree (Honours) level and who*:

- Makes professionally autonomous decisions for which he or she is accountable
- Receives patients with undifferentiated and undiagnosed problems and makes an assessment of their health care needs, based on highly developed nursing knowledge and skills, including skills not usually exercised by nurses, such as physical examination
- Screens patients for disease risk factors and early signs of illness
- Makes differential diagnosis using decision-making and problem-solving skills
- Develops with the patient an ongoing nursing care plan for health, with an emphasis on preventative measures
- Orders necessary investigations, and provides treatment and care both individually, as part of a team, and through referral to other agencies
- Has a supportive role in helping people to manage and live with illness
- Provides counselling and health education
- Has the authority to admit or discharge patients from their caseload, and refer patients to other health care providers as appropriate
- Works collaboratively with other health care professionals and disciplines
- Provides a leadership and consultancy function as required (RCN 2008)

In keeping with the 'meme' concept, the toolkit recognized that the rapid and plural development of practitioner, specialist and advanced roles in nursing had been an organic process reflecting different strategic, operational, professional and philosophical drivers and enablers. When viewed collectively, these could be seen as a genuine shift in both the perception and practice of nursing. However, the degree of variation between different elements of this whole meant that it was impossible to

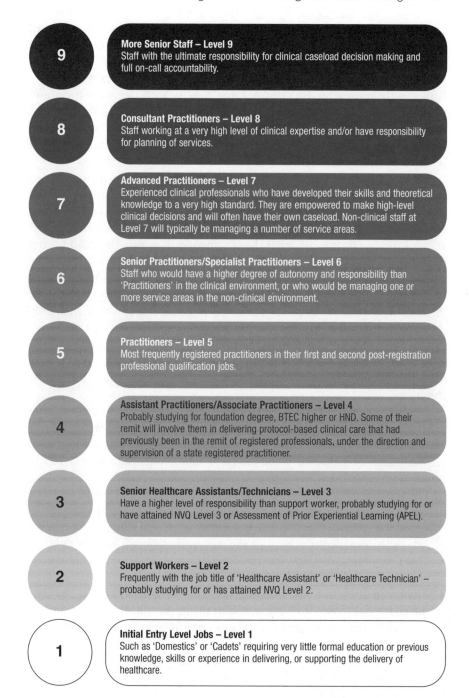

Figure 4.3 The Career Framework for Health
Source: Skills for Health (2006).

capture, measure, promote or defend this shift. The profession had unwittingly generated a 'chimera', a dream that was not likely to come true.

Recognizing that an inability to define advanced nursing practice consistently represented a considerable risk to both the profession and those with whom we practise, the toolkit aimed to establish a benchmark for advanced nursing practice. The use of the word 'benchmark' is important, since this is defined as an agreed point of reference against which something can be measured.

MNC and the Advanced Nursing Practice Toolkit provided an opportunity to gather together the outputs from writing, discourse and practice in this area and create a model that would allow commissioners, educators, regulators, practitioners and the public to better understand, utilize and support what that defined level of practice could bring to modern healthcare. Importantly, while the establishment of the benchmark for advanced-level practice sought to create some level of uniformity of understanding, it did not seek to advocate that all the different roles should become advanced practice roles, rather that only those roles that matched the benchmark should be known by this appellation. This allows for continued responsiveness within nursing practice, where roles can be structured to meet service need, but also real clarity around which of those roles are advanced level and which are something else.

Furthermore, the toolkit did not seek to freeze advanced nursing practice at a particular point in its development – to do so would surely render it quickly irrelevant – but to capture it as a 'waymarker' that would guide us until we were ready to benchmark again at a future point.

The toolkit achieved a great deal of consensus and clarified a number of key principles around advanced practice in the UK. For example:

- Advanced practice is a level of practice rather than a role or title.
- The Career Framework for Health (Figure 4.3) describes advanced practitioners across professional boundaries.
- Advanced practice in nursing can be broadly defined by the International Council of Nurses' definition (Box 4.4).
- The NMC definition outlines the clinical advanced nurse practitioner role within the UK context.
- Advanced practice is shown across four key themes:
  o advanced clinical/professional practice
  o facilitating learning
  o leadership/management
  o research.

- These themes are underpinned by autonomous practice, critical thinking, high levels of decision making and problem solving, values-based care and improving practice.
- The skills and knowledge base for advanced practice are influenced by the context in which individuals practise.
- Advanced practice is *not* simply a broad term that refers to all practice roles at a level above that of initial practice, including under its umbrella both specialist and consultant roles.
- Advanced practice and specialist practice are different. Specialist should be considered as one pole of the 'specialist–generalist' continuum, rather than on the developmental continuum from 'novice' to 'expert'. This approach defines specialist practice as that which is particular to a specific context, be it a client group, a skill set or an organizational context.
- Nurses may function at an advanced level in roles that are not necessarily predominantly clinical, for example education, research or leadership roles.
- Master's-level descriptors for practice and 'autonomy, accountability and working with others' are particularly characteristic of advanced practice competence, and master's-level education is therefore appropriate for this level of practice.

However, while the toolkit has been endorsed by all four Chief Nursing Officers and integrated into subsequent implementation models (most directly in Scotland and Wales), it could be argued that a number of key issues remain on which there are differing perspectives among key stakeholders, and that such dissonance risks even the temporary consensus that the toolkit has achieved.

Certainly, the recent experience of the global financial crisis, and its subsequent impact on health spending, has led to some review and retrenchment regarding advanced practice posts as part of an overall shrinkage in the nursing workforce. However, one might argue that financial constraints would provide a positive driver for the development of advanced practice roles, although only if those roles substitute for existing, more expensive or less efficient delivery models and team structures.

In the current context, enhancement models based on expansion of nursing provision seem unlikely to prosper unless there are clear efficiencies to be achieved, or robust evidence of the sustainability of a key service or of success in delivery of a key strategic priority (safety, effectiveness or person centredness).

Where we are today

Following the publication of the Advanced Nursing Practice Toolkit and completion of the work on *Modernising Nursing Careers*, the Scottish Government and the Welsh Assembly Government have published guidance for advanced nursing practice in their respective countries that is based on the principles contained within the toolkit (Scottish Government 2010; NHS Wales 2010). In Scotland, health boards are expected to have formal processes in place to identify, record and govern their advanced nurse practitioners, with data being collated nationally each year. Similar responsibilities are placed on Welsh NHS organizations to maintain audit trails of local decision making around the identification of ANPs.

The Department of Health (2010) in England has produced a position statement on advanced-level nursing that recognizes that it is 'well beyond initial registration', but does not go quite as far as the Scottish or Welsh documents in defining it. A decision on the NMC proposal to regulate advanced practice was delayed due to wider work on the regulation of health professionals. In 2007, a White Paper was published, *Trust, Assurance and Safety – The Regulation of Health Professionals in the 21st Century*. This proposed that regulation should be proportionate to risk and tasked the Council for Healthcare Regulatory Excellence (CHRE) to examine this area. In 2009, the CHRE published its first report on the matter and recommended that 'additional statutory regulation' was unnecessary. Subsequent reports (CHRE 2010a, b) strengthened the case for improving governance arrangements in the workplace rather than statutory registration. While not everyone is in support of this position (RCN 2009; NMC 2010; Prime Minister's Commission on the Future of Nursing and Midwifery 2010), the Department of Health's Command Paper, *Enabling Excellence: Autonomy and Accountability for Healthcare Workers, Social Workers and Social Care Workers* (DoH 2011), states that regulators who wish to introduce registers for advanced practice must provide compelling evidence that it is an appropriate move and the best use of registration fees.

Analysis and discussion

While the development of advanced practice roles in nursing could be viewed as a huge success, moving our professional practice forward in ways that could not have been imagined even 20 years ago, the result of rapid and uncontrolled variation of the original nurse practitioner meme has been that this concept is simultaneously widely known and inconsistently understood.

In the UK, even with the introduction of the toolkit, a wide variety of roles at different levels co-exist uncomfortably under this umbrella term. This variation is even more significant when reviewing the educational and research dimensions of advanced practice globally (Gardner et al. 2007; Chang et al. 2010; Zahran et al. 2012). Lowe et al. (2012) emphasize that clear definitions of advanced practice roles will lead to standardized measures that can verify efficiency, cost effectiveness and patient outcomes. Recommendations include further research; continued work by the ICN to drive consistency in defining AP roles; and assistance with professional regulation (Lowe et al. 2012).

Although most countries now have clear definitions and competency standards for nurse practitioners, no such clarity exists for many advanced practice nursing roles (Bryant-Lukosius et al. 2004; Chang et al. 2010). The Strong Model Delineation tool, which describes the dimensions of practice of the advanced practice role in an international contemporary health service context, has been validated in a few studies. Consequently, this has the potential to optimize the utilization of the advanced practice nursing workforce (Chang et al. 2010).

Impact

Progress over the last 20 years has been significant in advancing nursing practice, but developments have often been focused on individual or specific practitioner roles such as clinical nurse specialists or in specific operational areas such as emergency services or Hospital at Night. These areas have provided opportunities for innovation, growth and evaluation, but impact has been restricted to an operational level. Consensus was achieved at a policy level with Modernising Nursing careers (DoH 2006b; Scottish Government 2006), but has not been transferred into universal practice at an operational level. These developments are an important contribution to healthcare, but they have not addressed the risks of rapid replication, variation and strategic fit, particularly given the changing health needs of the population.

It is useful to consider progress in this area from the perspective of professional impact, clinical contribution, academic development and leadership (see Table 4.1).

Strategic leadership of advanced practice from health boards and commissioning bodies has concentrated on areas such as reducing waiting times; improving diagnostic targets, which are often a consequence of short-term political targets; and support for specific patient groups.

Table 4.1 The focus of advanced practice, 1990–2012

Professional	Clinical
Aspirant	Emergency services
Dependent on team	Out of hours
Limited independent roles	Specialist areas
Academic	**Leadership**
In house	Operational focus
Individual champions	Opportunistic funding
	No joint planning but growth
	Not systematic

Workforce planning for this cohort of staff is limited, despite the number of staff in such roles and the overall costs associated with them.

Professional governance of advanced practice has been at a local operational level, clinically focused but also influenced by other professional groups, who have been critical in providing clinical credibility and overall support. Evidence suggests that developments are at times dependent on key individuals. This approach brings benefits in innovation, but challenges in terms of overall sustainability.

There is good evidence that consensus exists in relation to the academic framework required for advanced practice, with many higher education institutions offering similar approaches in programmes that include the theory of advanced practice, research, critical decision making and an applied element for an area of specific practice. Despite this, there are few examples of strategic commissioning of education for advanced practice, with many programmes being purchased by individuals. The low number of doctoral-level practitioners in clinical practice is a risk that must be addressed, as without an increase in capacity building the generation of new knowledge and evidence to support advanced practice will be difficult to achieve.

Despite the variation, tensions and challenges to sustainability, advanced nursing practice has made significant progress over the last 20 years. The challenge is now to consider how to realize the potential further so that health outcomes can be improved.

Future focus: Consolidation and collaboration

The next phase of development for advanced practice will depend on a different set of conditions, as roles will require to be replicated, variation reduced and interventions targeted to improving health outcomes and population health. The progress made during the early years and the growth phase of advanced practice form an important platform on which to move to the next phase of consolidation and collaboration.

Advanced nursing practice is now well placed to be able to make a unique contribution to improving population health outcomes. The health and social care challenge as a result of the changing demographic profile can be addressed and improved by maximizing the potential of advanced nursing practice. However, this depends on consideration of three criteria to enable sustainable progress to be made.

First, commissioners and policy makers must have a strategic approach to designing workforce solutions, including the development of a sustainable business case for advanced practice. Nurses must influence commissioning (RCN 2011) and appreciate that the economic arguments and costs of advanced practice need to be understood.

Secondly, healthcare organizations must ensure that practitioners who are operating at an advanced practice level have the knowledge and skills to practise at that higher level. Investment will be required to ensure that advanced practice moves from an opportunistic postgraduate pathway to being organized at a systematic level, with master's-level preparation becoming the essential criterion for practice. It is also vital that investment is made in increasing capability at a doctoral level, as recommended in Choices and Challenges (Scottish Executive Health Department 2002), so that the generation of new knowledge for advanced practice is supported.

Thirdly, the contribution of advanced practice to improving health outcomes must be subject to scrutiny and investment made in developing the evidence base. The focus for advanced nursing practice (see Table 4.2) should change to address population health and in particular

Table 4.2 Future focus of advanced nursing practice

Focus	Location	Aim
Population health Early years Inequalities	Primary/community care Long-term conditions Complexity Health/social care	Health improvement Millennium Development Goals
Joint planning	**Academic**	**Impact**
Workforce planning Transferability Business case	Competency based Master's/doctoral level Interprofessional Joint system	Evidence base Translational research

early years, inequalities and long-term conditions. There should be an emphasis on working with families and in communities. There are glaring gaps and inequalities in healthcare that require a fundamental redesign of professional health education (Frenk et al. 2010). That will need to rest on a preventive and anticipatory model of care.

Conclusion: Lessons learnt and future challenges

Nurse practitioner and advanced nurse practitioner roles will continue to be shaped by internal and external forces. These can inhibit or promote variation, mutation, competition and inheritance. Nurse practitioner roles have found fertile ground in the UK in the service gaps created by changing policy decisions as well as demographic shifts, but the forces that created these gaps will continue to operate. The current challenging financial environment is a seismic event that will have a significant impact on nurse practitioner roles, as will trends in population demographics. The nurse practitioner and advanced nurse practitioner roles will flourish if they continue to adapt to the changing environment.

References

Asbridge, J. (2012) Foreword. In L. Cox, M.C. Hill and V.M. Lack, *Advanced Practice in Healthcare, Skills for Nurses and Allied Health Professionals*. Abingdon: Routledge.

Beckett, D.J., Gordon, C.F., Paterson, R. et al. (2009) Improvement in out-of-hours outcomes following the implementation of hospital at night. *QJM: International Journal of Medicine* 102: 539–546.

Booth, B. (1992) Autonomy in A&E. *Nursing Times* 88: 19.

Brook, S. and Rushforth, H. (2011) Why is the regulation of advanced practice essential? *British Journal of Nursing* 20: 996–1000.

Brooten, D., Youngblut, J.M., Deosires, W., Singhala, K. and Guido-Sanz, F. (2012) Global considerations in measuring effectiveness of advanced practice nurses. *International Journal of Nursing Studies* 49: 906–912.

Brown, S.A. and Grimes, D.E. (1995) A meta-analysis of nurse practitioners and nurse midwives in primary care. *Nursing Research* 44: 332–339.

Bryant-Lukosius, D., DiCenso, A., Browne, G. and Pinelli, J. (2004) A framework for the introduction and evaluation of advanced practice nursing roles: Development, implementation and evaluation. *Journal of Advanced Nursing* 48: 519–529.

Burgess, K. (1992) A dynamic role that improves the service: Combining triage and nurse practitioner roles in A&E. *Professional Nurse* 7: 301–303.

Burgoyne, S. (1992) Emergency nurse practitioners. *Nursing Standard* 6: 12–13.

Burnip, R., Erickson, R., Barr, G.D., Shinefield, H. and Schoen, E.J. (1976) Well-child care by pediatric nurse practitioners in a large group practice: A controlled study in 1,152 preschool children. *American Journal of Diseases of Children* 130: 51–55.

Byrne, G., Richardson, M., Brunsdon, J. and Patel A. (2000) Patient satisfaction with emergency nurse practitioners in A&E. *Journal of Clinical Nursing* 9: 83–93.

Carnwell, R. & Daly, W.M. (2003) Advanced nursing practitioners in primary care settings: An exploration of the developing roles. *Journal of Clinical Nursing* 15: 630–642.

Chambers, L.W. and West, A.E. (1978) The St John's randomized trial of the family practice nurse: Health outcomes of patients. *International Journal of Epidemiology* 7: 153–161.

Chang, A.M., Gardner, G.E., Duffield, C. and Ramis, M.-A. (2010) A delphi study to validate an advanced practice nursing tool. *Journal of Advanced Nursing* 66: 2320–2330.

Clark, S. and Paul, F. (2012) The role of the nurse practitioner within the Hospital at Night service. *British Journal of Nursing* 21: 1132–1137.

Coombs, M., Chaboyer, W. and Sole, M.L. (2007) Advanced nursing roles in critical care – a natural or forced evolution? *Journal of Professional Nursing* 23: 83–90.

Cooper, M.A., Hair, S., Ibbotson, T.R., Lindsay, G.M. and Kinn, S. (2001) The extent and nature of emergency nurse practitioner services in Scotland. *Accident and Emergency Nursing* 9: 123–129.

Cooper, M.A., Lindsay, G.M., Kinn, S. and Swann, I.J. (2002) Evaluating Emergency Nurse Practitioner services: A randomized controlled trial. *Journal of Advanced Nursing* 40: 721–730.

Council Directive 93/104/EC (1993) of 23 November 1993 concerning certain aspects of the organisation of working time. Brussels: European Council.

Council for Healthcare Regulatory Excellence (2010a) *Managing Extended Practice: Is There a Place for 'Distributed Regulation'?* London: CHRE.

Council for Healthcare Regulatory Excellence (2010b) *Right-Touch Regulation*. London: CHRE.

Cox, C. (2012) Professionalism in advanced practice: The professional role. In C. Cox, M.C. Hill and V.M. Lack, *Advanced Practice in Healthcare: Skills for Nurses and Allied Health Professionals*. London: Routledge.

Currie, K. and Grundy, M. (2011) Building foundations for the future: The NHS Scotland advanced practice succession planning development pathway. *Journal of Nursing Management* 19: 933–942.

Dawkins, R. (1976) *The Selfish Gene.* Oxford: Oxford University Press.

Delamaire, M. and Lafortune, G. (2010) Nurses in advanced roles: A description and evaluation of experiences in 12 developed countries. *OECD Health Working Papers,* No 54. Paris: OECD Oublishing. http://www.oecd-ilibrary. org/social-issues-migration-health/nurses-in-advanced-roles_5kmbrcfms5g7- en (accessed 1 October 2012).

Department of Health (1992) *The Extended Role of the Nurse/Scope of Professional Practice.* PL/CNO(92)4. London: DoH.

Department of Health (2003) *Dispelling the Myths.* London: HMSO.

Department of Health (2004a) *Modernising Medical Careers: The Next Step. The Future Shape of Foundation, Specialist and General Practice Training Programmes.* London: DoH.

Department of Health (2004b) *National Health Services (General Medical Services Contract) Regulations 2004.* London: DoH.

Department of Health (2005) *Supporting People with Long Term Conditions: Liberating the Talents of Nurses Who Care for People with Long Term Conditions.* London: DoH.

Department of Health (2006a) *The Competence and Curriculum Framework for the Physician Assistant.* London: DoH.

Department of Health (2006b) *Modernising Nursing Careers: Setting the Direction.* London: DoH.

Department of Health (2010) *Advanced Level Practice: A Position Statement.* London: DoH.

Department of Health (2011). *Enabling Excellence: Autonomy and Accountability for Healthcare Workers, Social Workers and Social Care Workers* (Cm. 8008, 2011). London: DoH.

Donald, F., Martin-Misener, R., Bryant-Lukosius, D. et al. (2010) The primary healthcare nurse practitioner role in Canada. *Nursing Leadership* 23: 88–113.

Duffield, C., Gardner, G., Chang AM. and Catling-Paull, C. (2009) Advanced nursing practice: A global perspective. *Collegian* 16: 55–62.

Eddy, A. (2008) Advanced practice for therapy radiographers: A discussion paper. *Radiography* 14: 24–31.

Elsom S., Happell, B. and Manias, E. (2005) Mental health nurse practitioner: Expanded or advanced? *International Journal of Mental Health Nursing* 14: 181–186.

Fotheringham, D., Dickie, S. and Cooper, M. (2011) The evolution of emergency nurse practitioner services in Scotland: A longitudinal survey. *Journal of Clinical Nursing* 20(19–20): 2958–2967.

Frenk, J., Chen, L., Bhutta, Z.A. et al. (2010) Health professionals for a new century: Transforming education to strengthen health systems in an independent world. *Lancet* 376: 1923–1958.

Gardner, G., Chang, A. and Duffield, C. (2007) Making nursing work: Breaking through the role confusion of advanced practice nursing. *Journal of Advanced Nursing* 57: 382–391.

Gerrish, K., Guillaume, L., Kirshbaum, M. et al. (2011) Factors influencing the contribution of advanced practice nurses to promoting evidence-based practice among front-line nurses: Findings from a cross sectional survey. *Journal of Advanced Nursing* 67: 1079–1090.

Gilfedder, M., Calder, C. and James, L. (2010) Advanced nursing practice roles: Concurrent presentation. In *NHS Education Scotland: Developing Acute Mental Health Services and Care in Scotland – Sharing Progress.* http://www.mendeley.com/profiles/ayrshire-mhs-nurses/publications/ conference_proceedings/ (accessed 7 November 2012).

Gooding, L. (2004) A hard day's night. *Nursing Management* 11: 24–26.

Goolsby, M.J. (2011) 2009–2010 AANP national nurse practitioner sample survey: An overview. *Journal of the American Academy of Nurse Practitioners* 23: 266–268.

Head, S. (1988) Nurse practitioners: The new pioneers. *Nursing Times* 84: 27–28.

Hinchliff, S. and Rogers, R. (2008) *Competencies for Advanced Nursing Practice.* London: Hodder Arnold.

Hoekelman, R.A. (1975) What constitutes adequate well-baby care? *Pediatrics* 55: 313–326.

Horrocks, S., Anderson, E. and Salisbury, C. (2002) Systematic review of whether nurse practitioners working in primary care can provide equivalent care to doctors. *British Medical Journal* 324: 819–823.

Hoskins, R. (2011) Evaluating new roles within emergency care: A literature review. *International Emergency Nursing* 19: 125–140.

Iliffe, S., Drennan, V., Manthorpe, J. et al. (2011) Nurse case management and general practice: Implications for GP consortia. *British Journal of General Practice* 61(591): e658–e65.

International Council of Nurses (2002) Definition and Characteristics of the Role. Geneva: International Council of Nurses Advanced Practice Network. http://icn-apnetwork.org/ (accessed 27 April 2011).

Jennings, N., O'Reilly, G., Lee, G., Cameron, P., Free, B. and Bailey, M. (2008) Evaluating outcomes of the emergency nurse practitioner role in a major urban emergency department, Melbourne, Australia. *Journal of Clinical Nursing* 17(8): 1044–1050.

Jones, N.P., Hayward, J.M., Khaw, P.T., Claoué, C.M.P. and Elkington, A.R. (1986) Function of an ophthalmic accident and emergency department: Results of a six month survey. *British Medical Journal* 292: 188–190.

Kilpatrick, K., Lavoie-Tremblay, M., Ritchie, J.A., Lamothe, L. and Doran, D. (2012) Boundary work and the introduction of acute care nurse practitioners in healthcare teams. *Journal of Advanced Nursing* 68: 1504–1515.

Kleinpell, R.M. (2009) *Outcome Assessment in Advanced Practice Nursing*, 2nd edn. New York: Springer.

Laurant, M., Reeves, D., Hermens, R. et al. (2004). Substitution of doctors by nurses in primary care. *Cochrane Database of Systematic Reviews*, Issue 4. Art. No.: CD001271. doi: 10.1002/14651858.CD001271.pub2. Revision published online 2009.

Livesley, J., Waters K. and Tarbuck, P. (2009) The management of advanced practitioner preparation: A work-based challenge. *Journal of Nursing Management* 17: 584–593.

Lowe, G., Plummer, V., O'Brien, A.P. and Boyd, L. (2012) Time to clarify: The value of advanced practice nursing roles in health care. *Journal of Advanced Nursing* 68: 677–685.

Marsden, J. (2003) Educational preparation for ENP roles. *Emergency Nurse* 10(10): 26–31.

Mason, S., Wardrope, J. and Perrin, J. (2003) Developing a community paramedic practitioner intermediate care support scheme for older people with minor conditions. *Emergency Medicine Journal* 20: 196–198.

Medicinal Products: Prescription by Nurses Act. 1992 (c.28) London: HMSO.

Modernisation Agency (2004) *Findings and Recommendations from the Hospital at Night Project*. London: Modernisation Agency.

Morris, F., Head, S. and Holkar V. (1989) The nurse practitioner: Help in clarifying clinical and educational activities in Accident & Emergency Departments. *Health Trends* 21: 124–126.

National Audit Office (1992) *NHS Accident and Emergency Departments in England*. London: HMSO.

National Prescribing Centre (2010) *Non-medical Prescribing*. http://www.npc. nhs.uk/non_medical/ (accessed 9 November 2012).

NHS Education for Scotland (2012) Advanced Nursing Practice Toolkit. http://www.advancedpractice.scot.nhs.uk/ (accessed 7 November 2012).

NHS Management Executive (1992) *Junior Doctors: The New Deal*. London: NHS Management Executive.

NHS Wales (2010) *Framework for Advanced Nursing, Midwifery and Allied Health Professional Practice in Wales*. Llanharan: National Leadership and Innovation Agency for Healthcare.

Nieminen, A.-L., Mannevaara, B. and Fagerström, L. (2011) Advanced practice nurses' scope of practice: A qualitative study of advanced clinical competencies. *Scandinavian Journal of Caring Sciences* 25: 661–670.

Nursing and Midwifery Council (2005) NMC Council Agendum 27.1 December 2005/c/05/160.

Nursing and Midwifery Council (2006) *Standards of Proficiency for Nurse and Midwife Prescribers*. London: NMC.

Nursing and Midwifery Council (2010) *Regulation of Advanced Nursing Practice*. London: NMC.

Norton, C. (2012) The future of gastroenterology nursing. *Frontline Gastroenterology* 3(Supp 1): 16–18.

Parish, C. (2007) Nurses 'best people' to lead NHS Hospital at Night Teams. *Nursing Standard* 21: 7.

Por, J. (2008) A critical engagement with the concept of advancing nursing practice. *Journal of Nursing Management* 16: 84–90.

Prime Minister's Commission on the Future of Nursing and Midwifery (2010) *Front Line Care: The Future of Nursing and Midwifery in England*. London: Prime Minister's Commission on the Future of Nursing and Midwifery in England.

Ramsden, S. (1986) Accident and Emergency Department: Nurse practitioner evaluation report. Barking: Barking, Havering and Brentwood Health Authority.

Read, S.M., Jones, N.M.B. and Williams, B.T. (1992) Nurse practitioners in accident and emergency departments: What do they do? *British Medical Journal* 305: 1466–1469.

Read, S., Jones, M., Collins, K. et al. (1999) *Exploring New Roles in Practice: Implications of Developments within the Clinical Team (ENRiP)*. Executive Summary. Sheffield: School of Health and Related Research (ScHARR), University of Sheffield.

Royal College of Nursing (2008) *Advanced Nurse Practitioners: An RCN Guide to the Advanced Nurse Practitioner Role, Competencies and Programme Accreditation*. London: RCN.

Royal College of Nursing (2009) *RCN's Position on Advanced Nursing Practice*. London: RCN.

Royal College of Nursing (2011) *Commissioning Health Services: A Guide for RCN Activists and Nurses*. London: RCN.

Sackett, D.L., Spitzer, W.O., Gent, M. and Roberts, R.S. (1974) The Burlington randomized trial of the nurse practitioner: Health outcomes of patients. *Annals of Internal Medicine* 80: 137–142.

Sakr, M., Angus, J., Perrin, J. et al. (1999) Care of minor injuries by emergency nurse practitioners or junior doctors: A randomised controlled trial. *Lancet* 354: 1319–1326.

Scottish Executive Health Department (2002) *Choices and Challenges: The Strategy for Research and Development in Nursing and Midwifery in Scotland*. Edinburgh: NHS Scotland.

Scottish Government (2006) *Modernising Nursing Careers: Setting the Direction*. Edinburgh: Scottish Government.

Scottish Government (2010) *Advanced Nursing Practice Roles: Guidance for NHS Boards*. Edinburgh: Scottish Government.

Sheer, B. and Wong, F.K.Y. (2008) The development of advanced nursing practice globally. *Journal of Nursing Scholarship* 40: 204–211.

Skills for Health (2006) *Key Elements of the Career Framework.* Bristol, Skills for Health. http://www.skillsforhealth.org.uk/component/docman/doc_download/301-career-frameworkkey-elements.html (accessed 15 March 2011).

Spitzer, W.O., Sackett, D.L., Sibley, J.C. et al. (1974) The Burlington randomized trial of the nurse practitioner. *New England Journal of Medicine* 290: 251–256.

Thompson, W. and Meskell, P. (2012) Evaluation of advanced nurse practitioner (emergency care): An Irish perspective. *Journal for Nurse Practitioners* 8: 200–205.

United Kingdom Central Council for Nursing and Midwifery (1992) *The Scope of Professional Practice.* London: UKCC.

Walsh, M. (1989) The A&E department and the nurse practitioner. *Nursing Standard* 4: 34–35.

Walsh, R. (2001) Patient satisfaction with emergency nurse practitioners. *Emergency Nurse* 8(10): 23–29.

West, L. (2006) Physical assessment: Whose role is it anyway? *Nursing in Critical Care* 11: 161–162.

Whitaker, L. (2006) The developing role of the night nurse practitioner: The impact of nurse prescribing. *Nurse Prescribing* 4: 161–164.

Wiseman, H. (2007) Advanced nursing practice: Influences and accountability. *British Journal of Nursing* 16: 165–172.

Woolwich, C. (1992) A wider frame of reference. *Nursing Times* 88: 34–36.

Yates, D.W. (1987) Nurse practitioners for A&E? *British Journal of Accident and Emergency Medicine* 2: 10–11.

Zahran, Z., Curtis, P., Lloyd-Jones, M. and Blackett, T. (2012) Jordanian perspectives on advanced practice: An ethnography. *International Nursing Review* 59: 222–229.

CHAPTER 5

Advanced nursing practice: Regulation, governance and professionalism

Sue First and Lucy Tomlins

Chapter outline

- Introduction
- History and regulation
- Governance
- Professionalism
- Accountability and clinical governance
- Advanced practice title and identity
- Regulation, registration and control?
- Future debate

Introduction

In the current climate we are seeing advanced nurse practitioners being used increasingly in the Health Service. In this chapter the long and turbulent history of regulation and registration, its implications and the need for governance will be explored in depth. This will include a detailed review of the regulator (NMC and previous incarnations) and how Health Service employers are responding to the demands of governance. In addition, the concept of professionalism will be tied to these key issues, since the conduct of the advanced practitioner sets a standard for the profession as a whole.

History and regulation

Throughout history, regulation has been synonymous with control. Not surprisingly, some of the first documented attempts at nursing regulation emerged through the newly formed Obstetric Society in 1825 (Park 2005), where doctors claimed midwifery practice as a medical specialty. The driving force to regulate midwifery practice stemmed from a desire to exclude unskilled and potentially dangerous practitioners, in an attempt to protect the women in their care. Midwifery education (as a precursor to nursing practice) was controlled to some extent by 1872 through the Royal College of Surgeons, although it was not until later in the nineteenth century that midwifery certification was granted to females, young ladies of 'good moral character' (Park 2005: 9). As can be seen from these embryonic beginnings, moral and professional behaviour was already a requirement.

The Midwives' Institute fought for over 20 years before the Midwives Act of 1902 was passed, which led to the development of central boards that were able to govern midwifery education and practice. The nursing profession followed on its heels by the passing of the Nurses Registration Act of 1919 and additional subsequent Acts (Park 2005). The original nursing professional body, the General Nursing Council (GNC), stipulated standards of education, training and character as prerequisites for consideration of acceptance onto the register. These were early indicators of regulation being linked to professionalism and the philosophy of governance setting standards for the profession.

An overwhelming number of nursing applications to join the Council almost led to its demise, but eventually the GNC established itself as the 'curator' of nursing practice and the body undertaking regulation. Following the Second World War, increasing numbers of nurses with diverse wartime experiences swelled the employment statistics for the newly formed NHS. Changes were therefore made to complement the evolving roles and emerging technological improvements in professional education and training. The Nurses, Midwives and Health Visitors Act of 1979 saw the creation in 1983 of the United Kingdom Central Council for Nursing, Midwifery and Health Visiting (UKCC). Its function was to create a register of nurses and associated practitioners in the UK, a role that was subsumed into the Nursing and Midwifery Council (NMC) in 2002. Division of the register into three parts occurred in 2005, distinguishing between nurses, midwives and specialist public health nurses. In its *Post-Registration Education and Practice* report (PREP) in 1994, the UKCC set new standards for the post-registration development of nurses, midwives and health visitors, which were designed to improve patient and client care through matching changing healthcare needs with flexible, responsive educational provision. All practitioners were expected to demonstrate that they were continually maintaining and developing their professional knowledge and competence in order to remain on the register. However, despite its best intentions, the ambitious aspirations of this report never came to fruition.

The PREP report also identified two different levels of practice beyond registration: specialist and advanced. Explicit standards were set for specialist practice. In 1996 the UKCC undertook a project to explore advanced practice and consider the feasibility and desirability of regulating this level. This year-long consultation with key stakeholders concluded that the Council should not set standards for advanced practice, but should reaffirm the importance of all practitioners on the register advancing their practice. It also recommended that the issue of specialist practice be re-examined (UKCC 2002: 4).

Over the following two decades, advanced nursing practice was acknowledged as a discrete role, prompting consultation within the profession and its governing body. Concurrent with the decision to make nursing an all-graduate profession, ANPs required degree-level education; subsequently master's-level thinking and minimum competency standards were demanded that would enable their role's admittance to the register. ANPs meeting the NMC's criteria were expecting to see their own sub-part of the register by 2006. This failed to materialize, however, in part due to the government's response to growing public distrust of the professions following the Shipman Inquiry (2005), which led to postponement of this final legislative move.

Towards the end of the 2000s, the Council for Healthcare Regulatory Excellence (CHRE) was commissioned as an independent body to investigate health workers' roles. Although in 2010 the NMC was motivated to address the ANP competency framework, by 2011 the project was again in jeopardy, as the CHRE was demanding evidence that regulation was indicative of the best use of fees. To date the future of ANP registration remains undecided, but the growing number of ANPs means that their stance is gathering momentum.

Table 5.1 offers a quick reference guide and consolidates the timeline outlining the progress of ANP regulation.

Governance

In 2002 the NMC became responsible for education, training and performance of its members, with the overarching aim of 'safeguarding and protecting the health and wellbeing of the public' (Willis 2009: 19). Regulation through registration has long been associated with protection

Table 5.1 Timeline: Regulating and governing advanced practice

1994	1996
UKCC agrees on post-registration education and practice arrangements. The regulatory body pinpoints two levels of post-registration practice.	UK taskforce set up to look at regulation of new nursing roles.
1997	**1998**
UKCC decides not to set standards for advanced practice.	UKCC launches consultation document *A Higher Level of Practice*, looking at how registrants can be assessed and recognized as advanced practitioners. It proposes that all applicants should hold a UK degree or equivalent and have practised for a minimum of three years full time. When the consultation ends, the UKCC's governing body agrees regulation is needed.
2002	**2004**
Nursing and Midwifery Council (NMC) takes over from the UKCC as nurses' regulatory body.	NMC launches consultation into how nurses in advanced roles should be known and regulated. It proposes that advanced nurses should have 'master's-level thinking'. The consultation sets out competencies that advanced nurse practitioners need to reach, covering management of patient illness, health promotion and disease prevention. It says nurses who attain the competencies will have their advanced status recorded on the NMC register.
2005	**2007**
NMC agrees to open a further sub-part of the nurses' register for advanced nurse practice (ANP), but has to seek permission from the Privy Council so that legislation can	The UK-wide White Paper *Trust, Assurance and Safety: The Regulation of Health Professionals* is launched following the government's response to recommendations set

be drawn up. The earliest anticipated date for legislation to be in place is estimated as August 2006. Only nurses who have achieved NMC-set competencies for a registered advanced nurse practitioner will be permitted to use the title advanced nurse practitioner.	out in the Fifth Report of the Shipman Inquiry.
2008	**2009**
Department of Health commissions health regulator umbrella body the Council for Healthcare Regulatory Excellence (CHRE) to put together evidence on the changing roles of health workers.	The CHRE publishes calls for a risk-based approach to the use of job titles.
2010	**2011**
The Commission on the Future of Nursing and Midwifery recommends that advanced practice is regulated. The NMC sets up a project group to examine ANP competencies.	The Command Paper says regulators who wish to introduce registers for advanced practice must provide compelling evidence that it is an appropriate move and best use of fees.

Source: AANPE, www.aanpe.org.

of the public through driving up standards and promoting best evidence-based practice. The link to governance is a natural one, which culminated in the exercising of more government control with the introduction of the Department of Health White Paper *Trust, Assurance and Safety* (DoH 2007), which sought to make councils like the NMC more accountable.

Governance emerged in the UK in the 1990s as a result of US influence, which encouraged public employees to embrace accountability and personal responsibility for success and excellence in their work (Flynn 2002). Various systems had been implemented throughout the history of the NHS in order to attempt to regulate quality and standards in clinical practice. Financial governance emerged in the 1980s to help manage resources. In 1998, it became a statutory duty of NHS Trusts to demonstrate quality assurance and improvement by addressing these areas through the concept of clinical governance.

Clinical governance can be defined as:

A framework through which NHS organisations are accountable for continuously improving the quality of their services and safeguarding high standards of care by creating an environment in which excellence in clinical care will flourish. (DoH 1998)

The clinical governance movement demanded devolution of responsibility, through occupational management of employee performance monitoring, resulting in staff appraisals linked to performance management and personal objectives. This ensured that quality standards were maintained. It also emerged as a tool for professional self-surveillance, which in post-modern organizations has evolved into audits of registration status by operational managers, coupled with an expectation that professional bodies maintain responsibility for individual professionals' 'fitness to practise'.

The requirement for clinical governance intensified in response to medical failures such as that at the Bristol Royal Infirmary (Bristol Royal Infirmary Inquiry 2001), which found excessively high death rates in a paediatric cardiac unit. The aim was to improve quality through, among other interventions, individual accountability for clinical practice via professional self-regulation. Self-regulation refers to a profession setting and maintaining standards such as the conduct and discipline demanded of its members:

Professional self-regulation is a contract between the public and the nursing, midwifery and health visiting professions. It allows the professions to regulate their own members in order to protect the public from poor or unsafe practice. (UKCC 2001: 10)

The resurgence of governance criteria in response to various current socio-political agendas has been prompted in part by significant events such as high-profile cases of missed child abuse (Laming 2003), failing hospital standards, vulnerable adult abuse and unmet targets (Francis 2013). These events have caused corresponding anxiety and anger in the public domain, which has engineered a culture of 'competency dependency'.

Although minimum standards are important, the system has its flaws. One can only be deemed competent at the point of assessment, and the assessment is only as good as the assessor. It would be pertinent for professionals to acknowledge that task-oriented styles of assessment to satisfy a risk-averse culture also have a tendency to stifle innovation. As with other areas of popular political policy, the current trend demands that evidence of quality be demanded by transparent, tick box-style targets in order to tabulate the efficiency and efficacy (or other specified criteria) of the Trust in league tables that can be scrutinized by the public. Governance is a serious business that demands set standards of its employees, one of which is current professional registration, demanded both for protecting the public and for safeguarding the interests of Trusts through litigation. According to the CHRE (2009), primary responsibility for the governance of new roles designed to meet the needs of the service provision environment should rest with employers and commissioners. Employers and commissioners should ensure that there are robust organizational governance arrangements surrounding all types of practice that those they employ undertake. This provides the most effective means of controlling for risks to patient safety from an individual professional's practice and provides a proportionate local response. Additional intervention by regulatory bodies would only contribute to public protection if the arrangements in place were inadequately controlling the types of practice that professionals were undertaking.

Therefore, governance is employer controlled and deals with maintaining standards, quality and reducing risks, putting public protection firmly in the hands of the employers. In contrast, regulation is professional body led and deals with individual competency and fitness to practice in relation to protection of the public.

Once a practitioner is registered, theoretically the safeguarding aspect of registration ought to have been addressed. This satisfies the demands of governance, although maintenance on the register is a separate issue. The profession's requirements for continuing professional development (CPD) are measured through evidence of updated competency, which mitigates the CHRE's questioning of the need for a separate part of the register. As ANPs symbolize achievement on the career pathway and role modelling for the profession, the behavioural aspect of professionalism need not be confused with the elevation of professional status that registration might be perceived to deliver. This is not a separate profession (as which for example midwifery could be classified), since in terms of its self-regulation it will always be affiliated to nursing as an extension of the profession.

What do ANPs perceive to be the benefits of having their own part of the register? At the RCN Congress in 2010, 80% of RCN members passed a resolution asking the RCN Council to lobby and support the NMC in resolving the lack of regulation of ANPs. RCN members speaking for the resolution cited the reasons outlined in Table 5.2, among which patient safety and public protection feature most prominently.

The culmination of ANPs' desires for regulation, registration and professional recognition materialized in the DoH White Paper *Trust Assurance and Safety – The Regulation of Health Professionals in the 21st Century* (2007), which addressed the issues of regulation. This

Table 5.2 Threads of arguments put forward by proposers and supporters of the resolution

Governance and control
The Prime Minister's Commission on the Future of Nursing and Midwifery in England recommended that there must be regulation in front-line care (DoH 2011b)
Patient safety and public protection were key issues, which should be monitored through measuring competency and reducing the risk of incidents through robust governance
Standardized level of education agreed
Professionalism and accountability
Accountability for and transparency of nursing
Progressing of the nursing career pathway
Remuneration
Career structure (elitist role)
Role clarity and internationalization
Lack of clarity regarding roles as well as patient confusion
Internationally transferable: USA, Japan, Australia, New Zealand, Netherlands
UK lagging behind as ANPs are regulated on an international level.

Source: RCN Congress 2010.

attempted to dispel the public's perception of covert activity by professionals to protect their members within professional bodies, and encouraged transparency (Willis 2009). However, the contradictory message from the CHRE and inconsistencies in the definition of an ANP (Brook and Rushworth 2011) appear to have negatively influenced the government's commitment to maintaining support for registration (DoH 2011b). In contrast, the RCN, nursing's largest supporting union, has remained steady and forthright in its determination to resolve the issue of a separate ANP register and maintain the profile of ANPs. Not until the debate on professionalism is brought into the arena, however, can one pursue the notion of the motivation for registration.

Professionalism

References to professionalism and professional identity date as far back as medieval universities, but not until the eighteenth century was there a distinction between 'professions' and 'occupations' (Abbott and Meerabeau, 1998). In 1711 Addison mentioned '[t]he three great professions of divinity, law and physic' (quoted by Carr-Saunders, 1928, cited in Abbott and Meerabeau, 1998: 4). Not until the nineteenth century did the first definitions of a profession appear, the key traits encompassing the need to be based around a body of knowledge, members having specialized skills and competence in application of this knowledge, and a code of ethics guiding the conduct of the professional, usually demanding professional autonomy. This elevated professionals in a hierarchy of superiority of occupational status. Furthermore, they exclude unskilled and unqualified occupations to obtain an advantageous monopoly of power in the labour market. According to Freidson (1994), professions and professionalism have largely been criticized in terms of economic self-interest, status and control of the poor.

Interestingly, nursing has always been the 'poor relation' to the original professions and would be classed as a 'demi-profession'. However, education reform and increasing competency levels within the nursing profession provided the impetus to challenge this inferior status and to demand more recognition. It is no wonder, then, that recognition features so highly on the ANP agenda.

Stacey (1992, cited in Abbott and Meerabeau, 1998: 1) draws a distinction between professionalism (behaviour) and professionalization (money and status). This provides an important means of identification, as professionalism helps differentiate between claims to the title by a paid occupation and a job that is motivated by ethical/moral behaviour. Professionalizing an occupation would have involved applying trait theory, in which motivation was associated with self-governance, expertise and financial remuneration, along with respect. However, current trends have shifted the focus to performance and contemporary thinking appears to promote the generalized professionalization of the health and social care workforce, thus redefining the terminology in respect of its social standing. One aim of this could be to satisfy the public perception of security that is often synonymous with the title 'profession' and therefore should demand a widespread, robust system of governance and regulation.

Accountability and clinical governance

The NHS Plan (DoH 2000) profiled a 10-year reform in which professional roles were targeted for change to meet the demands of a focus on consumers (Jones-Devitt and Smith 2007). Professionals are now

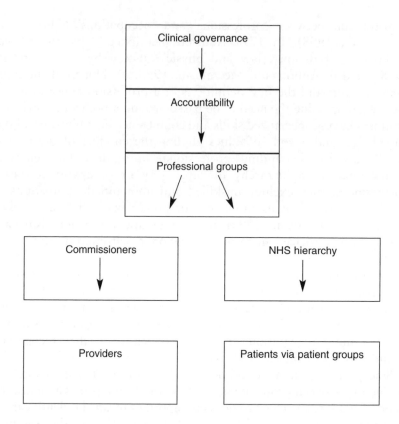

Figure 5.1 Regulation of professional groups

accountable not only to their patients and registering bodies, but to their employers in more ways than ever before through a range of National Occupational Standards, implementation of the Knowledge and Skills Framework (DoH 2004), development of professional portfolios, and evidence of CPD and competency. Professional accountability is at the heart of clinical governance for both individuals and professional groups, and a model for multiple accountability has long been advocated (Allen 2000; see Figure 5.1).

In the model in Figure 5.1, professional groups are held accountable by stakeholders along a continuum of intersecting axes. The NHS places demands on organizations, and on professionals within those services, to achieve targets as evidence of a quality service; they who will be penalized for failures, thereby regulating their activities. Horizontal accountability is to those peer professionals and local commissioning groups who will include sanctions for failure in the commissioning process, thereby holding such professional groups accountable for their activities and their practice. This will have a direct impact on the delivery of patient interventions and care.

In the vertical representation of accountability, all NHS organizations and GP practices are required to respond to the demands and needs of their local communities and to consult with them on a regular basis using local patient groups and expert patients. Professional groups to which the practitioners belong are bound to be collectively accountable through the application of clinical governance and therefore the law. Organizations have been charged with being accountable for their practice to patients, the public and users of the service, by involving users in all levels and aspects of NHS process and delivery, as stipulated in much of the Department of Health guidance (DoH 2001b). This regulatory function provides a powerful safety net in terms of political appeal.

The regulation of individuals can be portrayed in a similar model of accountability to the one for professional groups (see Figure 5.2). In a

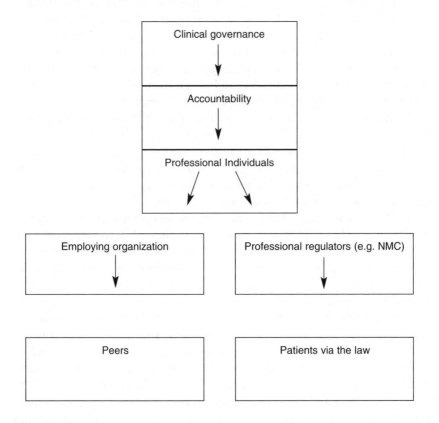

Figure 5.2 Regulation of individuals

vertical downward direction, individual professionals are held account-able for their practice both through the case or common law of negligence, under which patients can sue for compensation if a practitioner's intervention has been found to be sub-standard, and the criminal law of assault and battery, under which practitioners can be charged and found guilty of a criminal act. However, individuals are protected from personal indemnity by the legal doctrine of vicarious liability, according to which the employing organization accepts liability for the practice of its employees. Individuals are held to account for their practice by their employer via contract and employment law, as they are bound to adhere to their employer's policies, practices and procedures as part of their employment contract. The regulation of individual nurses via codes of conduct and practice has been devolved by parliament to the NMC, as part of the Nurse, Midwives and Health Visitors Act, 1997.

However, the Department of Health (2011a) has expressed caution over the confusion about where the responsibility lies for 'poor practice'. Employers' response to the demands for governance may lead to duplicated efforts by employing organizations and professional governing bodies. The Department of Health suggests that too much reliance on centralized national regulatory systems weakens the potential for prompt and effective local responses to problems, and that a balance therefore needs to be sought. As can be seen from this model of accountability, regulation is not solely responsible for patient safety.

A practitioner is accountable to much more than merely the professional governing body. The importance of accountability and its topical profile are partly explained by the progressive increase in skills-based competency, responsibility and decision making required at all levels of nursing, in response to the modernization agenda (DoH 1997) of upskilling the health and social care workforce.

In 2009, when the CHRE opposed the development of a separate register in its UK-wide report, it concluded that ANP was not a regulatory issue, as patient safety and governance were the roles and responsibilities of employers, commissioners, professional and regulatory bodies (CHRE 2009). It proposed that skill advancement is a natural outcome of career progression and that advancing practice ought not to require additional statutory regulation. Conversely, it further comments that regulatory bodies ought to consider some sort of assurance through action, where nursing practice appears to have gone so far beyond its fundamental scope that it poses a significant risk to the public. Therefore, the rationale for a separate part of the register, to fulfil the notion of action and assurance in protecting the public, would require evidence by ANPs of sufficient advancement in skill and competency beyond their base that they pose a risk to the public without statutory intervention. Thankfully, to date no legal cases involving ANPs have hit the press and given rise to discussion regarding the evidence of risk. This issue is currently being addressed through the move towards some form of national governance framework, as is occurring in NHS Wales (All Wales Guidelines for Advanced Practice, 2010).

Advanced Practice Title and Identity

Professions have been defined in the past by their members' specialist knowledge and skills (Goode 1969, cited in Freidson 1994). Knowledge has therefore been seen as an essential element in the professional repertoire, a situation that stands firm in today's changing professional climate. When the UKCC recognized the three different levels of professional, specialist and advanced nursing practice (UKCC 2002), the advanced level was seen as the most complex. At that time the UKCC envisaged progression up the career ladder to correspond with equivalent academic advancement, such that advanced nurse practitioners were to be educated to master's level (Woods 2000). There is also a perception that advanced nurse practitioners are 'associating themselves with a different identity' (Woods 2000). Undertaking master's-level education requires the student to 'reinvent' themselves, leading to an initial identity crisis and consequently resulting in a desire to develop a new identity as an ANP. This is a prolonged process under the influence of factors such as higher education, philosophy, socialization, professional relationships and the nature of clinical practice (Maguire et al. 1995: 54, cited in Woods 2000).

Advanced clinical status provides some of the impetus for ANPs to strive towards a new professional identity and recognition for such on a separate part of the register. Case study research (Woods 2000) suggests that far from it devaluing their nursing origins and being an elitist move, ANPs' desire for a separate part of the register is merely an acknowledgement and recognition of their individualized role. This enhances the traditional argument for a register for governance, quality and standards purposes, because ANPs' level of competency and scope of practice go beyond the boundaries of those of a traditional nurse. However, as Brook and Rushforth (2011) point out, the title 'advanced' infers expertise, and the word 'expertise' implies no additional risk, since one is purporting to practise with greater competency and knowledge. Therefore, the CHRE would argue that there is insufficient justification for regulation and its additional expense. However, Woods (2000) suggests that recognition of ANP status is fundamental in establishing a new nursing identity, which is partially achieved through the national recognition that registration would provide. Adding to the complexity of this debate regarding the protection of the advanced practice title is the fact that many ANPs do not hold a master's degree, and therefore do not fulfil the conditions for acceptance onto a separate part of the register should it exist.

The status of ANP regulation on the international scene was established in 2008 by a survey carried out by Pulcini and Gul (2010). Of the 32 member countries of the International Council of Nurses International Nurse Practitioner/Advanced Practice Nursing Network, 23 reported formal recognition of the role. These represented an amalgam of professional organizations, hospitals, healthcare agencies and others, such as nursing, midwifery, medical and dental councils. Surprisingly, of the 76% who reported requiring registration or licensure, less than half demanded licensure renewal for maintaining this professional regulation. Arguably, an internationally recognized title and role allow for more potential transferability through the recognition of minimum standards and an agreed level of education, which was alluded to at the RCN Congress (2010).

Regulation, registration and control?

Although the nursing profession in the UK and abroad has successfully protected the title of advanced nursing practitioner (DoH, 2010), it continues to seek further recognition through educational elevation of the profession to graduate status. Evetts (2010) affirms this view and summarizes an alternative interpretation of professionalism as a developing discourse of occupational change and control. Colyer (2004) argues that professional bodies' responses to government demands have been an attempt to self-manage their development and career evolution, but that the Department of Health remains in control. In addition, governmental influence to 'professionalize' the workforce has further diluted the status of the profession and challenged its attempts at self-management. Indeed, the skills escalator (DoH 2001a) introduced the concept of role development, with a 'non-registered professional' assistant practitioner progressing to post-registration, advanced and consultant-level practitioner roles.

The irony in this debate is the counterintuitive stance of the demand for recognition of an advanced or expert status by regulation and the resultant control through surveillance that such registration proposes. This poses a conflict particularly for nurses (ANPs), whose historical roots have left them in a default position of deference and subservience. Walshe (2002) exposes the paradigms of regulation as deterrence (coercion to behave well through strict enforcement of demanding standards) versus compliance (well meaning and willing to comply – a supportive and advisory mechanism), where the regulatees (nurses) have an expectation of support advice and protection from the regulator if they comply with regulations, but accept the coercive nature of conforming to standards. As such, the regulatee is by definition obliged to uphold the discipline of the regulating body, the nature of which fails to encourage, in fact actually deters, the lateral thinking, questioning and critical analytical abilities evolved through master's-level education, and subsequently stifles the innovation, trail blazing and risk taking desired in an ANP. In essence, the element of calculated risk that leads to innovative and evolving practice is at risk of being contained through increased bureaucratic processes of governance and regulation (Weber 1987). This highlights the contradiction between restraining regulations and the expression of tacit knowledge and expertise in complex situations, which Flynn (2002) reminds us is the province of 'profession and professionalism'.

Future debate

In the debate about regulation, the historical roots of professionalism continue to influence current motivation to pursue the issue of registration. The argument regarding governance and safety is limited in its impact as a robust rationale for demanding a separate part of the nursing and midwifery register. It has been suggested that advanced practice should be recognized as a 'level of practice' (Barton et al, 2012) and not defined as a specific role. This level needs to be identified with national standards defined within a national governance framework. Consequently, this could remove the need for a separate part of the register. The governance issue is addressed by the assessment of attainment at advanced level, which provides adequate safety assurance.

Irrespective of this, however, the debate remains vibrant, requiring a clear and honest appraisal of the benefits and advantages that registration would bring. The approach that may provide a more successful outcome might include focusing on level of practice, maintaining international recognition and remuneration with career progression, which are topics that the RCN highlights as influential. Nevertheless, a substantial argument for registration will have to gain credit in order to receive the input of finances and resources that devising and maintaining a separate part of the register would demand.

It is clear that the current climate is forcing a re-evaluation of notions of professionalism and that our future workforce will be obliged to adapt to new ways of working, new roles and a shift of professional power and autocracy. Interprofessional education will register at the heart of these reforms, encouraging the move towards a more cohesive interprofessional collaborative effort. The professions as we know them will be radically different and will have to relinquish their personal issues to embrace those of the wider professional world. As we enter this new phase in the delivery of health and social care, the dilemma regarding professionalization is likely to revolve around ensuring that health-care workers are able to behave professionally as opposed to gaining a professional title. Embedding such principles will remain challenging, but will be greatly enhanced through interprofessional education and collaborative working. Embracing the concept of IPE might provide the ANP with a generally accepted view that natural professional boundaries will be dissolving, and therefore provide a natural progression to the opportunity to work outside of these boundaries.

References

Abbott, P. and Meerabeau, L. (eds) (1998) *The Sociology of the Caring Profession*, 2nd edn. London: UCL Press.

All Wales Guidelines for Advanced Practice (2010) National Leadership and Innovation Health Care. Accessed at http://www.wales.nhs.uk/

Allen, P. (2000) Clinical governance in primary care. Accountability for clinical governance: Developing collective responsibility for quality in primary care. *British Medical Journal* 321: 608–611.

Barton, B.D., Bevan, L. and Mooney, G. (2012) The Development of Advanced Practice (Part 1). *Nursing Times* 108: 24, 18–20.

Bristol Royal Infirmary Inquiry (2001) *Learning from Bristol: The Report of the Public Inquiry into Children's Heart Surgery at the Bristol Royal Infirmary 1984-1995*. London: HMSO.

Brook, S. and Rushworth, H. (2011) Why is the regulation of advanced practice essential? *British Journal of Nursing* 20(16): 996–1000.

Carr-Saunders, A.M. (1928) *Professions: Their Organisation and Place in Society*. The Herbert Spencer Lecture. Oxford: Clarendon Press.

Colyer, H.M. (2004) The construction and development of health professions: Where will it end? *Journal of Advanced Nursing* 48(4): 406–412.

Council for Healthcare Regulatory Excellence (2009) *Advanced Practice: Report to the Four UK Health Departments*. 17/2008. London: CHRE.

Department of Health (1997) *The New NHS: Modern, Dependable*. London: HMSO.

Department of Health (1998) *A First Class Service: Improving Quality in the New NHS*. London: HMSO.

Department of Health (2000) *The NHS Plan: A Plan for Investment, a Plan for Reform.* London: DoH.

Department of Health (2001a) *Working Together, Learning Together: A Framework for Life Long Learning in the NHS.* London: HMSO.

Department of Health (2001b) *Shifting the Balance of Power.* London: HMSO.

Department of Health (2004) *The NHS Knowledge and Skills Framework (NHS KSF) and the Development Review Process.* London: HMSO.

Department of Health (2007) *Trust, Assurance and Safety: The Regulation of Health Professionals in the 21st Century.* White Paper. London: HMSO.

Department of Health (2010) *Position Statement on Advanced Practice.* London: HMSO.

Department of Health (2011a) *Enabling Excellence, Autonomy and Accountability for Healthcare Workers, Social Workers and Social Care Workers.* London: HMSO.

Department of Health (2011b) *The Government's Response to the Recommendations in Front Line Care: The Report of the Prime Minister's Commission on the Future of Nursing and Midwifery in England.* London: DoH.

Evetts, J. (2010) Advisory Board member Julia Evetts visits Ljubljana – Interview with Julia Evetts. http://www.hegesco.org/index2.php?option=com_content&do_pdf=1&id=41 (accessed 12 January 2013).

Flynn, R. (2002) Clinical governance and governmentality. *Health, Risk and Society.* 4(2): 155–173.

Francis, R. (2013) *Report of the Mid Staffordshire NHS Foundation Trust Public Inquiry: Executive Summary.* London: HMSO.

Freidson. E. (1994) *Professionalism Reborn: Theory, Prophecy and Policy.* Oxford: Polity Press.

Goode, W.J., Jr (1969) The theoretical limits of professionalization. In A. Etziono (ed.), *The Semi-professions and Their Organization.* New York: Free Press.

House of Commons (1902) *Midwives Act 1902.* Londo: HMSO.

House of Commons (1979) *Nurses, Midwives and Health Visitors Act 1979.* London: HMSO.

Jones-Devitt, S. and Smith, L. (2007) *Critical Thinking in Health and Social Care.* London: Sage.

Laming, W. (2003) *Report of the Inquiry into the Death of Victoria Climbié.* London: Department of Health.

Morrin, N. (1992) Unequal partners. *Nursing Times* 88(22): 58–60.

Park, L. (2005) Who's regulating who? *Midwifery Matters* 105: 9–12.

Pulcini, J. and Gul, R. (2010) Clinical scholarship: An international survey on advanced practice nursing education, practice and regulation. *Journal of Nursing Scholarship* 42(1): 31–39.

RCN Congress (2010) *Caring Together*. Resolution submitted by the RCN Emergency Care Association. 25–29 April. http://www.rcn.org.uk/ newsevents/congress/2010/congress_2010_resolutions_and_matters_for_ discussion/20._advance_regulation_for_advanced_nursing (accessed 17 December 2012).

Stacey, M. (1992) *Regulating British Medicine: The General Medical Council.* Chichester: Wiley.

The Shipman Inquiry (2005) http://webarchive.nationalarchives.gov.uk/ 20090808154959/http://www.the-shipman-inquiry.org.uk/home.asp (accessed 1 March 2015).

UKCC (2002) *Report of the Higher Level of Practice Pilot and Project. London: UKCC.* http://www.nmc-uk.org/Documents/Archived%20Publications/ UKCC%20Archived%20Publications/Higher%20Level%20of%20Practice%20 Report%20-%20Chapter%202%20January%202002.PDF (accessed 1 March 2015).

UK Central Council for Nursing, Midwifery and Health Visiting (2001) Professional Self-Regulation and Clinical Governance. London: UKCC.

Walshe, K. (2002) The rise of regulation in the NHS. *British Medical Journal* 324: 967–970.

Weber, S. (1987) The limits of professionalism. In S. Weber, *Institution and Interpretation: Theory and History of Literature*. Minneapolis, MN: University of Minneapolis Press.

Willis, R. (2009) 90 years strong. *Nursing Standard* 24(14): 18–19.

Woods, L.P. (2000) *The Enigma of Advanced Nursing Practice*. Salisbury: Quay Books.

CHAPTER 6

Advanced assessment and clinical decision making

Wendy Mashlan, Julie Hayes, Sue Wakefield-Newberry, Pippa Hutchings, Louise Roberts, Shiree Bissmire, Simon Williams, Ceri Thomas and Jane Whittingham

Chapter outline

- Introduction: Case histories
- An independent prescriber
- An advocate for the patient in secondary care
- A perspective on stroke care
- Working within care of the elderly rehabilitation
- A practice focus on gastroenterology
- The dilemmas in non-medical prescribing
- Continence assessment and management of the older person
- A practice focus on respiratory medicine

Introduction: Case histories (Julie Hayes)

This chapter has been compiled by a team of advanced nurse practitioners working in a secondary care hospital setting. That team manages patient care services for elderly rehabilitation and works autonomously under the direction of medical consultants, clinically managing patient care from admission to discharge.

The chapter seeks to provide insights into the everyday clinical life and decision-making challenges of advanced nurse practitioners through eight diverse clinical case histories, written by members of the advanced nurse practitioner team. Advanced practice is an extremely rewarding career choice, but it comes with increased risk and demands on the individual practitioners. Front-line care (Prime Minister's

Commission on the Future of Nursing and Midwifery 2010) actively promotes and encourages an 'entrepreneurial spirit' within 'radical shifts in service delivery', which is encapsulated in the ethos of advanced practice nursing. Many of the patients clinically managed by our team of advanced nurse practitioners have complex disease patterns that can be difficult to manage. Clinical guidance is used when possible, but such guidance does not help with the multiplicity of signs and symptoms that do not conform to the 'textbook' presenting complaints that we are all taught. Thus, the responsibility to provide clinical care ultimately rests with the treating clinician – that is, the advanced nurse practitioner.

Within healthcare empirical knowledge is valued above all other forms of knowledge, but its practical application is intimately linked to clinical experience, intuition and reflexive practice in the clinical arena (Billay et al. 2007). As advanced nurse practitioners, our decision-making skills have been shaped by a multi-faceted approach to knowing and learning. Years of exposure to clinical situations have enabled our clinical experience to develop alongside our equally important educational, research and leadership roles. This exposure has facilitated us in taking on the responsibility of clinical autonomy and decision making. In a secondary care setting, advanced nurse practitioners tend to be a stable part of the medical workforce alongside the medical consultant. This stability can be viewed as a valuable commodity in terms of workforce planning and succession planning for clinical roles within nursing.

There are four 'pillars of advanced practice' (NHS Education for Scotland 2007; NLIAH 2010) – clinical, educational, leadership and research – and these themes are interwoven throughout the chapter. Each of the eight clinical case histories is written by an experienced advanced nurse practitioner, and together they seek to illustrate the complexity and diversity of the advanced nurse practitioner's daily decision-making challenges. Each case history is divided into three sections: the clinical scenario, a critical analysis and a conclusion.

Case history 1: An independent prescriber (Wendy Mashlan)

Case scenario

I was asked by my colleague (a nurse practitioner without an independent prescribing qualification) at 4 p.m. on a Friday to review one of their patients whose international normalized ratio (INR) was considered to be sub-therapeutic. The patient, Mr M, had been on warfarin for many years following a prosthetic heart valve replacement, and he was also found to be in atrial fibrillation, two key conditions that require anticoagulation to prevent thrombus formation in a bid to reduce the risk of a patient having a cerebro-vascular accident, myocardial infarction or pulmonary embolus.

I reviewed his current INR, which was 1.3; the required range according to local guidelines is 2.5–3.5. I wondered why his INR had dropped from his previous result of 2.6. I noticed he had recently been started on nutritional supplements as his appetite had been quite poor. The supplements contain a number of vitamins, including vitamin K, which can block the effects of warfarin and cause a low INR reading. I decided to omit the supplements and ask the staff to refer Mr M to the dietician for advice. On review, Mr M showed a significantly undertherapeutic INR and required additional anticoagulant cover until his INR was within an acceptable range. My treatment of choice at this time was enoxaparin. However, in order to ensure that Mr M was treated appropriately, I consulted the British National Formulary (BMA/RPS 2012). On doing so I found that there was no guidance to use a low molecular weight heparin to cover a sub-therapeutic INR for either atrial fibrillation or an existing prosthetic valve replacement.

I proceeded to contact the hospital cardiology pharmacist for advice, who asked what sort of valve the patient had, as this would dictate the type of covering treatment he would require. At this point I was unaware that there was no documentation in the patient's notes and the valve had not been identified on the warfarin management chart. I told the pharmacist that I needed to clarify this position before the decision about management could be made.

I approached Mr M and explained the concern over his INR and the need to establish whether he had a metallic valve or tissue valve replacement, as this would determine his necessary treatment. Mr M appeared sensible and orientated in his manner and he confirmed that he had a metallic heart valve. To support his response, I asked whether he minded if I examined his heart; he gave his consent. On review of Mr M he appeared well, his vital signs showed that he was haemodynamically stable and he complained of no new symptoms. On examination I found that he had audible metallic-type heart sounds, which were irregularly irregular, with no obvious added heart sounds through the cardiac cycle. Given these findings, I felt confident that the covering treatment to ensure optimum anticoagulation should be managed against his prosthetic valves being metallic.

I telephoned the pharmacist to confirm that we would need to prescribe anticoagulant cover for metallic heart valves. The pharmacist advised that a heparin infusion as per hospital protocol should be commenced. This was a new situation for me as an independent prescriber. I downloaded the protocol from the hospital intranet and followed the prescribing regime in the absence of contraindication such as renal or hepatic impairment: 5000 units of heparin bolus over 3–5 minutes, followed by an infusion of 20,000 units (20 ml of 1000 units/ml) heparin sodium to run at 1000–1400 units/hour (1–1.4 ml/hr). To ensure that Mr M was receiving the correct amount of heparin, continued monitoring was necessary. He required blood for APTT ratio 6 hours post-commencement to ensure control. The protocol establishes whether the infusion rates need to be increased or decreased in accordance with the APTT ratio result. A repeat blood test for INR would be required the morning after commencing the heparin infusion.

I explained to the staff on the ward the purpose of heparin infusion and how the therapeutic intervention should be managed. I also contacted the out-of-hours/weekend medical team to explain the need for close monitoring as per protocol until the INR was within an acceptable range. Because bleeding may occur when a patient receives heparin, as a precaution I also prescribed the heparin antidote, protamine sulphate, on the PRN (when needed) side of the drug chart and ensured that staff observed for this possible side effect.

I visited Mr M on the Monday after the weekend. He had been managed very well by the staff and on-call medical teams. His INR was found to be within an acceptable range, so the heparin infusion had been stopped. A handover of events was given to the patient's regular senior doctor so that Mr M's further management could be continued.

Critical analysis

More often than not we rely on intuitive knowledge within our clinical practice (Carper 1978). As advanced nurse practitioners we often work at an expert level that ensures that everyday problems are easily resolved with little analysis or in-depth questioning. Benner (1984) supports this understanding by suggesting that the expert practitioner is able to home in on the accurate region of the problem without wasting too much time on alternative solutions.

As an advanced nurse practitioner in an independent prescribing role within this scenario, I felt that I applied the principle of this way of thinking. Even though I did not have all the information to hand, I knew where to access it in a prompt and proficient manner and acted on the necessary requirements for this patient, not the unnecessary ones. Use of reflexive thinking allowed previous experiences to be brought to the forefront of my mind. Schön (1983) describes the reflexive practitioner as one who 'reflects in action' to bring together thinking and doing in one act. It is this critical way of thinking that allowed me to manage Mr M efficiently and effectively.

Many of the patients I manage are on warfarin and require close monitoring. I am aware that if an INR becomes unstable then there may be several different reasons for this, including drug interaction, concurrent illness and dietary changes, all of which could potentially increase or decrease the patient's level of coagulation. In this case all those potential causes were reviewed and acted on accordingly. In Mr M's case I felt that the recent addition of diet supplements may have caused the INR to fall through the interaction of vitamin K, which is a known antidote of warfarin.

In relation to Mr M's required management and treatment, as an experienced advanced nurse practitioner I knew how to access the most up-to-date and evidence-based information about the most appropriate therapeutic intervention. This position underpins the necessity that the advanced nurse practitioner has to ensure that all risks to the patient have been managed, in essence ensuring that a 'duty of care' is provided to patients through a process of beneficence balanced by the need to ensure non-maleficence (Rich and Parker 1995; Tingle and Cribb 1996).

The realization of how I came to make these decisions did not occur until after the event. This is not unusual, as for many advanced nurse practitioners the process of reflection in practice is not realized until they reflect on the clinical scenario, a process of intuitive thinking as alluded to by Benner (1984). Schön (1987) reviews the process of reflection and defines it in terms of reflection both in action and on action, suggesting that practitioners not only think on their feet during a key event, but also look back on the situation to review what was good and bad about the decisions made. The process of reflection on action is not dissimilar to the learning loop described by Dewey (1933, cited by Rich and Parker 1995), a process of feedback between experience and its relationship to the event.

Conclusion

If I were faced with a similar clinical scenario again, I would feel quite confident in dealing with it safely and effectively. The use of reflective and critical analysis has allowed me to unravel key events that exposed me to myself as an advanced nurse practitioner and revealed my ability to make decisions within my clinical practice (Berragan 1998; O'Callaghan 2005). This in turn ensures that I am as safe and competent with my clinical decision making as possible, an essential component of an advanced practice role (Rich and Parker 1995).

Case history 2: An advocate for the patient in secondary care (Sue Wakefield-Newberry)

Case scenario

The clinical setting is an advanced nurse practitioner-led frailty clinic that takes place twice weekly at a small community hospital. The majority of patients attending the clinic are older adults with multiple chronic diseases and disabilities; the aim is to manage the patient within their own environment and to avoid hospital admissions. I was contacted one morning by a local general practitioner (GP), who asked if I would assess one of his patients who was of particular concern to him. After hearing his description of the pattern of events, I arranged an appointment for this patient as a matter of urgency.

Mrs S was a 72-year-old woman who was escorted by two friends to our frailty clinic. She had difficulty giving a history and so the help of her friends was required to understand what had been happening. Approximately 12 weeks before, Mrs S had been seen by her GP complaining of falls, confusion and wandering; his impression was that this was early-onset dementia. As time passed the symptoms got worse and the GP tried to arrange admission to the larger general hospital for further investigations, but to his dismay Mrs S refused. Eventually, after another fall causing a head injury and constant headache, he managed to convince her to come to the frailty clinic. Mrs S had a past medical history of ischaemic heart disease, hypertension, hyperlipidaemia and neurasthesia. She lived alone in a house and was totally independent and healthy three months ago.

On examination, her vital signs were within normal range, and her respiratory, cardiac and abdominal examinations were all unremarkable. Neurological examination reported a Glasgow Coma Scale score of 15/15; cognition was assessed using an adapted mini-mental test in which she scored 8/10. Examination of the cranial nerves showed hemianopia, facial palsy, neglect and weakness on the left side. Ataxia and slight dysarthria were also noted. Lower motor examination continued to show abnormalities, with arm drift and weakness in her left upper and lower limbs. Reflexes were decreased, with normal tone and sensation. Her plantars were equivocal. Assessment of coordination showed dysdiadochokinesia and dysmetria also on the left, which was not in keeping with the rest of her neurological findings. My differential diagnosis at this time was a chronic subdural haemorrhage, cerebro-vascular accident or space-occupying lesion.

I then began to explain my findings to Mrs S, trying not to appear too insensitive, but explaining the need for investigations in order to treat her in an optimal manner. Again Mrs S reiterated that she would not be admitted to the general hospital and reassured me that she knew the consequences, and that she had thought about what should happen to her should she decline in health. Mrs S had decided not to receive any life-prolonging interventions and had discussed this with her friends many times in the past. The main problem at that time was that I felt she was not safe to go home alone. We spent much time deliberating options, some of which she rejected immediately and some she thought about for a while. Eventually, she decided to allow me to admit her to the community hospital ward, where she could be near her friends, and she agreed to a visit to the general hospital for a head CT, with the understanding that whatever the diagnosis, she would return that day. At this time I felt that I had no reason to question her capacity to make an informed choice about her future treatment.

The following day she returned after having a CT, which showed a large right-sided parietal tumour with significant oedema. Discussions with the neurosurgeons concluded that it was inoperable. Mrs S was relieved to be transferred back to the community hospital, where treatment to reduce symptoms commenced as well as occupational therapy and physiotherapy assessments. She was determined to go home and, after multi-disciplinary input, was discharged home with social services, district nurse and GP support. Many weeks later she died at home with her friends present. They recalled a peaceful death where she was happy and comfortable.

Critical analysis

Nurse practitioner-led clinics have been found to have a positive influence on the quality of care (Loftus and Weston 2001). Being honest with the patient when the prognosis is poor can be difficult, but effective communication skills are fundamental to the patient's autonomy (Thorns 2010). Autonomy is the ability for self-rule and can only occur in the absence of controlling interferences, therefore it is important to give the options to patients without bias (Billings and Krakauer 2011). Not all patients have the same end-of-life wishes, therefore each must be treated as an individual case. There should be no rigid approach and custom should not replace clinical decision making (Thorns 2010).

I cannot say that I felt comfortable discussing all the complications and future progression of the illness with Mrs S as these remained uncertain, but the more we discussed issues that may arise, the more confident I felt that she was completely in control of her decisions and was certain of the way in which she wanted to spend the remainder of her days. In the past, capacity has been assessed by psychiatrically trained health professionals. However, since the implementation of the Mental Capacity Act 2005, this should be done by the professional who is most involved in the care of that patient. At no point did I feel that Mrs S lacked capacity, so I believed that her wishes should be met to the best of our abilities.

NICE guidelines (2004) recognize the significance of focusing on patients' needs and preferences, and the later 'Preferred Priorities for Care' (National Preferred Priorities for Care Review Teams 2007) accentuated this. The paper inspires the sharing of information, communication and documentation of patients' options for care. This approach allows multi-disciplinary teams to plan appropriate admission and reduce interventions, and for patients to plan ahead and think about their values and beliefs.

Conclusion

Although nurses are not required generally to develop the skills to manage end-of-life decision making, nurse practitioners working in nurse-led clinics need to have the capabilities to respect patients' autonomy and choice of treatment and to act as a patient advocate. On reflection, I feel that this patient was regarded with the respect and dignity that were her fundamental right. My only concern is that not all patients will have this opportunity to convey their wishes due to personal limitations such as dementia, delirium or critical illness, or even due to lack of resources. This is why it is essential for the advanced nurse practitioner to act as an advocate to arrange the necessary care to support the end-of-life decisions that their patients make.

Case history 3: A perspective on stroke care (Pippa Hutchings)

Case scenario

'An earthquake in the brain, the shockwaves of which leave a profound impact on how people move, see, speak, feel or understand their world.' This was how the Secretary of State for Health, Alan Johnson MP, described the effects of stroke (DoH 2007). While stroke can result in devastating and irreversible disability, the introduction of drug treatments such as thrombolysis offers a 'window of opportunity' to maximize patients' recovery. Evidence indicates that, for patients who meet inclusion/exclusion criteria (between 18 and 80 years of age, definite onset of symptom time known, no haemorrhage confirmed by CT), if thrombolysis is performed within three hours of symptom onset, 32 out of every 100 patients treated will have improved outcomes and only 3 will have a worse final global disability outcome as a result of therapy (Saver and Kalafut 2011). With approximately 110,000 people every year suffering a first or recurrent stroke, the possibility to reduce the severity of stroke in a proportion of these patients should not be under-estimated. This case describes a practice focus on a post-thrombolysis patient and his care throughout his stay in hospital.

A 58-year-old man presented to the Accident and Emergency Department with the sudden onset of a dense left-sided hemiparesis with significant left-sided neglect. He had a previous history of dyslipidaemia and was a current smoker. On arrival his observations were Glasgow Coma Scale (GCS) 15/15; blood pressure 159/92; heart rate 78 sinus rhythm; glucose 5.0 mmol; temperature 36.4 °C; National Institute of Health Stroke Scale (NIHSS) score 17.

The Stroke Care Pathway was initiated and the consultant contacted me on the stroke unit, explaining that the patient may be a possible thrombolysis candidate. I asked the consultant to continue to check the thrombolysis inclusion/exclusion criteria and immediately arranged for the patient to be taken to the CT scanner. I then liaised with the ward manager to ensure that a monitoring bed could be made available.

The CT scan of the head showed an evolving right parietal infarct with no haemorrhage. Alteplase 0.9 mg/kg was then administered, the first 10% as a bolus and the remaining dose as an infusion over the course of one hour. At present, alteplase is the only thrombolytic drug licensed for use in the treatment of stroke in the UK (Lawson and Gibbons 2009). Later that day the patient was transferred to an acute care bed on the stroke unit.

Post-thrombolysis the treatment aims are to keep the patient's systolic blood pressure below 185 mmHg, oxygen saturation above 95% and blood glucose levels between 4 and 11 mmol, and to monitor hourly neurological observations and assess the patient's swallow.

When this patient arrived on the stroke unit, I reviewed the notes and then went to assess him to ensure that the appropriate drugs were prescribed and to monitor his condition. Stroke guidelines state that aspirin 300 mg once daily (OD) should be given 24 hours post-thrombolysis for the next 14 days. I also prescribed simvastatin 40 mg OD, to start 48 hours post-thrombolysis. I performed a bedside swallow assessment (NICE 2008a), which the patient passed, and I prescribed paracetamol as he had a headache. Neurological observations are carried out hourly for the first 24 hours, and his GCS was 15/15, power to the left upper and lower limb remained 0/5 on the MRC scale, his sensation was absent on the left upper and lower limb and he remained dysarthric.

Aspiration pneumonia is a risk in stroke patients, therefore it is important to continue to monitor speech and swallow for improvements as well as deterioration. On auscultation the patient's chest was clear, with no added sounds noted. On examination of his abdomen he was tender over his suprapubic area and a palpable bladder could be felt. A bladder scan then revealed a residual volume of 850 ml, so I inserted a urinary catheter.

A repeat NIHSS was performed immediately after thrombolysis and I performed another 24 hours later. At 24 hours the patient showed a slight deterioration on the scale. As per protocol, a repeat head CT was requested. The repeat scan confirmed two infarcts in the right posterior frontal lobe, with no haemorrhage visible. I initiated amlodipine 5 mg OD due to a systolic blood pressure remaining above 185 mmHg, and on subsequent days I added perindopril 2 mg OD and then chlortalidone 25 mg OD. I also requested an echocardiogram to assess left ventricular function and to exclude any structural defect such as a patent foramen ovale, and an ultrasound carotid doppler to assess for carotid stenoses.

The patient is currently in his rehabilitation phase and is receiving ongoing therapy. During this phase my role focuses on monitoring his physical condition and liaising with other healthcare professionals. Weekly multi-disciplinary meetings are held to discuss progress and set goals. In addition, maintaining communication with family members is vital. Monitoring psychological health is another key element of the rehabilitation process. A referral was made to the dietetic service due to weight loss while in hospital. It was also recognized that the patient may require input from the mental health team due to a low mood.

Critical analysis

Even before I meet the patient, my role often involves preparing for their arrival by ensuring that I have a monitored bed in the acute care area of the ward, or giving advice on what needs to be organized to ensure that the patient receives the best care and, most importantly in the case of possible thrombolysis patients, that there are no time delays in receiving treatment.

When a patient arrives in the emergency department they are immediately taken to the CT scanner. A scan 24 hours post-thrombolysis is also a requirement; additionally, if there is any change in their neurological status a CT scan is a priority to arrange. Being able to perform a full neurological examination and detect any changes is vital and prompt action is crucial.

Advanced nurse practitioners must discuss any requests for scans with a radiologist and it is important to know your patient's history and current status. Being prepared to argue your case and also listen to other experts' advice is an important element of the role. Post-thrombolysis, any drop in a patient's level of consciousness could be due to a cerebral bleed and the only way of detecting this is through scanning.

As a non-medical prescriber I feel confident in prescribing the necessary medications for stroke patients. In addition, I liaise directly with other nursing staff to ensure that there are no delays in patients receiving the medications.

Conclusion

Summers et al. (2009) suggest that coordinated care of acute ischaemic stroke patients results in improved outcomes, decreased lengths of stay and decreased costs, and that nurses play a pivotal role in all phases of stroke patient care. Within this coordinated care setting, the role of the advanced nurse practitioner provides the ability to practise autonomously and to help in the expedient delivery of complex, comprehensive stroke care.

Case history 4: Working within care of the elderly rehabilitation (Louise Roberts)

Case scenario

Mrs T was an 87-year-old woman who was initially admitted with vomiting and lethargy. She was diagnosed with a urinary tract infection and mild renal impairment. The infection was treated with oral antibiotics, alongside which she received intravenous fluid therapy to correct the renal derangement.

The admission assessment also identified an ischemic right foot, and as this was a new issue for the patient a CT angiogram was carried out. The results indicated narrowing of the right common iliac artery, so during the scan a 'stent' was inserted as a means of increasing the blood flow to the foot. A diagnosis of peripheral vascular disease was made by the vascular surgeon, who felt that no further intervention was required.

Mrs T had a limited medical history that consisted of rheumatic fever as a child, hypertension and rheumatoid arthritis. She lived alone in a bungalow and was normally independent and self-caring. Her family lived near and were always willing to help her out if need be. Her drug history consisted of steroid use, which had been stopped years before, and antihypertensive medication.

In the initial stages after admission Mrs T appeared to make good progress. The physiotherapist had been working with her and had reported a good level of mobility, so discharged her from their care. A few days after, the staff noticed that she had become immobile and could just about transfer from bed to chair. Mrs T complained of a new onset of pain over her hip area, which concerned both her and staff.

As an advanced nurse practitioner working within rehabilitation, I am involved in assessing patients prior to transfer to the care of elderly wards. I was asked to assess Mrs T for suitability for rehabilitation input. Given that her pre-morbid status dictated a state of independence and her ability had suddenly declined, I felt it would be advantageous to accept the patient and transfer her to a bed under my care. I placed Mrs T on the rehabilitation waiting list and she was transferred the following day.

I undertook a full assessment of the patient. My main concern was with the acute onset of pain over both hip joints with no associated radiation, and sudden reduction of ability to mobilize and transfer. Her foot necrosis looked stable with no clear signs of infection, and there was no history of a recent fall or other related trauma. On examination there were no signs of hip deformity, bruising, swelling or shortening of either limb, and no obvious pain on palpation over the hip joints or shaft of femur. She had difficulty in performing a straight leg raise with either leg and there was a significantly decreased range of movement on both sides actively and passively because of increased pain. I knew the patient had a history of rheumatoid disease; however, knowing that this pathology normally affects smaller joints with a specific presentation, I did not feel that it related to her current presentation. My impression at this point was that Mrs T may have underlying osteoarthritis, possible atraumatic fracture or a muscle strain. Given her overall presentation, I decided to organize a plain X-ray of her hips and pelvis.

I reviewed the X-ray, where I identified stable fractures of the inferior and superior pubic rami on the left side. These types of fracture can cause referred pain to the hips and become increasingly worse with movement and mobility. I made a referral to the on-call trauma and orthopaedic team to advise on treatment and management. They reviewed Mrs T that afternoon and advised conservative management (non-operative treatment), optimization of pain control and mobilization as pain allowed. Mrs T was prescribed a fentanyl patch at 25 mcg/hr over 72 hours with regular paracetamol 1 g QDS (four times a day).

My main concern with this patient was that she had sustained an atraumatic fracture and this would need to be investigated. I requested a number of bone profiling bloods to help identify the cause, which included liver function tests, full blood count, thyroid function tests, urea and electrolytes, erythrocyte sedimentation rate, immunoglobulins/electrophoresis and a specimen of urine for Bence Jones protein. The causes of atraumatic or low trauma fractures can include possible underlying osteoporosis, myeloma or bone metastasis. In conjunction with the above tests, I also requested a DEXA scan that would allow evaluation of bone density. This is the gold standard investigation to determine osteoporosis.

Mrs T's bloods were pretty unremarkable except for a borderline low corrected calcium; the DEXA scan confirmed the likelihood of osteoporosis. In the absence of renal impairment on her repeat bloods, she was commenced on alendronate 70 mg once per week, a bisphosphonate that is used to decrease bone turnover. In tandem with this a calcium and vitamin D tablet was also prescribed, as recommended by the NICE guidelines (2008b) for the treatment of osteoporosis. To ensure concordance with this regime, patient education is essential to explain how and when to take the treatment, side effects and the risk of further fractures if the treatment and dosing regime is not adhered to. Mrs T fully understood the need to take the medication, so I did not feel that compliance would be an issue.

Mrs T made good progress, became more mobile and experienced less pain over a three-week period. Her analgesia was revised and her fentanyl patch stopped, and following full assessment by the occupational and physiotherapists she was deemed fit for discharge home.

Critical analysis

Atraumatic or low trauma fractures have been associated with high mortality and morbidity in the elderly population (National Osteoporosis Society 2006). The impact on their physical function can be catastrophic (Johansen et al. 2010). This type of presentation provides an opportunity for health professionals to establish an underlying cause, raise awareness of the future risks of re-fracture and implement preventive measures (Chen et al. 2011). This was a key part of my role as an advanced nurse practitioner while clinically managing Mrs T.

The cause of the patient's fracture was secondary to underlying osteoporosis. One in three women and one in twelve men over 50 years of age will suffer a fracture as a result of osteoporosis (National Osteoporosis Society 2006). This was a key differential diagnosis to consider with Mrs T, who had not had a recent fall or other related trauma to sustain pubic rami fractures. In total osteoporosis causes 310,000 fractures in the UK each year, the estimated cost of which is

£1.7 billion (Rutherford 2010). However, the cost to the patient is significantly more in terms of quality of life. This can be evidenced in Mrs T's case, as she was clearly affected by the pain and associated reduced mobility. Her reliance on the nursing staff became more obvious, whereas she had been completely independent prior to the event.

Conclusion

The majority of people will not have known that they have osteoporosis before breaking a bone. This was an important consideration in my management of Mrs T. I felt that I needed to ensure that the correct diagnosis was made in order to provide the most effective treatment for her. Initially it was essential to manage her pain to be able to increase her overall abilities and then the treatment of her osteoporosis was imperative to prevent further fractures occurring. Overall, I felt that I carried out a comprehensive assessment of the patient that allowed for the most appropriate investigations, treatment and management to be prescribed.

Case history 5: A practice focus on gastroenterology (Shiree Bissmire)

Case scenario

The ward staff requested that I review a 43-year-old man at 4.30 p.m. The nursing staff suggested that the patient, Mr W, had become progressively drowsy over the course of the day. He had been initially admitted to the gastroenterology ward five days previously with jaundice, malaise and poor oral intake. He reported significant alcohol consumption over the past 16 years, which had increased recently following the death of his mother (reported increase from 15 to 40 units of alcohol per day). The initial diagnosis was severe alcoholic hepatitis and treatment of pentoxyffyline was commenced.

The nursing staff again noted that Mr W was increasingly drowsy, associated with worsening abdominal distension that had progressively deteriorated over the past four days. When the patient was awake he had little oral intake and reported ongoing vague abdominal pain, for which there was little relief after analgesia.

On receipt of this information, I undertook a full clinical assessment. Mr W was asleep, but rousable to voice; his speech was slow when responding to questions. Clinical observations were low-grade pyrexia (37.8 °C), blood pressure 104/54 mmHg, pulse 83 bpm, saturations 96% on room air (self-ventilating). He was icteric with multiple tattoos.

An initial neurological assessment identified that Mr W was orientated to time and place, but disorientated to person, offering limited insight into his current clinical situation and poor concentration. Asterixis was present on examination.

Clinical assessment highlighted a distended abdomen with the presence of ascites and shifting dullness. Mr W was tender on palpation of the abdomen; I was unable to palpate organomegaly given the presence of fluid. There was also a suggestion of rebound tenderness. Bilateral pitting oedema was noted up to mid-calf, with a documented weight gain of 4 kg over the past 2 days.

Due to the sudden deterioration in Mr W's clinical condition and the presence of ascites, I performed multiple investigations including full blood count, renal and liver profile, coagulation screen and blood cultures; a chest X-ray and mid-stream urine were also requested. Given that the ascites was a new clinical finding, I performed a diagnostic ascitic tap to exclude infection by requesting a white cell count and microscopy, culture and sensitivity of the ascitic fluid.

Review of the nursing care plan identified no bowel action for three days; this had not been reviewed by the medical team earlier in the day. A review of the prescription chart showed that diazepam had been prescribed by the on-call night team the evening before, at the request of the nursing staff, for agitation, despite Mr W being in hospital for five days with no objective evidence of alcohol withdrawal. Closer inspection of the drug chart also showed three separate doses of codeine phosphate 60 mg given for ongoing abdominal pain. I stopped both of these medications and prescribed an antibiotic (cephalosporin) as prophylaxis pending the availability of the white cell count from the ascitic fluid. Given Mr W's encephalopathy, I also prescribed regular doses of lactulose and ensured adequate nutritional supplements to sip were prescribed. Handover was given to the medical registrar on call to review the patient with the results of the investigations requested.

Critical analysis

The circumstances described above can be a common finding when responsible for the care of patients with liver disease; deterioration may be sudden and in some cases inexplicable. The circumstances of this particular case raised the possibilities of varied potential diagnoses. As the only member of the team available, it was my responsibility competently to assess, diagnose and implement treatment for Mr W.

Many contributory factors could have influenced the sudden deterioration. It was noted that Mr W had not had his bowels opened for a number of days, which, in association with poor concentration, drowsiness and asterixis, may indicate hepatic encephalopathy, and this may have been precipitated by the prescription of codeine phosphate given for abdominal pain. Constipation can increase the production and absorption of ammonia from the gut, and treatment of encephalopathy assumes that ammonia is mainly produced by colonic bacteria in the gut, therefore there is a therapeutic effect of bowel cleansing to help reduce encephalopathy by lowering ammonia levels with the use of lactulose (Shawcross and Jalan 2005).

Also pertinent to the clinical context is the development of abdominal pain in the presence of ascites in a patient with stigmata of chronic liver disease. Cardenas and Gines (2005) suggest that bacterial infections are one of the most feared problems that complicate the course of patients with advanced liver disease. The prevalence of spontaneous bacterial peritonitis in cirrhotic hospitalized patients with ascites ranges between 10% and 30% (Caly and Strauss 1993), with a significant proportion of patients with spontaneous bacterial peritonitis having symptoms including fever, mild abdominal pain and confusion, all symptoms that Mr W exhibited.

A theory practice deficit had previously been identified in the context of management of patients with cirrhosis and ascites. To address this, a protocol was developed that enabled me to perform diagnostic ascitic sampling, with the ability to perform a total therapeutic abdominal paracentesis if required. The development of this skilled intervention is required to offer patient-focused care, as a diagnostic paracentesis is mandatory in all patients with cirrhosis requiring hospital admission (Rimola et al. 2000).

Conclusion

As an advanced nurse practitioner with a non-medical prescribing qualification, I am able to utilize advanced clinical assessment skills with the integration of current knowledge into practice, while providing diagnostic and interventional decision making, by utilizing my clinical judgement to diagnose and adequately treat Mr W and other patients. Redelmeier et al. (2001) suggest that clinical judgement is the exercise of reasoning under uncertainty when caring for patients while combining scientific theory, personal experience, patients' perspectives and other insights. This was earlier suggested by Benner et al. (1996, cited in Rashotte and Carnevale 2004) and Facione and Facione (1996), who believe that clinical judgement, clinical thinking, diagnostic reasoning and clinical decision making may describe similar cognitive activities that nurses perform in making choices about patient care options. This statement is relevant in the role of the advanced nurse practitioner.

It is often impossible to determine causation in many cases of clinical deterioration. In the case of Mr W, it was impossible to determine whether his altered state of consciousness was due to hepatic encephalopathy or the use of opiate medication. By reviewing my clinical decision-making skills on a regular basis and by implementing clinical reasoning, I feel comfortable in managing patients with complex liver disease.

Case history 6: The dilemmas in non-medical prescribing (Simon Williams)

Case scenario

Joan, an 85-year-old female, was a patient on the rehabilitation ward following a subarachnoid haemorrhage. A subarachnoid haemorrhage is a condition when the blood vessels in the brain haemorrhage into the subarachnoid space, the area between the brain and the thin membrane that covers it (NHS Choices n.d.). Her past medical history included osteoporosis, hypertension and recurrent deep vein thrombosis that had, prior to this diagnosis, been treated with warfarin. Warfarin had been omitted due to the subarachnoid haemorrhage, as this drug potentially thins the blood and this can cause more haemorrhage in the brain. Porth (2005) notes that warfarin acts by decreasing prothrombin and procoagulation factors, and therefore acts as a vitamin K antagonist.

Since the haemorrhage, Joan had become very confused and experienced several falls prior to and during admission. During a ward visit, her daughter noted that her right calf was slightly swollen and suspected that it was a familiar picture of a deep vein thrombosis (DVT), as recurrent DVTs were evident in her past medical history. An ultrasound doppler scan of her leg was organized and the result was conclusive of a DVT. Goldhaber and Piazza (2011) note that recurrent venous thromboembolisms (VTE) occur with surprising frequency after discontinuing anticoagulation therapy.

Under normal prescribing conditions there would generally be no issue in prescribing anticoagulation therapy. The British National Formulary (BMA/RPS 2012) recommends enoxaparin 1.5 mg/kg once daily and then warfarin for three months, both treatments until the international normalized ratio (INR) is 2 or more.

Low molecular weight heparin (LMWH) has been evaluated in a large number of randomized clinical trials and has shown to be safe and effective for the prophylaxis and treatment of thromboembolic disorders (Symes 2008). The Drug Bank (2010) goes on to explain that enoxaparin binds to and accelerates the activity of antithrombin III. By activating antithrombin III, enoxaparin preferentially potentiates the inhibition of coagulation factors Xa and IIa. Factor Xa catalyses the conversion of prothrombin to thrombin, so enoxaparin's inhibition of this process results in decreased thrombin and ultimately the prevention of fibrin clot formation.

Since Joan's provisional diagnosis was a subarachnoid haemorrhage, as an advanced practitioner my initial decision was not to treat the DVT and I anticipated that the thrombus would disperse by itself. Four days later the leg was re-reviewed and remained swollen, so the decision was made to commence Joan on the prophylactic dose of 40 mg, as per British National Formulary guidelines, rather than the treatment dose.

Munson (2008) comments that while many people think that prescribing is a simple and mechanistic skill, in reality standardized therapies and regimes will not always work for everyone, as exemplified in this scenario. Thus, selecting the correct treatment for Joan could have a huge impact on her condition.

This had been a time of great anxiety for the family. Ultimately, and regrettably, Joan was at risk of dying due to the subarachnoid haemorrhage and now the thromboembolic event. Making a decision as to whether the thrombus will eventually result in pulmonary emboli as a result of not treating the DVT, or possibly having a further significant haemorrhage by treating the thrombus, was not something that would be taken lightly.

Nonetheless, as healthcare professionals we must act as the patient's advocate. Cowley and Lee (2011) cite Action for Advocacy's (2002) definition of advocacy: 'Taking action to help people say what they want, secure their rights, represent their interests and obtain services they need.' In this instance it is representing Joan's 'health interests'. Furthermore, talking to the family about enoxaparin would have given them some understanding of why we had prescribed the drug.

Concordance within prescribing gives a holistic approach to care. Jones (2003) suggest that concordance means shared decision making and arriving at an agreement that respects the patient's wishes and beliefs. Courtenay and Griffiths (2005) view concordance as a partnership approach to interactions about medicines between healthcare professionals and patients.

As a result of the subarachnoid haemorrhage, Joan's mental capacity was deemed impaired; consequently, the decision to treat or not rested with me and the family. Mental capacity is required for an adult to make autonomous treatment choices (Hotopf 2005). The Mental Capacity Act

(2005) provides a framework to empower and protect people who may lack capacity (Office of the Public Guardian 2005). The Act defines when someone lacks capacity and it supports people with limited decision-making ability to make as many decisions as possible for them. The Act lays down rules for substitute decision making. Someone taking decisions on behalf of the person lacking capacity must act in the best interests of the person concerned (Johnston and Liddle 2006).

Critical analysis

I reflected on the situation and saw no reason to believe that as Joan's healthcare professionals we could have done anything different. The initial plan to 'watch and wait' was an appropriate judgement, as the thrombus may have dispersed on its own. Michelson (2007) affirms that platelet aggregation in itself is not an irreversible process, which is an important characteristic allowing for the intervention of regulatory mechanisms capable of preventing excessive and potentially dangerous propagation of thrombosis. Nonetheless, due to Joan's previous history of deep vein thrombosis, added to the fact that her condition had left her less mobile than previously, the probability of this happening was less likely.

Effective use of communication skills is an integral part of advanced nursing practice (DoH 2000a, b; National Institute for Clinical Excellence 2004). Transparency through communication is essential, as it could prevent a complaint from occurring or, as in this incident, be vital when discussing complex medical treatment.

Conclusion

It is important to note that within an independent prescribing role the situation is never simply 'black or white'. As this case shows, there are a number of grey issues with which one has to deal on a patient-to-patient basis. Furthermore, this situation highlighted to me the fact that I will face many similar situations in the course of my prescribing life.

Case history 7: Continence assessment and management of the older person (Ceri Thomas)

Case scenario

Mrs X was a 77-year-old woman who had been admitted to hospital following a fall, increased confusion and double incontinence. She was living alone with no input from social services. It was established on admission that incontinence had been an issue for the past three months, with diarrhoea up to six times a day. Her family were not coping, as they were having to call on her and help to change her after these episodes every day. She was also having occasional urinary incontinence.

Mrs X had sought advice from her GP, who had prescribed loperamide and referred her to the hospital as an outpatient for a surgical review regarding her altered bowel habit. On this acute admission she had been diagnosed and treated for a urinary tract infection and an abdominal X-ray had revealed faecal loading. Her diagnosis at this time was overflow diarrhoea and a urinary tract infection. She had been commenced on a laxative regime, the loperamide and co-codamol stopped, and she had been transferred to a care of the elderly/rehabilitation ward for discharge planning and review of her social situation.

I reviewed Mrs X shortly after transfer to my ward and it soon became evident that incontinence was still an issue. Discussion with her revealed that it was clearly a distressing situation, significantly affecting her quality of life, and an interview with the family highlighted the extent of their concern. They feared that they would not be able to continue to care for their mother with her current incontinence. I proceeded to carry out an assessment of her problem.

The history around the problem and the presenting complaint were clarified with both the patient and the family. Her current medication and medical history were reviewed, as certain conditions can be linked with incontinence and certain medications can exacerbate the situation. It was noted that Mrs X had hypothyroidism, therefore a thyroid function test was carried out to ensure that she was taking the prescribed dose of levothyroxine, as hypothyroidism can cause constipation. Her thyroid function was within normal range. Her diuretic prescription was also reviewed. There was no evidence of cardiac failure and her blood pressure was the lower end of normal, therefore I discontinued it. Her BMI was within normal range. My impression was that the urinary incontinence at this time was probably secondary to the constipation, with a possibility of an ongoing urinary tract infection.

The urinary incontinence was difficult to categorize, as the patient denied symptoms of urgency, frequency and stress. A physical examination took place in the form of an abdominal examination, examination of the perineum and rectal examination. The abdomen was noted to be slightly distended with no tenderness, and normal bowel sounds. There was no evidence of haemorrhoids or rectal/vaginal prolapse. Rectal examination revealed normal tone and sensation around the perineum and a rectum loaded with hard faeces. A post-void bladder scan was carried out that demonstrated no significant residual volume. A repeat abdominal X-ray showed that the colon was still loaded despite laxatives. A repeat mid-stream urine sample was sent to exclude ongoing urinary tract infection, which revealed no significant growth.

Neurological examination was grossly normal apart from some cognitive problems in the form of poor short-term memory. The family were concerned that Mrs X's cognitive function had declined over the past 10 months and expressed concerns around drug compliance. A CT scan of her head was requested and performed, which was grossly normal for a patient of Mrs X's age, so a referral was made to old age psychiatry for an opinion regarding her confusion and poor memory. Mrs X was seen and diagnosed with mild cognitive impairment.

I prescribed a new laxative regime, and a stool chart and fluid balance chart were initiated to promote and monitor sufficient fluid intake. Mrs X was reviewed by a physiotherapist to ensure that there were no problems with her mobility and a full functional assessment was carried out by the occupational therapist. Over a period of two weeks, Mrs X's constipation was eliminated and she was passing normal type 4 stools regularly. Her faecal incontinence and urinary incontinence resolved completely and on discharge she was continent. Her cognition also improved. Mrs X was given advice on diet and fluid intake. A social worker was allocated to her and a social care package of two calls a day was put together to assist with personal care and to prompt medication. A referral was made to the community continence adviser to review Mrs X at home.

Critical analysis

Managing continence is complex and challenging. As nurses are usually the first point of contact in relation to continence problems, assessment and management of this syndrome are predominantly considered a nursing role (Winder 2001). Within my three years of student training, my following years as a staff nurse and even as a ward sister, I was not equipped to carry out a full continence assessment. A *Nursing Times* survey (2009) revealed significant gaps in nurses' training and education in continence management. More than one third of over 1000 respondents had not received any education about caring for incontinent patients in their nurse training and over half had had no training post-registration. In order for patients to experience an improvement in their incontinence and overall quality of life, a comprehensive assessment and management plan need to take place (Thomas 2001).

An assessment of the abdomen, external genitalia and a digital rectal examination should be performed with the focused aim of palpating for masses or an enlarged bladder and assessment for pelvic floor dysfunction (NICE 2006, 2010). Within the context of an assessment for urinary incontinence, an assessment of general medical history to identify possible causes and comorbidities, including a review of all current medication that may be contributing to the problem, should be offered (NICE 2010). Medical conditions that may be relevant to urinary incontinence need to be reviewed and optimized as a result of that review (NICE 2006). A focused baseline assessment in relation to faecal incontinence should include a relevant medical history, a general examination, an anorectal examination and, if appropriate, a cognitive assessment (NICE 2007). A cognitive assessment would include the higher mental processes of the brain and the mind, including memory, thinking, judgement, calculation and visual spatial skills. Cognition is relevant as it forms part of not only a diagnostic assessment but also tailoring the treatment plan to the patient's needs (DoH 2001).

Conclusion

While nurses provide invaluable contributions to this area, advanced skills such as physical examination, medical and medication reviews, arguably essential in continence management, are not conventional nursing practices. The target of advanced practice is to ensure that advanced nurse practitioners are prepared as expert clinicians, change agents, consultants, educators, researchers and collaborators (RCN 2010). The introduction of non-medical prescribing has enhanced the quality of incontinence assessments due to the added understanding of medications and the conditions they are used to treat. I have completed a three-year MSc in Advanced Clinical Practice, gained a non-medical prescribing qualification and worked closely alongside consultant geriatricians and members of the multi-disciplinary team within a care of the elderly arena for the past 15 years. I am confident that advanced nurses working with older people are in a prime position to improve the assessment and management of incontinence overall.

Case history 8: A practice focus on respiratory medicine (Jane Whittingham)

Case scenario

Mrs A was assessed following presentation to her GP with breathlessness and had been feeling generally unwell for one month. Her GP arranged a chest X-ray, which was abnormal; local policy automatically informs the respiratory team of all such chest X-rays. Mrs A's chest X-ray indicated potential pleural effusion, therefore she was referred to the respiratory team.

It was possible to offer Mrs A an appointment in the nurse-led pleural outpatient clinic within three days of the referral. At this point a full clinical history was taken along with a detailed clinical examination. Mrs A had a background of breast cancer ten years previously that had been treated with curative intent. She was extremely anxious throughout the consultation, particularly given her previous cancer history.

From the chest X-ray a right-sided effusion was suspected and the clinical findings concurred with this differential diagnosis. Thoracic ultrasound was performed at the consultation and confirmed the presence of a large right-sided effusion; at this point aspiration of fluid is indicated (BTS 2010). This may be purely diagnostic or both diagnostic and therapeutic in nature to improve symptoms. In this case therapeutic aspiration was also indicated, and advanced clinical and decision-making skills were used to decide which action to take. In this clinic I work autonomously in making these decisions based on the clinical picture presented and the risks involved in the procedure.

Mrs A was not at all keen for aspiration, so advanced negotiation and communication skills backed up with expert knowledge were required to discuss the need for intervention. Informed consent to any intervention is key, and this must be obtained prior to any invasive procedure, therefore further training has been undertaken for an advanced nurse practitioner to be able to perform this activity.

A further part of the role is to inform the patient of the next stages in their pathway. With pleural effusion this is dependent on the results of the specimens of fluid sent to the laboratory for analysis. When the results are available, I organize any further imaging or investigations required, prior to discussion of the case at the multi-disciplinary team (MDT) meeting where a treatment plan is discussed. The patient then attends an outpatient clinic to discuss treatment options, along with any results available to the team.

Mrs A's effusion was found to be exudative in origin, therefore a staging CT was indicated. At initial consultation Mrs A was informed that if this was the case she would be contacted with an appointment for a scan, which duly happened. She was then discussed at the weekly MDT when all the results were available. Unfortunately, her pleural fluid was found to contain malignant cells and the histology indicated this to be from a breast origin. She attended clinic that day to discuss these results and agree a treatment plan with the respiratory consultant and oncologist in the orthopaedic 'joint' clinic.

Following assessment, patients with pleural effusion have 'open-door' access to the service if their symptoms worsen. This allows further assessment of the effusion and speedy treatment if required. I have the autonomy to refer on to other services such as thoracic surgeons or interventional radiologists if their input is required. The 'open-door' policy also allows patients to have contact with me to discuss their concerns and to allay psychological issues without the need to attend an outpatient setting if they prefer. Mrs A had experienced symptomatic relief from the therapeutic aspiration and did not require further intervention for her pleural effusion.

Critical analysis

There are many recent guidelines directed at ensuring that patients with a suspected diagnosis of cancer are assessed and treated in a timely manner. The current targets state that these patients should be seen by a member of the specialist team within 10 days (WAG 2005; NICE 2011). Nurse practitioners working in nurse-led clinics have been found to provide efficient outpatient care while cutting waiting times to help meet these targets (Lipley 2001; Lane and Minns 2010). One criterion within the guidelines for urgent referral to respiratory services is suspected pleural effusion. The discovery of malignant cells in pleural fluid signifies disseminated or advanced disease and therefore indicates a reduced life expectancy. Median suvival following diagnosis ranges from 3 to 12 months and is dependent on the stage and type of the underlying malignancy. It is therefore imperative to obtain a specimen of fluid for means of diagnosis (BTS 2010).

British Thoracic Society guidelines strongly recommend that all pleural procedures for pleural fluid should be guided by thoracic ultrasound (RCR 2005; BTS 2010). This has had a big impact on both the delivery of respiratory services and the training of junior doctors to meet this standard.

Conclusion

The challenges outlined in this case created a need for change in the way in which patients are assessed and treated within respiratory medicine. These included implementing changes in the role of the respiratory advanced nurse practitioner (RANP) in order to take on additional new skills, which included Royal College of Radiologists Level 1 ultrasound and the ability to perform thoracentesis. Part of the role has evolved into being the first contact for all patients with chest X-rays where an abnormality is presumed to be due to pleural effusion. The patient can be assessed, treated and monitored by me. This has created a 'one-stop clinic' that frees up time for the respiratory consultants to focus on other areas of more complex patient diagnosis and treatment, and prevents patients having to make multiple outpatient visits. Patients also perceive that I have more time to spend with them and are able to discuss their anxieties around the procedures, potential diagnoses and treatment pathways.

This innovation in care ensures that patients are assessed, diagnosed and treated within specified waiting times, thus striving to meet national targets. Patients also make fewer hospital visits and have one point of contact, resulting in an improved patient journey.

Reflective questions

1. What was your impression of the advanced practice role in clinical practice prior to reading this chapter?
2. Discuss the reflective models applicable to advanced practice and how you can apply them to evaluate your own practice.
3. From a service provision point of view, how does the advanced practice service model compare to the medical model?
4. Has this chapter influenced your clinical practice and development?

References

Action for Advocacy (2002) *The Advocacy Charter: Defining and Promoting Key Advocacy Principles.* London: Action for Advocacy.

Benner, P. (1984) *From Novice to Expert: Excellence and Power in Clinical Nursing Practice.* Menlo Park, CA: Addison-Wesley.

Berragan, L. (1998) Nursing practice draws upon several ways of knowing. *Journal of Clinical Nursing* 7(3): 209–217.

Billay, D., Myrick, F., Lutranga, F. and Yonge, O. (2007) A pragmatic view of intuitive knowledge in nursing practice. *Nursing Forum* 42(3): 147–155.

Billings, A.J. and Krakauer, E.L. (2011) On patient autonomy and physician responsibility in end-of-life care. *Archives of Internal Medicine* 171(9): 849–853.

British Medical Association and Royal Pharmaceutical Society of Great Britain (2012) *British National Formulary,* 63rd edn. London: BMA/RPS.

British Thoracic Society (2010) *Pleural Disease Guideline.* London: BTS.

Caly, W.R. and Strauss, E. (1993) A prospective study of bacterial infections in patients with cirrhosis. *Journal of Hepatology* 18(3): 353–358.

Cardenas, A. and Gines, P. (2005) Management of complications of cirrhosis in patients awaiting liver transplantation. *Journal of Hepatology* 42: S124–S133.

Carper, B. (1978) *Fundamental Patterns of Knowing in Nursing.* Rockville, MD: Aspen Systems.

Chen, S.J., Cameron, I.D., Simpson, J.M. et al. (2011) Low trauma fractures indicate increased risk of hip fracture in frail older people. *Journal of Bone Mineral Research* 46(2): 428–433.

Courtenay, M. and Griffiths, M. (2005) *Independent and Supplementary Prescribing: An Essential Guide,* 2nd edn. Cambridge: Cambridge University Press.

Cowley, J. and Lee, S. (2011) Safeguarding people's rights under the Mental Capacity Act. *Nursing Older People* 23(1): 19–23.

Department of Constitutional Affairs (2005) *Code of Practice Mental Capacity Act.* London: DCA.

Department of Health (2000a) *The NHS Plan.* London: HMSO.

Department of Health (2000b) *The NHS Cancer Plan.* London: HMSO.

Department of Health (2001) *The National Service Framework for Older People.* London: HMSO.

Department of Health (2007) *National Stroke Strategy.* London: DoH. http://webarchive.nationalarchives.gov.uk/20130107105354/http://www.dh. gov.uk/en/Publicationsandstatistics/Publications/PublicationsPolicyAnd Guidance/DH_081062 (accessed 21 February 2012).

Drug Bank (2010) Enoxaparin. http://www.drugbank.ca/drugs/DB01225 (accessed 26 March 2011).

Facione, N. and Facione, P. (1996) Externalizing the critical thinking in knowledge development and clinical judgement. *Nursing Outlook* 44: 129–136.

Goldhaber, S.Z. and Piazza, G. (2011) Optimal duration of anticoagulation after venous thromboembolism. *Circulation* 123(6): 664–667.

Hotopf, M. (2005) The assessment of mental capacity. *Clinical Medicine* 5(6): 580–584.

Johansen, A., Mansor, M., Beck, S., Mahoney, H. and Thomas, S. (2010) Outcome following hip fracture: Post-discharge residence and long-term mortality. *Age and Ageing* 39(5): 653–656.

Johnston, C. and Liddle, J. (2006) The Mental Capacity Act 2005: A new framework for healthcare decision making. *Journal of Medical Ethics* 33: 94–97.

Jones, G. (2003) Prescribing and taking medicines. *British Medical Journal* 327: 7419.

Lane, L. and Minns, S. (2010) Empowering advanced practitioners to set up nurse led clinics for improved outpatient care. *Nursing Times* 106(13): 14–15.

Lawson, C. and Gibbons, D. (2009) Acute management of stroke in the emergency department. *Emergency Nurse* 17(5): 30–34.

Lipley, N. (2001) NAO backs nurse-led clinics to ease outpatient waiting. *Nursing Standard* 15(46): 6.

Loftus, L.A. and Weston, V. (2001) The development of nurse-led clinics in cancer care. *Journal of Clinical Nursing* 10(2): 215–220.

Michelson, A.D. (2007) *Platelets*, 2nd edn. Waltham, MA: Academic Press.

Munson, E. (2008) Passion for prescribing. *Nursing Standard* 22(28): 24.

National Institute for Health and Clinical Excellence (2004) *Improving Supportive and Palliative Care for Adults with Cancer.* London: NICE.

National Institute for Health and Clinical Excellence (2006) *Urinary Incontinence: The Management of Urinary Incontinence in Women.* London: NICE.

National Institute for Health and Clinical Excellence (2007) *Faecal Incontinence: The Management of Faecal Incontinence in Adults.* London: NICE.

National Institute for Health and Clinical Excellence (2008a) *Stroke: Diagnosis and Initial Management of Acute Stroke and Transient Ischaemic Attack.* London: NICE.

National Institute for Health and Clinical Excellence (2008b) *Alendronate, Etidronate, Risedronate, Raloxifene, Strontium ranelate and Teriparatide for the Secondary Prevention of Osteoporotic Fragility Fractures in Post Menopausal Women* (amended). TA161. London: NICE.

National Institute for Health and Clinical Excellence (2010) *Lower Urinary Tract Symptoms: The Management of Lower Urinary Tract Symptoms in Men.* London: NICE.

National Institute for Health and Clinical Excellence (2011) *Lung Cancer: The Diagnosis and Treatment of Lung Cancer.* London: NICE.

National Leadership and Innovation Agency for Healthcare (2010) *Framework for Advanced Nursing, Midwifery and Allied Health Professional Practice in Wales.* Llanharan: NLIAH. www.wales.nhs.uk/sitesplus/documents/829/NLIAH%20Advanced%20Practice%20Framework.pdf (accessed 20 February 2015).

National Osteoporosis Society (2006) Osteoporosis Facts and Figures v1.1. Camerton: NOS. http://nos.org.uk/Document.Doc?id=47 (accessed 20 February 2015).

National Preferred Priorities for Care Review Teams (2007) *Preferred Priorities of Care.* Leicester: National End of Life Care Programme.

NHS Choices (n.d.) Subarachnoid haemorrhage. http://www.nhs.uk/Conditions/ Subarachnoid-haemorrhage/Pages/Introduction.aspx (accessed 1 March 2015).

NHS Education for Scotland (2007) *Advanced Nursing Practice Toolkit.* Edinburgh: NHS Scotland. http://www.advancedpractice.scot.nhs.uk (accessed 20 February 2015).

Nursing Times (2009) Nurses must receive sufficient continence education and training. *Nursing Times* 105(1): 32–33.

O'Callaghan, N. (2005) The use of expert practice to explore reflection. *Nursing Standard* 19: 39.

Office of the Public Guardian (2005) *Mental Capacity Act.* Birmingham: OPG.

Porth, C.M. (2005) *Pathophysiology: Concepts of Altered Health States*, 7th edn. London: Lippincott, Williams and Williams.

Prime Minister's Commission on the Future of Nursing and Midwifery in England (2010) *Front Line Care.* London: PMC.

Rashotte, J. and Carnevale, F.A. (2004) Medical and nursing clinical decision making: A comparative epistemological analysis. *Nursing Philosophy* 5: 160–174.

Redelmeier, D.A., Ferris, L.E., Tu, J.V., Hux, J.E. and Schull, M.J. (2001) Problems for clinical judgement: Introducing cognitive psychology as one more basic science. *Canadian Medical Association* 164(3): 358–360.

Rich, A. and Parker, D.L. (1995) Reflection and critical incident analysis: Critical and moral implications of their use within nursing and midwifery education. *Journal of Advanced Nursing* 22: 1050–1057.

Rimola, A., Garcia-Tsao, G. and Navasa, M. (2000) Diagnosis, treatment and prophylaxis of spontaneous bacterial peritonitis: A consensus document. *Journal of Hepatology* 32: 142–153.

Royal College of Nursing (2010) *Advanced Nurse Practitioners: An RCN Guide to the Advanced Nurse Practitioner Role, Competences and Programme Accreditation.* London: RCN.

Royal College of Radiologists (2005) *Ultrasound Training Recommendations for Medical and Surgical Specialities.* London: RCR.

Runyan, B.A. (2004) Management of adult patients with ascites due to cirrhosis. *Hepatology* 39: 841–856.

Rutherford, D. (2010) Osteporosis. Netdoctor. http://www.netdoctor.co.uk/ diseases/facts/osteoporosis.htm (accessed 29 February 2012).

Saver, J.L. and Kalafut, M. (2011) Thrombolytic Therapy in Stroke. Medscape. http://emedicine.medscape.com/article/1160840-overview (accessed 20 March 2012).

Schön, D.A. (1983) *The Reflective Practitioner: How Professionals Think in Action.* London: Temple Smith.

Schön, D.A. (1987) *Educating the Reflective Practitioner: Toward a New Design of Teaching and Learning in the Professions.* London: Jossey-Bass.

Selim, M. (2007) Stroke: Historical perspectives and future directions. In D.M. Greer (ed.), *Acute Ischemic Stroke: An Evidence-Based Approach.* Toronto: Wiley.

Shawcross, J. and Jalan, R. (2005) Dispelling myths in the treatment of encephalopathy. *Lancet* 365: 431–434.

Summers, D., Leonard, A., Wentworth, D. et al. (2009) Comprehensive overview of nursing and interdisciplinary care of the acute ischaemic stroke patient. *Stroke* 40: 2911–2944.

Symes, J. (2008) Low molecular weight heparins in patients with renal insufficiency. *CANNT Journal* 18(2): 55–61.

Thomas, S. (2001) Continence in older people: A priority for primary care. *Nursing Standard* 15(25): 45–53.

Thorns, A. (2010) Ethical and legal issues in end-of-life care. *Clinical Medicine* 10(3): 282–285.

Tingle, J. and Cribb, A. (1996) *Nursing Law and Ethics.* Oxford: Blackwell Science.

Welsh Assembly Government (2005) *National Standards for Lung Cancer Services.* Cardiff: WAG.

Winder, A. (2001) Devising an effective general nursing continence assessment tool. *British Journal of Nursing* 10(4): 935–947.

CHAPTER 7

Non-medical prescribing

Helen Ward and Amanda Armstrong

Chapter outline

- Introduction
- Historical background to non-medical prescribing
- Non-medical prescribing education
- Professional and legal accountability
- Maintaining competence in practice and CPD
- Principles of prescribing
- Clinical skills for prescribing
- Competencies for prescribers
- Impact of prescribing on clinical practice
- Conclusion

Introduction

The road to prescriptive authority for nurses has been a long and complicated one. This chapter focuses on non-medical prescribing for nurses and discusses the historical background, the professional, legal and ethical issues, the principles for safe and competent prescribing and the clinical skills required. The competencies for prescribing (NPC 2012) are discussed, and the chapter concludes by considering the impact of prescribing on modern clinical practice.

The Department of Health (DoH 2003, 2006, 2012) and several changes to the Medicines Act 1968 have enabled the prescribing of prescription-only medicines by professionals other than doctors and dentists. Some nurses have had the authority to prescribe from a limited Nurse Prescribers' Formulary since 1994. However, since 2006 this has been extended to give independent prescribing rights to nurses, pharmacists, physiotherapists and podiatrists, and supplementary prescribing rights to radiographers (DoH 2003a). This led to the term 'non-medical prescribing'.

Modern management of disease often involves drug treatments and as a consequence many healthcare professionals contribute to medicines management, a broad concept described as 'a system of processes and behaviours that determine how medicines are used by the NHS and patients' (NPC 2001). If implemented correctly, this system will enable patients to profit from medicines that provide maximum benefit with minimal side effects, meaning that they will receive evidence-based, safer care.

The terms prescribing, supply and administration of medicines all relate to each other. However, they are not synonymous and the distinctions should be clearly understood. When prescribing, the prescriber makes a choice to prescribe a medication to be taken or used by the patient based on an accurate and comprehensive assessment of that patient. Medicines should be prescribed in concordance with the patient and informed by best available current evidence. A prescription is a legal order requesting the supply of a medicine(s) and giving instructions on its administration (by a patient, carer or healthcare professional). The medicine is then made available to a patient, carer or other healthcare professional so that it can be administered. A further distinction can be made between the supply and dispensing of medicines. Dispensing includes supply, but also encompasses other activities aimed at ensuring safe and effective use of medicines. Administration is the means of giving a medicine to a patient, either into the body (tablets, capsules, liquids, suppositories, pessaries or injections) or topically onto the body (external preparations). Medicines can be administered by a healthcare professional, carer or patient (self-administration). A healthcare professional who supplies and/or administers medicine(s) does so as instructed by a prescriber, or as directed by patient group directions (PGDs).

Currently there are three prescribing options for nurses:

- Nurse prescribing
- Nurse independent prescribing
- Nurse supplementary prescribing

Nurse prescribing is an accurate description for nurses prescribing from the Nurse Prescribers' Formulary (NPF) only. This formulary is for community nurse prescribers who have completed the V100 or V150 Nurse Prescribing programmes. These nurses have different-coloured prescription pads and are able to prescribe from a limited range of medicines and medicinal products only.

The Department of Health (DoH 2006) defines independent prescribing as 'prescribing by a practitioner responsible and accountable for the assessment of patients with undiagnosed or diagnosed conditions and for decisions about the clinical management required, including prescribing'. Independent nurse prescribers are able to prescribe any drug from the British National Formulary (BNF), provided that they are clinically competent to do so. This is on the same basis as medical prescribers (DoH 2012).

Supplementary prescribing is described as 'a voluntary prescribing partnership between an independent prescriber and a supplementary prescriber, to implement an agreed patient-specific clinical management plan with the patient's agreement' (DoH 2003).

Historical background to non-medical prescribing

In 1986, a committee headed by Baroness Cumberledge stated: 'The Department of Health and Social Security (DHSS) should agree a limited list of items and simple agents which may be prescribed by nurses as part of a nursing care programme, and issue guidelines to enable nurses to control drug dosage in well-defined circumstances' (DHSS 1986). After eight years of political and professional negotiation, district nurses (DNs) and health visitors (HVs) began prescribing in 1994. Specific recommendations to the government on prescribing by DNs and HVs had been made by the Advisory Group on Nurse Prescribing in 1989 (DoH 1989). The necessary legislation enabling nurse prescribing was provided in the Medicinal Products: Prescribing by Nurses etc. Act 1992, implemented in 1994. DNs and HVs have since been able to prescribe a limited range of products approved by the Department of Health and listed in the British National Formulary as the Nurse Prescribers' Formulary. In developing the non-medical prescribing agenda, the government has built on the prescribing experience acquired by nurses who possess DN and HV qualifications.

Towards independent prescribing

The Nurse Prescribers' Formulary (NPF) for DNs and HVs, or 'limited' NPF, was quickly criticized by nurse prescribers as well as doctors as being too restricted, and despite having prescribing rights very few nurses were actually prescribing (Luker 1997). These reactions led to recommendations to extend nurse prescribing (DoH 1999). After a lengthy consultation process, a formulary was drawn up from four areas of clinical practice – minor injury, minor ailments, health promotion and palliative care – with 80 medical conditions and 180 prescription only medicines (POMs) selected for nurses to prescribe from the Nurse Prescribers' Extended Formulary.

The government's strategy document *The NHS Plan* (DoH 2000a) integrated the main principles of NHS modernization. The principal aim of the reform was to provide high-quality, accessible healthcare, designed and delivered around the needs of its users. An important part of the reform, and one of the tools designed to achieve its aims, was the goal to redesign the NHS workforce to develop and utilize their skills and abilities. Within this document the Chief Nursing Officer defined ten key roles for the profession, one of which included prescribing (DoH 2000a). Following *The NHS Plan*, the Department of Health, in collaboration with professional bodies, detailed changes to the NHS workforce in a range of specific documents (DoH 2000b, 2001, 2002). Nurses and other allied health professionals were encouraged to expand their clinical roles, particularly in chronic disease management, and were empowered to prescribe medicines (DoH 2000c).

In 2003, alterations were made to the NHS regulations and POMs in order to allow implementation of supplementary prescribing by nurses and pharmacists (DoH 2003). Supplementary prescribing is based on a voluntary agreement between a medical independent prescriber (doctor/dentist), the patient and the supplementary prescriber (nurse; DoH 2003). This agreement is recorded as a clinical management plan (CMP), a legal document that has to be agreed to and signed by both the independent prescriber and the supplementary prescriber before supplementary prescribing can take place. Each patient for whom supplementary prescribing is used has to have their own CMP, although each CMP can encompass a number of disease states.

Several key factors have to be incorporated into the CMP to fulfil the legal requirements, including clinical outcomes, name(s) of the medication(s), when the patient should be referred back to the independent prescriber, review dates and plan for reporting adverse drug reactions. The ideal CMP should consider evidence-based prescribing, clinical governance and the supplementary prescriber's level of competency. The CMP can be cancelled at any time, by the independent prescriber, supplementary prescriber or patient.

However, while giving nurses the opportunity to prescribe any medicine within their area of clinical competency, nurses viewed supplementary prescribing as being time consuming and offering them limited autonomy (Courtney et al. 2007). Restrictions within the CMP often meant that nurses were unable to manage patients comprehensively without having to refer back to the doctor.

In 2006 the Nurse Prescribers' Extended Formulary was discontinued and all independent nurse prescribers received prescriptive authority to prescribe any drug from the BNF (including some controlled drugs), provided that it was within their scope of professional practice (DoH 2006). This development, which was welcomed by the nursing profession, enabled nurses to become autonomous and responsible for their prescribing decisions and in many cases to complete a package of care for the patient without having to liaise with a doctor. From this time on, the only restrictions were schedule 4 and 5 controlled drugs.

Subsequently, legislative changes to the Misuse of Drugs Regulations 2012 enabled independent nurse and pharmacist prescribers to prescribe, administer and give directions for the administration of schedule 2, 3, 4 and 5 controlled drugs (DoH 2012). This means that all nurses with the appropriate prescribing qualification can now prescribe any medicine from the BNF on the same terms as a doctor.

Non-medical prescribing education

Nurses wishing to gain prescriptive authority as an independent/ supplementary or community nurse prescriber are required by the Nursing and Midwifery Council (NMC) to undertake a specific programme of education and training. There are currently three separate programmes for nurse prescribers: V300 for independent/ supplementary prescribing; V100 for specialist community practice nurses; and V150 for community nurses wishing to prescribe from the Community Practitioner Formulary, but who do not have a specialist practice qualification. The standards for all three are set by the NMC and can be found in the *Standards of Proficiency for Nurse and Midwife Prescribers* (NMC 2006). The differences in the formulary from which nurses can prescribe reflect the different practice needs, although there are significant overlaps.

V100

The first programme developed for training nurse prescribers was implemented in 1993 as a short course comprising 15 taught hours, an open learning pack and a final examination (Culley 2005). It was delivered by selected accredited higher education institutions (HEIs) and prepared nurse prescribers in eight NPF pilot sites. The programme content had been stipulated by the UKCC in 1991.

Following the success of the pilot study, a programme was initially designed to prepare DNs and HVs to prescribe from a limited NPF and was delivered as a stand-alone module. This programme was formally introduced in 1994 and then rolled out nationally. It is now available as V100 and is offered as part of the Specialist Community Public Health Nurses qualification, comprising 5 days of study.

V150

In 2007, the NMC approved the Standards of Proficiency for nurse prescribers without a specialist practice qualification to prescribe from the Community Practitioner Formulary. In order to undertake this programme, known as the V150, nurses must have been practising as a registered nurse for a minimum of two years and identify an area of clinical need where prescribing from the NPF will improve patient care and service delivery. In addition, they must be able to study at a minimum of degree level and have employer support to undertake the programme.

Nurses undertaking V150 also need to identify a practising community practitioner nurse prescriber who will agree to provide clinical supervision for the duration of the programme. It is the responsibility of the sponsoring trust to ensure that the student has an identified nurse prescriber who has agreed to support the student and provide 65 hours of supervised training.

V300

The NMC Standards of Proficiency for Nurse and Midwife Prescribers (NMC 2006) form the structure of a generic non-medical prescribing programme known as V300. This is offered by most universities as an integrated programme with other non-medical prescribers such as pharmacists, physiotherapists, podiatrists and radiographers. The programme is also approved by all the relevant professional bodies, including the NMC, to ensure educational quality assurance (NMC 2006). It can be offered at undergraduate or postgraduate level, although the competencies for prescribing practice are the same. Educational programme providers are required to meet with local key stakeholders to ensure that nurse prescribers are meeting the healthcare needs of the local population.

Undertaking a non-medical prescribing programme

Department of Health guidance (DoH 2006) requires nurse prescribers to fulfil the following criteria:

- Study at least at degree level.
- Three years' post-registration experience, with one year in the area in which they will be prescribing.
- Competent to undertake a history and clinical assessment and make a diagnosis.
- A designated medical practitioner (DMP) willing to supervise the 12 days (78 hours) of learning in practice.
- An identified 'need and opportunity' to act as a nurse prescriber.
- Access to a budget to meet the cost of prescriptions.
- Access to continuing professional development (CPD).
- Work within a robust clinical governance framework.

A number of key principles should be considered when selecting nurses to undertake the non-medical prescribing programme: patient safety, benefit to patient in terms of quicker and more efficient access to medicines and a better use of the nurse's skills (DoH 2004).

Educational programmes for non-medical prescribing can be delivered as either a taught or a distance learning programme. The taught programme consists of a minimum of 26 study days with an additional 12 days (78 hours) of supervised learning in the clinical area, and for distance learning programmes there must be a minimum of 8 taught days with an additional 12 days (78 hours) of supervised learning in clinical practice.

All educational preparation for prescribing programmes must be completed within one academic year and all nurses undertaking the programme must complete it within one year, unless there are exceptional circumstances and then it must be completed with two years. If a registrant does not successfully complete all the assessment components, both independent and supplementary, within this timeframe, the whole programme, including the assessments, must be undertaken again.

Throughout the programme all students are required to apply the principles of prescribing to their practice and reflect on this through a learning log or portfolio. However, they may not prescribe until they have successfully completed the programme and the relevant qualification has been recorded with the NMC (NMC 2006).

Supervision in practice as part of education

Supervised clinical practice is a crucial element of the non-medical prescribing educational programme. Each student is required to identify a DMP (doctor or dentist) who will provide them with supervision, support and opportunities to develop the competencies required to become a safe, cost-effective and competent prescriber.

The time spent with the DMP and the range of activities undertaken within the 78 hours of supervised clinical practice will depend on the individual student and their relevant experience. However, as guidance, time should be spent observing consultations with patients, discussion of differential diagnoses, clinical reasoning in relation to the patient presentation, and discussion and analysis of the patient management plan using a case study approach.

Nurse prescribers who have achieved prescriptive authority must aim to maintain their standard of competence through CPD.

Prescribing for children

In 2006 the NMC issued a statement stipulating that only nurses with the relevant knowledge, competence, skills and experience in nursing children should prescribe for children. This is important for primary care services such as out-of-hours provision, walk-in centres and GP practices, as children are frequent attendees of these services. Anyone prescribing for children must be able to demonstrate competence to do so or refer to another prescriber (NMC 2006). In 2007, the NMC then stipulated that all non-medical prescribing programmes must incorporate additional learning outcomes to ensure that all nurses undertaking the programme can take a history, undertake a clinical assessment and make an appropriate diagnosis or refer, having considered the legal, cognitive, emotional and physical differences between children and adults. Any nurse planning to prescribe for children must ensure that they have adequate training in the assessment of children. If not, it is advised that they seek further training. The DMP is required to confirm demonstration of competence.

Professional and legal accountability

There are several components to the English legal system that must be understood, as all non-medical prescribers are accountable for their prescribing decisions. As a prescriber you are accountable to the public through criminal law, to the patient through civil law, to the employer through your contract of employment and to your profession through the professional code of conduct (Armstrong 2011).

Prescribing within the area of competence

All nurses are accountable to civil law with regard to the scope of their practice and must prescribe only in areas in which they are deemed to be competent. In cases where a nurse may want to expand the scope of their clinical practice by increasing their area of competence, it is important that this is done within the framework of clinical governance.

Consent

Patient consent is a fundamental principle of healthcare law and is based on the legal and ethical principle that a patient has a right to decide what will happen to their body. Provision of information is core to the consent process and it is the nurse prescriber's responsibility to provide the patient with correct information regarding any treatment that is prescribed (Dimond 2009). Nurse prescribers should confirm that their patients know and understand what their treatment is for, how it works and any risks or possible adverse reactions. Patients should also be given advice about what to do if they experience any adverse reactions.

Record keeping

Nurse prescribers are encouraged to adopt good record keeping practice and maintain records that are 'unambiguous and legible' (DoH 2006). Records should contain details of the prescription as well as a documented record of the consultation. Ideally, any information given to the patient should be documented in the patient's notes. Neighbour (1987) describes this as 'safety netting' and considers it to be an integral part of the consultation process. The information should include advice given to patients about when and how to seek further medical attention if symptoms deteriorate. Records should be written immediately after the consultation or as soon as possible subsequently (NMC 2009).

Professional indemnity

Vicarious liability means that healthcare professionals have legal exemption from liability for damages or claims made by patients and resulting from performing duties specified in their job description. Despite this, many professional organizations now insist that practitioners have their own professional indemnity insurance. The NMC Code of Conduct (2010) suggests that while employers have vicarious liability for their employees' acts of omission or negligence, this would not cover independent practice and some areas of advanced practice. It is the individual's responsibility to establish their insurance status and take appropriate action, so nurses should ensure that they have personal professional indemnity insurance through organizations such as the RCN and that their job description reflects any extended role, including prescribing.

Although indemnity protects the prescriber in the case of legal claims by patients, any claims would be reviewed with respect to contractual law. This demands that practitioners adhere to all policies and procedures laid down by their employer. Practitioners must then act within the context of these policies and within the parameters of their employment contract and job description.

Prescriptive authority is a good example of how advanced nursing is developing. However, through the expansion of responsibility there is also a risk of the expansion of liability.

Maintaining competence in practice and CPD

Healthcare professionals have a duty of care and are responsible for the well-being of their patients. Clinical governance is a tool that can be used to achieve this and to provide safe, effective and high-quality, patient-centred care. The Department of Health defines clinical governance as a 'system through which NHS organisations are accountable for continuously improving the quality of their services and safeguarding high standards of care, by creating an environment in which clinical excellence will flourish' (DoH 2004b). Organizations and their employees are responsible for ensuring that their work conforms to the principles of clinical governance. This has clear implications for non-medical prescribing practice.

Clinical governance principles can be well integrated into prescribing practice by the provision of high-quality education and training, followed by continuous professional development. Non-medical prescribing practice should also be subject to regular audits and evaluations and be part of risk assessment frameworks established by employer organizations (DoH 2004). Audit departments in trusts are available and utilized by practitioners whose high standards of clinical excellence can only be achieved by a non-medical prescriber who is competent in their area of practice and who is able to achieve and maintain appropriate skills and knowledge, supported by the organization.

All NHS organizations and healthcare providers have a duty to support their staff in expanding and maintaining their clinical competence. Halligan (2006: 7) calls clinical governance the 'organisational conscience'. There should be a partnership between employer and employee that strives to maintain professional competencies and improve care, based on evidence-based practice. This is very important in prescribing practice where new evidence is emerging constantly and the influence of cost is becoming increasingly important.

Non-medical prescribers have the opportunity to reflect on their clinical practice both as an individual and with their team. Structured reflection is a tool frequently used to facilitate this. Reflection facilitates the evaluation of individual practice, and identifies gaps in knowledge and areas for development. There are many models to choose from and practitioners need to select one that best meets their needs and personality (Burns and Bulman 2004; Johns 2004). Gaps identified can lead to the need for regular clinical supervision, which helps practitioners to expand their knowledge base, become clinically more proficient and gain confidence in their practice settings. Research studies exploring nurse prescribers' practice experiences suggest that workplace peer support, mentoring and clinical supervision are important factors in maintaining nurses' prescribing competence in practice (Anguita 2012; Basford 2003).

In order to maintain competence and keep abreast of current research, practitioners should implement the skills acquired during their prescribing course. Critical appraisal skills are particularly useful in evaluating the validity and usefulness of newly published research before considering its implementation. It is important also to join with other practitioners in prescribing forums, study groups and professional teams to assess evidence. Developing critical appraisal skills comes with practice and peer support is also valuable, as is sharing opinions and experience.

A variety of evidence-based resources exist for prescribers to use, including a range of National Service Frameworks that all support good practice. The National Institute for Health and Clinical Excellence (NICE) produces evidence-based guidelines for use by prescribers on a regular basis. On a more local level, Health Trusts produce formularies and clinical guidelines for practitioners to use. Once they become confident, non-medical prescribers can participate in the development of such tools as clinical guidelines (Chapman 2008). A pharmacy lead in a primary care or an acute trust can be very helpful in offering guidance on local prescribing issues, especially around local formulary usage. Financial data can be obtained in the form of PACT (prescribing analysis and cost tabulation) through the employing NHS organization. This provides information about individual prescribing patterns, trends and costs. PACT is also available electronically (ePACT.net), which gives non-medical prescribers access to their prescribing patterns and the opportunity to use tools to analyse the data through their NHS internet accounts (Garrett 2008).

Finally, the National Prescribing Centre also offers learning support to newly qualified practitioners. This is particularly important when practitioners are unable to gain peer or professional support easily.

Principles of prescribing

In 1999 the National Prescribing Centre published '*Seven Principles of Good Prescribing ... a Stepwise Approach* (NPC 1999). Although this tool was originally designed for nurse prescribing, it is still applicable to non-medical prescribing and is widely used as a guide for the principles of good prescribing on non-medical prescribing programmes. It is commonly known as the 'Prescribing Pyramid' (see Figure 7.1) and the NPC recommends that the prescriber consider each step carefully before approaching the next.

Step 1: Consider the patient

It is the prescriber's responsibility to ensure that a detailed and holistic history is taken from the patient. Patients will need to have a diagnosis established before prescribing a medicine can be considered, or, if they already have an established diagnosis, this may need to be reviewed before a prescription for medicine can be issued. In Step 1 the prescriber must consider the symptoms with which the patient is presenting and whether or not the patient has taken any over-the-counter medicine or has self-medicated with herbal or alternative medications. The potential

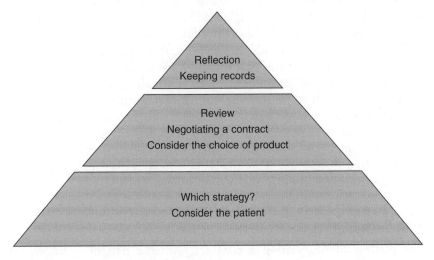

Figure 7.1 The Prescribing Pyramid

for drug interactions must always be considered. Patients should be asked whether they have experienced any allergic reactions to medicines previously taken and, if so, what the reaction was. Patients may mistake a mild side effect for an allergy to a medicine.

Step 2: Which strategy?

Step 2 advises the prescriber to consider whether or not other treatment options are appropriate before prescribing a medicine. The NMC states that nurse prescribers should only prescribe a medicine where there is a genuine need (NMC 2006). Should you undertake any further investigations or refer the patient for another opinion? It is worth remembering that patients may come to the consultation with an alternative agenda.

Step 3: Consider the choice of product

The range of products available is enormous. Some non-medical prescribers may find the mnemonic EASE a useful guide to what consider in Step 3 (NPC 1999):

E – how **E**ffective is the product?
A – is it **A**ppropriate for this patient?
S – how **S**afe is it?
E – is the product cost-**E**ffective?

Guidelines such as those produced by NICE should be consulted to ensure that the correct regimes are being followed. These should be considered alongside local guidelines; if there is any doubt the relevant pharmacy department will always provide advice.

When choosing the product, the prescriber must ensure that it is appropriate for the patient, and the dose, formulation and duration of the treatment should be tailored to the individual. Particular caution must be taken when prescribing for certain groups of patients, for example the very young and the very old, patients who have liver or kidney disease, or those who are pregnant or breastfeeding.

All medicines are associated with causing side effects or possible adverse drug reactions. The likely beneficial effect of a medicine prescribed should outweigh the potential harm (BPS 2010).

Step 4: Negotiating a contract

The process of negotiating a contract with the patient is known as concordance and is viewed as a shared decision between the patient and the prescriber. Patients' involvement in the prescribing process is known to improve adherence to medication (NICE 2009).

Step 5: Review

Patients need to be reviewed to establish whether or not the prescribed medication has been effective, safe and acceptable. Regular reviews are not usually carried out for acute medicines such as antibiotics, but by safety netting the patient the prescriber ensures that the patient returns if the prescribed medicine has not been effective. Medicines that are prescribed on a regular basis and need to be taken to manage long-term conditions should be reviewed by a prescriber at least every six months. The process is commonly known as a medicines review.

Step 6: Keeping records

All prescribers have a responsibility to keep accurate and up-to-date records of any medicines that have been prescribed. This should also include details of any advice given to the patient on how to manage their condition and any recommendations offered to the patient in regard to medicines that can be bought over the counter.

Step 7: Reflection

Step 7 encourages the prescriber to review and reflect on prescribing decisions. A team approach here can be very helpful to improve prescribing knowledge and practice.

The British Pharmaceutical Society also publishes ten principles of good prescribing (BPS 2010). These are similar to those advocated by the NPC, but there are two additional principles that prescribers should take into consideration:

- Be aware of the common factors that cause medication errors and know how to avoid them.
- Always seek to keep up to date with the knowledge and skills relevant to your clinical practice. Be prepared to seek advice if necessary.

Clinical skills for prescribing

The clinical skills required for prescribing are similar to those that underpin advanced practice generally. The prescriber needs to undertake an assessment of the patient before prescribing any medication (NMC 2006). For the purposes of this chapter, the clinical skills for prescribing have been divided into three areas: consultation, physical examination and clinical reasoning.

Consultation skills

Conducting an effective consultation is paramount for safe prescribing. The prescriber needs to ensure that a full and in-depth history is obtained from the patient. History taking enables the prescriber to formulate a diagnosis or re-establish an existing diagnosis; it helps to fill in any gaps and test hypotheses; it enables the prescriber to establish which systems need to be examined; and, most importantly, it establishes a relationship with the patient.

There are several models of consultation that the prescriber can use (Bryne and Long 1976; Pendleton et al. 2003; Neighbour 1987; Kurtz and Silverman 1996; Kurtz et al. 2005). These help the prescriber develop their own consultation skills and act as a guideline to ensure comprehensive history taking, but there is no one consultation model that is suitable for all consultations. It may be that an individual uses components from several different consultation models and adapts them to suit their own area of clinical practice.

Effective consultation skills are the cornerstone of prescribing. Without effective communication you will not be able to elicit sufficient or accurate information from your patient and without this your clinical decision making may be unsafe (Nuttall and Rutt-Howard 2011).

Physical examination skills

The development of physical examination skills underpins advanced practice and is often taught as a core module on advanced practice courses, rather than specifically as part of a prescribing programme. However, without physical examination skills the prescriber is unable to make accurate and informed clinical decisions for prescribing.

The extent to which the prescriber undertakes physical examination will depend on the patient's presenting symptoms and the prescriber's role. The rationale behind physical examination is to accept or refute any differential diagnoses generated during the history taking. It is not only the ability to perform a physical examination but the interpretation of the findings in relation to the patient's presenting symptoms that are key to a safe and effective consultation.

Clinical reasoning skills

Once history taking and physical examination have been undertaken, the prescriber needs to use their underpinning knowledge of pathophysiological principles to come to a decision about whether to prescribe or not. This is known as clinical reasoning and forms part of the overall problem-solving pathway.

It is important for nurses to have a good understanding of decision-making processes in order to identify when good decisions have been made (Buckingham and Adams 2000). Using a theoretical framework for clinical decision making enables the prescriber to structure the consultation to enhance patient care, providing transparency and therefore better protection against litigation. There are numerous theories related to the clinical reasoning process (Buckingham and Adams 2000; Higgs et al. 2008), but Barrows and Pickell's (1991) stages model of problem solving, although designed for medical students, provides an excellent framework for the overall prescribing process. The stages fit neatly into the Prescribing Pyramid and are as follows:

- Forming the initial concept.
- Generating hypotheses.
- Formulating an enquiry strategy.
- Applying appropriate clinical skills.
- Developing the problem synthesis.
- Laboratory and diagnostic findings.
- Diagnostic decision making.
- Therapeutic decision making.
- Reflection in and on practice.

This model allows the prescriber to take responsibility to make autonomous decisions in relation to prescribing, as it uses theory to underpin clinical practice. The process begins with the patient's presenting complaint and employs consultation skills to process the information gained from history taking and physical examination to reach a list of possible differential diagnoses. These are then tested further until a diagnosis is made and a management plan constructed. Occasionally no conclusion can be made regarding a diagnosis, in which case the practitioner may decide on a working diagnosis, which could be confirmed later following the results of further investigations. Reflection allows the prescriber to consider all aspects of the consultation process, building on what went well and revising the more challenging aspects.

Competencies for prescribers

In 2012, the National Prescribing Centre published a single competency framework for all prescribers. This consolidates existing frameworks for prescribing from each of the professional bodies. It was developed by a multi-professional steering group and validated by a focus group of prescribers. The aim of this framework is to implement a core set of competencies for prescribing regardless of profession. If these are acquired and maintained, the framework should enable healthcare professionals to be safe and effective prescribers (NPC 2012) and underpin the prescriber's personal responsibility for prescribing.

The single competency framework comprises of 72 individual competency statements under 9 competency dimensions, which form 3 prescribing domains (see Figure 7.2).

The consultation

1. **Knowledge:** Has up-to-date clinical, pharmacological and pharmaceutical knowledge relevant to own area of practice.

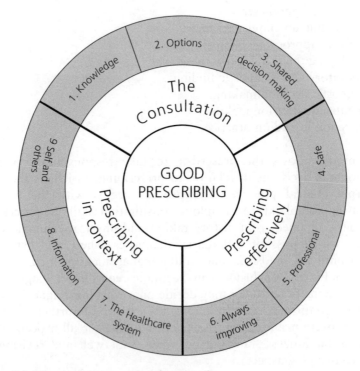

Figure 7.2 The single competency framework

2. **Options:** Makes or reviews a diagnosis, generates management options for the patient and follows up management.
3. **Shared decisions:** Establishes a relationship based on trust and mutual respect. Recognizes patients as partners in the consultation.

Prescribing effectively

4. **Safe:** Is aware of own limitations. Does not compromise patient safety.
5. **Professional:** Ensures prescribing practice is consistent with scope of practice, organizational, professional and regulatory standards, guidance and codes of conduct.
6. **Always improving:** Actively participates in the review and development of prescribing practice to optimize patient outcomes.

Prescribing in context

7. **Healthcare systems:** Understands and works within local and national policies, processes and systems that impact on prescribing practice. Sees how own prescribing impacts on the wider healthcare community.
8. **Information:** Knows how to access relevant information. Can use and apply information in practice.
9. **Self and others:** Works in partnership with colleagues for the benefit of patients. Is self-aware and confident in own ability as a prescriber. (NPC 2012)

The NPC envisages that the single competency framework will be used in several ways to ensure safe and effective prescribing for patients. For instance, it can be employed to achieve the following:

- Inform education curricula and the delivery of prescribing programmes.
- Provide the professional bodies with a basis for the development of levels of prescribing competency.
- Help prescribers in CPD through the identification of strengths and weaknesses in relation to prescribing.
- Stimulate discussions for prescribing within a multi-disciplinary team.
- Inform the development of organizational systems to ensure safe and effective prescribing.
- Inform organizational recruitment processes.
- Help healthcare professionals prepare to prescribe.

Impact of prescribing on clinical practice

Since 1994 the scope and practice of nurse prescribing have grown steadily (NPC 2012). Advances in prescriptive authority may have seemed slow and frustrating at times, but by 2012 the Medicines Act had been amended to enable independent nurse prescribers to prescribe all medicines in the same way as doctors (DoH 2012). It is now widely accepted that prescribing is a core component of the advanced practice role. With the advent of independent nurse prescribing, the principles for NHS reform set out in *The NHS Plan* (DoH, 2001a), to improve patient care, choice and access to health professionals, patient safety, better use of health professionals' skills and more flexible working, have been fulfilled. However, Stewart (2012, cited in Anguita 2012) suggests that although the published literature concludes that there is a high level of patient satisfaction regarding nurse prescribers, there must be more evidence for the success of nurse prescribing focusing on clinical, economic and human outcomes. Latter et al. (2011) conclude that nurse and pharmacist independent prescribing is becoming a well-integrated, established component of patient management. They also suggest that education for non-medical prescribing is fit for purpose and that prescribing by nurses is safe and clinically appropriate, with most Trusts having core clinical governance and strategies for prescribing.

There are now 54,000 nurse and midwife prescribers across the UK, and over 19,000 nurse independent and supplementary prescribers. Latter et al. (2011) found that 93% of nurse independent prescribers had used their prescribing qualification and that 86% were currently prescribing. At the time of their evaluation, the majority of independent nurse prescribers were working in primary care, although more recently nurses working in secondary care settings have been undertaking non-medical prescribing programmes.

Conclusion

Although prescribing is now firmly embedded within the advanced practice role, the future may see prescribing as an integral component of pre-registration nursing and becoming the norm for everyday nursing practice. However, before this can be achieved, the pioneers of nurse prescribing will need to have their prescribing habits evaluated and audited to ensure that nurse prescribing is improving the health outcomes and meeting the needs of patients (Anguita 2012; Latter et al. 2011).

Nurses have always been responsible for the administration of medicines, but it is the new role of nurse prescribing that is challenging. The different programmes and formularies that encompass non-medical prescribing are complex and have the potential to be very confusing for the patient. The added accountability and responsibility that nurses have as prescribers can also be daunting at first. However, with confidence develops competence and as the numbers of nurse prescribers increase, attitudes towards nurse prescribing will become more positive.

This is an exciting time for nurses as advanced practice roles develop in response to patient need, and nurses in the UK now have the most comprehensive prescribing authority in the world. These roles have clearly benefited patients and contributed significantly to promoting the image of nursing as a primary profession.

References

Anguita, M. (2012) More and better research into non-medical prescribing is needed. *Nurse Prescribing* 10(4): 162–164.

Armstrong, A. (2011) Legal considerations for nurse prescribers. *Nurse Prescribing* 9(12): 603–608.

Barrows, H. and Pickell, G. (1991) *Developing Clinical Problem-Solving Skills.* New York: W.W. Norton.

Basford, L. (2003) Maintaining nurse prescribing competence: Experiences and challenges. *Nurse Prescribing* 1(1): 40–45.

British Pharmaceutical Society (2010) *Ten Principles of Good Prescribing.* London: BPS.

Bryne, P. and Long, B. (1976) *Doctors Talking to Patients.* London: HMSO.

Buckingham, C. and Adams, A. (2000) Classifying clinical decision making: A unifying approach. *Journal of Advanced Nursing* 32(4): 981–989.

Burns, S. and Bulman, C. (2004) *Reflective Practice in Nursing,* 2nd edn. Oxford: Blackwell Science.

Chapman, S. (2008) Making decisions about prescribing in diabetes. *Practice Nursing* 19(3): 128–131.

Courtney, M., Carey, N. and Burke, J. (2007) Independent extended and supplementary prescribing practice in the UK: A national questionnaire survey. *International Journal of Nursing Studies* 44(7): 1093–1101.

Culley, F. (2005) Understanding developments in non-medical prescribing. *Nursing Times* 101(34): 30–33.

Department of Health (1989) *Report of the Advisory Group on Nurse Prescribing.* London: DoH.

Department of Health (1999) *Review of Prescribing, Administration and Supply of Medicines.* London: HMSO.

Department of Health (2000a) *Health Service Circular 2000/026*. London: DoH.

Department of Health (2000b) *Pharmacy in the Future: Implementing the NHS Plan*. London: DoH.

Department of Health (2000c) Lord Hunt announces proposals to extend prescribing powers for around 10 000 nurses. Press release 2000/0611. London: Media Centre, DoH.

Department of Health (2001) *The NHS Plan: An Action Guide for Nurses, Midwives and Health Visitors*. London: DoH.

Department of Health (2002) *Liberating the Talents: Helping Primary Care Trusts and Nurses to Deliver The NHS Plan*. London: DoH.

Department of Health (2003) *Supplementary Prescribing by Nurses and Pharmacists within the NHS in England: A Guide to Implementation*. London: DoH.

Department of Health (2004) *Extending Independent Nurse Prescribing within the NHS in England: A Guide for Implementation*, 2nd edn. London: DoH.

Department of Health (2006) *Improving Patients' Access to Medicines: A Guide to Implementing Nurse and Pharmacist Independent Prescribing within the NHS in England*. London: DoH.

Department of Health (2012) *Dangerous Drugs, England and Wales. Dangerous Drugs, Scotland. The Misuse of Drugs (Amendment No 2) (England Wales and Scotland) Regulations 2012*. London: HMSO.

Department of Health and Social Security (1986) *Neighbourhood Nursing: A Focus for Care (Cumberlege Report)*. London: HMSO.

Dimond, B. (2009) *Legal Aspects of Consent*, 2nd edn. London: Quay Books

Garrett, D. (2008) Non-medical prescribers in primary care: Practitioners or policemen? *Nurse Prescribing* 6(3): 106–109.

Halligan, A. (2006) Clinical governance: Assuring the sacred duty of trust to patients. *Clinical Governance* 11(1): 5–7.

Higgs, J., Jones, M., Loftus, S. and Christensen, N. (eds) (2008) *Clinical Reasoning in the Health Professions*, 3rd edn. London: Butterworth Heinemann.

Johns, C. (2004) *Becoming a Reflective Practitioner*, 2nd edn. Oxford: Blackwell.

Kurtz, S.M. and Silverman, J.D. (1996) The Calgary-Cambridge Referenced Observation Guides: An aid to defining the curriculum and organizing the teaching in communication training programmes. *Medical Education* 30(2): 83–89.

Kurtz, S.D., Silverman, J.M. and Draper, J. (2005) *Teaching and Learning Communication Skills in Medicine*. Oxford: Radcliffe Publishing.

Latter, S., Blenkinsopp, A., Smith, A. et al. (2011) *Evaluation of Nurse and Pharmacist Independent Prescribing*. London: DoH.

Luker, K. (1997) Patients' views of nurse prescribing. *Nursing Times* 93(17): 51–54.

National Institute for Health and Clinical Excellence (2009) *Medicines Adherence.* London: NICE.

National Prescribing Centre (1999) *Seven Principles of Good Prescribing … a Stepwise Approach.* Liverpool: NPC.

National Prescribing Centre (2001) *Maintaining Competence in Prescribing: An Outline Framework to Help Nurse Prescribers.* Liverpool: NPC.

National Prescribing Centre (2012) *A Single Competency Framework for All Prescribers.* London: NICE.

Neighbour, R. (1987) *The Inner Consultation: How to Develop an Dffective and Intuitive Consultation Style.* Lancaster: MTP Press.

Nursing and Midwifery Council (2006) *Standards of Proficiency for Nurse and Midwife Prescribers.* London: NMC.

Nursing and Midwifery Council (2009) *Guidelines for Records and Record Keeping.* London: NMC.

Nursing and Midwifery Council (2010) *Code of Conduct.* London: NMC.

Nuttall, D. and Rutt-Howard, J. (eds) (2011) *The Textbook of Non-Medical Prescribing.* Oxford: Wiley-Blackwell.

Pendleton, D., Schofield, T., Tate, P. and Havelock, P. (2003) *The new Consultation: Developing doctor patient communication.* Oxford: Oxford University Press.

CHAPTER 8

Public health and health promotion

Michelle Anderson

Chapter outline

- Introduction
- Current context
- Who are public health practitioners?
- Professional practice in public health
- The role of advanced nurse practioners in public health
- Theoretical underpinnings and models
- Conclusion

Introduction

This chapter aims to give the advanced nurse practitioner an under-standing of the multi-disciplinary nature of public health in the UK. It examines who public health practitioners are and professional practice in public health. It also cross-references the advanced nurse practitioner role attributes (RCN 2012a) related to public health and health promotion with the nine identified areas of public health activity defined by Skills for Health and the Public Health Resource Unit (2008).

The principles and practices of health promotion have not until recently been especially associated with the broader clinical concepts of advanced nursing practice. This is evidenced by the limited number of publications on this area, which may be seen as signifying that there is a limited relationship between the two concepts. However, I contend that this is not the case, but more simply that the relationship between health promotion, public health and advanced nursing is emergent and not yet fully explored. This chapter investigates how health promotion and its key contribution to public health are in fact intimately linked to

Table 8.1 Core areas of public health activity

Core areas	Defined areas in the advanced practice context
1. Surveillance and assessment of the population's health and well-being	5. Health improvement
	6. Health protection
2. Assessing the evidence of effectiveness of interventions, programmes and services to improve population health	7. Public health intelligence
	8. Academic public health
3. Policy and strategy development and implementation for population health and wellbeing	9. Health and social care quality
4. Leadership and collaborative working for health and well-being	

Source: UK Public Health Workforce Advisory Group (2013).

the emergence of the advanced nurse practitioner's role, their contribution to disease prevention and the strategic direction of service delivery and redesign.

There are four core areas of public health activity and five defined areas that relate specifically to the context in which the advanced practice nurse may practise (see Table 8.1; the numbering is for ease of reference later in the chapter). These areas were developed into the Public Health Skills and Knowledge Framework (PHSKF) in response to the growing public health workforce, changes in public health provision and a need for coherence.

Before discussing any activity related to public health or health promotion, it is necessary to provide working definitions. There are numerous explanations, ideals and subjective experiences applied to health promotion and public health, so I have given those that are most widely used. However, I would urge the reader to explore each area further to find definitions that reflect their own ideals and values.

The concept of public health was formulated in the early nineteenth century when disease epidemics led to pressure for both social and sanitary reform. It is defined as 'the science and art of preventing disease, prolonging life and promoting health through the organised efforts and informed choices of society, organisations, public and private communities and individuals' (Wanless 2004: 27). This not only recognizes the role of professionals in improving health and reducing inequalities, but also identifies both personal and community responsibility. The Faculty of Public Health (2009) further explains that public health should be population based, with collective responsibility for health, its protection and disease prevention, recognizing the key role of the state, socio-economic determinants of health and disease and partnership working.

Naidoo and Wills identify health promotion as 'one of the processes in securing public health' (2009: 55). There are numerous definitions, many of which come from opposing beliefs and ideals. Indeed, Tannahill (1985) says that health promotion is a meaningless concept because it is used so variously. The most widely quoted definition comes from the World Health Organization's (1986) Ottawa Charter, which defines health promotion as follows:

> the process of enabling people to increase control over, and to improve, their health. To reach a state of complete physical, mental and social well-being, an individual or group must be able to identify and to realize aspirations, to satisfy needs, and to change or cope with the environment. Health is, therefore, seen as a resource for everyday life, not the objective of living. Health is a positive concept emphasizing social and personal resources, as well as physical capacities. Therefore, health promotion is not just the responsibility of the health sector, but goes beyond healthy life-styles to well-being.

While this definition was seen as rather idealistic, it was important because it identified health as more than physical, and health promotion as something that was not only the responsibility of the healthcare sector. It highlighted it as an activity that depended on three actions: advocacy, enablement and mediation (WHO 1986).

Current context

The NHS has long been criticized as being a sickness-led service as opposed to a health-led one and there has been a concerted effort in recent years to begin altering this balance. The massive increases seen in diseases that are viewed as preventable and a result of individual lifestyle choices, coupled with a time of austerity within public spending, have resulted in a need to find new ways of working. Public health dominates the political agenda not only in the UK but in most of the Western world and has become a multi-agency concern. Health improvement through reductions in inequality and recognition of social responsibility is now the basis of numerous government policies. However, despite continual attention from policy makers, the King's Fund (2011) review of NHS performance from 1997 to 2010 identified the lack of progress in reducing health inequalities as the most significant health policy failure of that decade. Marmot (2010) highlighted the fundamental need to reduce inequalities as key if any changes were to be made to overall health status in the UK.

Furthermore, the World Health Organization (WHO 2011) identified that non-communicable diseases (NCDs) as a result of lifestyle were increasing, with 36 million of the 57 million annual deaths globally resulting from causes such as diabetes, cancers and coronary heart disease. It also stated that a large percentage of NCDs were preventable through reduction of the four main risk factors of tobacco use, insufficient physical activity, harmful use of alcohol and unhealthy diet. This means that once again attention has turned towards individual behaviours, perhaps at the cost of addressing socio-economic factors. Conversely, it could be argued that we all have some element of personal responsibility for our health and that until we recognize that fact, improvement in public health status will not happen.

Changes in the provision of public health services have also caused difficulties. The publication of new public health policies by the four countries of the UK (DOH 2010; WAG 2010; Scottish Government 2010; Department of Health, Social Services and Public Safety 2011) has led to massive reorganizations in an attempt to streamline service provision. While this has been necessary, changes in the roles of people 'at the coalface', such as dedicated public health workers and staff of health promotion units, has meant that their function has become somewhat strategic and lacking in face-to-face contact. There is thus a need for the wider multi-disciplinary providers of public healthcare to work in a cohesive and joined-up way in order to maximize their collective contribution (Skills for Health and Public Health Resource Unit 2008) at a time when resources are scarce and the effects of ill health and poverty are growing.

Who are public health practitioners?

The public health workforce is represented by numerous organizations and agencies from both within and outside the NHS (see Table 8.2 for examples), providing a multi-disciplinary approach to the population's health. There are three different levels of involvement (Douglas 2010): public health specialists from a variety of professional backgrounds, such as directors of public health and environmental health officers; public health practitioners, including nurses and health promotion specialists; and professionals whose work includes elements of public health, such as social workers, teachers and police officers.

Public health practitioners come from a variety of backgrounds, which may include medicine, nursing, health promotion, nutrition,

Table 8.2 The public health workforce – examples from within and outside the NHS

NHS	Agencies outside the NHS
Health promotion specialists	Environmental health officers
General Practitioners	Local Education Authorities
GP practice managers	Social services such as youth and
Community nurses, including	community workers, social workers,
district nurses, health visitors, school	Trading Standards and community
nurses, community mental health	safety officers
nurses, community midwives,	Police and probation officers
practice nurses, specialist nurses	Voluntary and community groups
Hospital nurses	Higher education
Dentists	Employers
Pharmacists	

Source: Scriven (2010).

pharmacy, public health intelligence, public health protection, health economics, environmental health, health psychology and academia. Practitioners may be working in the NHS, local authorities, the independent sector or the voluntary sector (Public Health Wales 2012).

The nurse's role within public health is a vital one working alongside other agencies and organizations. The role has at times appeared fragmented and sometimes hidden, and the RCN argues that there is a need to make the contribution of nurses more visible (RCN 2012a). Nursing practice within this field has traditionally been seen as the remit of community nurses (Ball 2006); the Nursing and Midwifery Council (NMC) specialist register for health visitors and school nurses (NMC 2004) acknowledges their role within public health. Although the service these nurses provide is quite rightly recognized, it is important not to overlook the contribution made by other nurses, working not only in primary but also secondary and tertiary care settings. Nurses have long provided invaluable information about their local population and case loads when assessing health needs, which has been assisted by their engagement with patients and their families and working knowledge of the service provision within a defined locality. Health promotion has been undertaken by nurses working in all fields, a role that features not only as a key role requirement for qualified nurses, but also as an integral part of competencies for pre-registration nurses (NMC 2010). Furthermore, nurses in all settings and specialties invariability support those with chronic disease to manage and live with their conditions.

Thus all nurses have varied aspects of a public health role within their job definition, including:

• Screening patients for disease risk factors and early signs of illness.
• Developing, with the patient, an ongoing nursing care plan for health, with an emphasis on preventive measures.
• Helping people to manage and live with illness.
• Providing counselling and health education.
• Working collaboratively with other healthcare professionals and disciplines.
• Providing leadership and consultancy. (RCN 2012b)

The RCN supports this position and states: 'Regardless of the environments nurses work in or their titles or individual roles, all nurses have a part to play in improving the health of local people' (2012b: 3).

These role attributes provide an 'upstream approach' to public health with the aim of prevention rather than cure; they also minimize the impact of illness, promote health and function, and help people maintain their roles in society. This is apt given the current burden of essentially preventable disease and the rise in those living with chronic conditions (RCN 2012b).

The importance of public health as part of all nurses' roles is especially relevant when considering the role and attributes of an advanced nurse practitioner. Advanced nurse practitioners often hold particular knowledge in relation to population health, condition-specific indicators, health promotion provision and leadership.

Professional practice in public health

There are several standard-setting bodies for public health. These include the Faculty of Public Health, which sets standards for consultants and some public health specialists. Occupational standards for other public health practitioners come under the remit of the Skills for Health Council (2008) and these will be outlined below.

National Occupational Standards

The multi-disciplinary nature of public health practice gave rise to a need for appropriate training and competencies. To this end, a competency-based framework for public health was developed by Healthwork UK in 2001 on behalf of a steering group comprising the Multidisciplinary Public Health Forum, Faculty of Public Health and the Royal Institute of Public Health and Hygiene, with support from the health departments of the four UK countries. Standards for public health specialists and practitioners (Skills for Health 2008) were developed that described good practice and aimed to improve the capacity and capability of the public health workforce.

UK Public Health Register (voluntary)

The development of standards provided a benchmark for practice, but to ensure that these measures were being utilized and observed, it was necessary to establish a register of practitioners. In 2006 the UK Public Health Register (UKPHR) was commissioned by the four UK governments to develop a regulatory framework for public health practitioners. A wide-ranging UK-wide consultation took place, including individuals and organizations working in the provision of public health medicine, government, academics and practitioners.

Two levels of registration were initially identified: practitioner and advanced practitioner. However, it is interesting to note that this was quickly changed to a single 'practitioner' level, after the Council for Healthcare Regulatory Excellence (CHRE) found that the 'advanced practice' levels were more in line with individual career progression. As such, the CHRE suggested that advanced practice should be recognized through professional accreditation (PHORCaST 2012), and on this basis UKPHR proceeded with a single level of practitioner registration.

UKPHR is currently supporting four local assessment and verification pilot schemes to set standards that are recognized throughout the UK. Registrants must meet these standards and maintain competence through CPD and revalidation with the aim of 'providing significant public protection from unprofessional or unethical behaviour as well as enhancing recognition for the public health professional' (PHORCaST 2012).

However, the development and implementation of standards and registration have not been without their problems. Indeed, changes in registration levels and practitioner requirements have meant that few have actually attained full registration to date.

The role of advanced nurse practitioners in public health

Advanced nurse practitioners' (ANPs) competencies (RCN 2012a) not only support the role of the ANP in public health, they provide specific competencies covering health promotion/health protection and disease prevention. The competencies listed in Table 8.3 are those with a direct

Table 8.3 Competencies relevant to public health

Domain 1: Assessment and management of patient health/illness status	Skills for Health Core/ Defined Activities
Health promotion/health protection and disease prevention	
1 Assesses individuals' health education/promotion related needs.	1, 5, 6, 9
2 Plans, develops and implements programmes to promote health and well-being and address individual needs.	4, 5, 6
3 Provides health education through anticipatory guidance and counselling to promote health, reduce risk factors, and prevent disease and disability.	5, 6
4 Develops and uses a follow-up system within the practice workplace to ensure that patients receive appropriate services.	1, 4, 9
5 Recognises environmental health problems affecting patients and provides health protection interventions that promote healthy environments for individuals, families and communities.	6
For health promotion/health protection and disease prevention, and management of patient illness	
17 Analyses the data collected to determine health status of the patient.	1, 7
18 Formulates a problem list and prioritised management plan.	1
19 Assesses, diagnoses, monitors, co-ordinates, and manages the health/illness status of patients during acute and enduring episodes.	1
22 Applies principles of epidemiology and demography in clinical practice by recognising populations at risk, patterns of disease, and effectiveness of prevention and intervention.	1
23 Acquires and uses community/public health assessment information in evaluating patient needs, initiating referrals, co-ordinating care and programme planning.	1
30 Evaluates results of interventions using accepted outcome criteria, revises the plan accordingly, and consults/refers when needed.	2, 3

Domain 1 *continued*	Skills for Health Core/ Defined Activities
31 Works collaboratively with other health professionals and agencies as appropriate.	4, 9
Domain 2: The nurse/patient relationship	
1 Creates a climate of mutual trust and establishes partnerships with patients, carers and families.	4, 5, 6
3 Creates a relationship with patients that acknowledges their strengths and knowledge, and enabling them to address their needs.	5, 6
6 Applies principles of empowerment in promoting behaviour change.	5, 6
7 Develops and maintains the patient's control over decision-making, assess the patient's commitment to the jointly determined plan of care, and fosters personal responsibility for health.	4, 5
Domain 3: The education function	
Timing	
1 Assesses the on-going and changing needs of patients, carers and families for education based on the following: A Needs for anticipatory guidance associated with growth and the developmental stage. B Care management that requires specific information or skills. C The patient's understanding of their health condition.	1
2 Assesses the patient's motivation for learning and maintenance of health-related activities using principles of change and stages of behaviour change.	2, 5
3 Creates an environment in which effective learning can take place.	5, 6
Eliciting	
4 Elicits information about the patient's interpretation of health conditions as a part of the routine health assessment.	1, 2
5 Elicits information about the patient's perceived barriers, supports, and modifiers to learning when preparing for patient's education.	1, 2, 7

Domain 3 *continued*	Skills for Health Core/ Defined Activities
6 Elicits the patient's learning style to facilitate an appropriate teaching approach.	2
7 Elicits information about cultural influences that may affect the patient's learning experience.	2
8 Enables patients, by displaying sensitivity to the effort and emotions associated with learning about how to care for one's health condition.	1, 2, 5

Enabling

9 Enables patients in learning specific information or skills by designing a learning plan that is comprised of sequential, cumulative steps, and that acknowledges relapse and the need for practice, reinforcement, support, and re-teaching when necessary.	5, 6
10 Enables patients to use community resources when needed.	2
11 Communicates health advice and instruction appropriately, using an evidence-based rationale.	5, 6

Providing

12 Negotiates a jointly determined plan of care, based on continual assessment of the patient's readiness and motivation, re-setting goals, and optimal outcomes.	4, 5, 6

Negotiating

13 Monitors the patient's behaviours and specific outcomes as a guide to evaluating the effectiveness and need to change or maintain educational strategies.	1

Coaching

14 Coaches the patient by reminding, supporting and encouraging, using empathy.	5, 6

Domain 4: Professional role	

Develops and implements the role

2 Functions in a variety of role dimensions: advanced health care provider, co-ordinator, consultant, educator, coach, advocate, administrator, researcher, role model and leader.	1, 2, 3, 4, 7, 8, 9

Domain 4 *continued*	Skills for Health Core/ Defined Activities
Directs care	
5 Uses sound judgement in assessing conflicting priorities and needs.	2
6 Builds and maintains a therapeutic team to provide optimum therapy.	4
8 Acts as an advocate for the patient to ensure health needs are met consistent with patients' wishes.	6
9 Consults with other health care providers and public/ independent agencies.	4
Provides leadership	
13 Evaluates implications of contemporary health policy on health care providers and consumers.	2
14 Participates in legislative and policy-making activities that influence an advanced level of nursing practice and the health of communities.	3
16 Evaluates the relationship between community/public health issues and social problems as they impact on the health care of patients (poverty, literacy, violence etc.).	3

relevance to public health and health promotion and have been cross-referenced with the Skills for Health core and defined activities from Table 8.1. For the full list of competencies see RCN (2012a).

While the ANP has a plainly recognized role in public health and health promotion, a study by Rash (2008) found that they spend less than 1% of their patient interactions involved in health promotion. Reasons given for this included lack of time, lack of importance attached to the promotion of health, working within a medical model, lack of knowledge and a perception that patients view it as boring, blaming and annoying. Despite these findings, both the American College of Nurse Practitioners and American Academy of Nurse Practitioners have identified health promotion as a primary function of advanced practice nurses (Berry 2006). Although traditionally focused disease treatment in healthcare is evolving towards health prevention and wellness promotion (Thomson and Kohli 1997), there is still a need for educators to address the lack of knowledge that ANPs say they face.

For ANPs to meet the RCN competencies fully, it is necessary for them to have an understanding of the theoretical underpinnings of health promotion, health psychology and models that guide both behaviour and practice. The rest of the chapter aims to give the reader a basic understanding of approaches to health promotion and their possible applications, as well as models of behaviour change and practical tools that can be utilized with patients. It is the ANP who will be leading the application and dissemination of these tools, and thus moving service delivery to be health oriented rather than based on crisis intervention.

Theoretical underpinnings and models

Promoting health is a complex, multi-faceted task. Health is not only dependent on individual choices about how we live our lives, it is also affected by numerous other variables such as social, demographic and psychological factors. If we were able to encourage individuals simply to live a healthier lifestyle, many of the non-communicable diseases we currently see would disappear. However, for an individual to make any change it is necessary to go through a complex psychological process that is affected by internal and external factors.

Health education has always been a mainstay of health promotion and involves a mix of behavioural advice and risk communication that aims to elicit behaviour change. In psychology this is described as a social cognitive approach, which assumes that behavioural choices are a reflection of how people see and view the world (Upton and Thirlaway 2010). Any decisions related to an individual changing their behaviour involve, at a fundamental level, a cost–benefit analysis. Thus an obese patient may see the cost involved in eating a healthy diet as not eating high-calorie, fat-rich foods that are enjoyable versus the benefit of being slimmer and healthier. Nevertheless, this is over-simplistic, since numerous other variables will affect that decision. A number of models of change have been developed that expand on this basic principle of the cost–benefit model.

Approaches to promoting health

Naidoo and Wills (2009) identify five main approaches that can be taken when promoting health with individuals, families, communities and populations:

• Medical
• Behavioural

- Educational
- Empowerment
- Social change

The differing aims and methods of these approaches will be discussed in turn.

Medical approach

As the name suggests, this approach is based around the traditional medical model prevalent in health services and aims to reduced mortality and premature morbidity. Its aim is the prevention of disease at three different levels:

- Primary: preventing onset of a disease state through risk education – immunization, encouraging healthy lifestyles.
- Secondary: preventing disease progression through early identification – screening for diseases such as cancer where it is still deemed to be treatable.
- Tertiary: preventing an illness reoccurring, reducing further disability or improving quality of life – palliation, rehabilitation.

The medical approach is expert led, often instigated as a result of epidemiological data. It has been used throughout public health and has resulted in large gains in population and individual health through immunization and screening. However, its shortcomings include that it ignores the socioeconomic determinants of health and can be deemed as victim blaming when those who do not take up the proferred services become ill.

Behavioural approach

Perhaps the most widely used health promotion method aims to encourage individuals to adopt healthy behaviours. It assumes that if they are provided with information individuals will choose to change their lifestyles. Nevertheless, as with the medical approach, it does not take into account the effect of socio-economic factors and the influence these will have on behaviour. The behavioural approach can be used with individuals (e.g. making changes in diet) or through mass media (e.g. smoking cessation campaigns).

Educational approach

The educational approach is sometimes confused with the behavioural approach because it involves the provision of information. However, its aim is not to elicit change in behaviour, but instead to provide the individual with knowledge so that they can then make a voluntary choice about their health. The approach works through helping individuals to develop the skills necessary to make informed decisions about health-related options. Again, it ignores the socio-economic determinants of health and also the psychological complexities of decision making, which will be discussed later in the chapter.

Empowerment approach

This approach works with individuals and communities to enable them to identify and meet their own perceived needs. The role of the health promoter here differs to the previous three approaches in acting as a facilitator only, withdrawing as the change grows and develops. Also unlike the previous approaches, the empowerment approach can be seen to be proactive and allows recognition of socio-economic factors that may affect the individual or community. It can be used very successfully, although it must be recognized that the issues identified are those perceived as important to the patient, so the process cannot be influenced by the healthcare practitioner.

Social change approach

Also known as radical health promotion, the social change approach aims to bring change in the physical, social and economic environment to promote health. Although it is often seen as beyond the remit of the nurse, there are times when it will be utilized, such as in the provision of health profiles, research and lobbying through professional organizations. The social change approach can also be used within organizations, for example providing healthy food in a staff canteen.

All of these approaches have advantages and disadvantages, so they are usually more successful when used in combination, as in the example in Box 8.1.

Models of behaviour change

There are numerous models that aim to explain the many complexities of behaviour change and how people move to healthy behaviours. Most come from the fields of health psychology or learning theory. While it is beyond the remit of this chapter to explore them all, the key models will be outlined that explain the intention to change and the actual change process.

Box 8.1 Combining approaches

Mr Davies has found that he is feeling quite chesty in the morning and getting breathless when walking upstairs. He has smoked 20 cigarettes a day for 25 years, relying on them to cope with the stress of his job. He would like to give up, but does not think he will be successful.

By using a combination of approaches Mr Davies would have a greater chance of changing his behaviour than using the approaches in isolation:

- **Medical approach** – prescribe nicotine replacement.
- **Behavioural approach** – provide information about smoking, dispel myths, reinforce benefits of cessation.
- **Educational approach** – develop skills through discussion of coping strategies, information about support groups, encourage, inform.
- **Empowerment approach** – counselling, identification of stressors.
- **Social change approach** – smoking ban.

Understanding why people behave in a particular way is central to planning health promotion interventions. Factors that can inhibit or encourage the intervention must be taken into account to enable the advanced nurse practitioner to support the individual fully. No one will make a change to their behaviour in isolation. There are both internal and external factors that will affect their decisions, such as education, culture, family, environment, income and peer pressure.

A number of theories have been developed to try to explain the different factors affecting health-related behaviours. They suggest that an individual's behaviour is determined by their attitude towards that behaviour. For example, an individual may smoke despite thinking that it is an unhealthy behaviour. Attitudes are developed from two parts: cognitive (knowledge and information) and affective (feelings and emotions). Attitudes to a certain behaviour are influenced by beliefs held about that action or intention. For example, a smoker may believe that smoking helps to calm them, but if they are then encouraged to believe that smoking is a stimulant, their belief may alter. This view of beliefs is identified in a relatively simplistic model known as knowledge–attitudes–beliefs (KAB), which views a change in behaviour as a result of information alone. However, as seen in numerous early health campaigns, simply giving information has proven to be ineffective and does not automatically lead to behaviour change (Naidoo and Wills 2009).

Other factors that influence behaviour include values, which are developed through socialization and are an emotional belief, and drives, which are described as strong motivating factors (Tones and Tilford 2001). The term 'drive' can also be used to describe addictions or factors such as hunger.

Health psychology theories and models

These theories come from models of cognition, social cognition and empowerment, all of which must be considered when helping a patient to change behaviour.

Health belief model

This is perhaps the most widely recognized model showing how beliefs affect decision making (Becker 1974). These beliefs in turn will affect the feasibility of the individual changing their behaviour and in many ways this takes the form of a cost–benefit analysis. When considering, for example, attending a screening appointment or making a health-related behaviour change, the individual will consider their perceived susceptibility to a disease and its severity against the costs and benefits of undertaking or altering behaviour. Often this model is used to predict protective health behaviour and compliance with medical advice.

The theory of reasoned action and planned behaviour

This theory suggests that individual behaviour is a result of two factors: attitudes and subjective norms (Ajzen and Fishbein 1980). These are influenced by beliefs, motivation and personal evaluations. The two factors combine to form a behavioural intention. Ajzen and Fishbein (1980) acknowledge that behavioural intention is not always consistent and may be affected by the stability of an individual's beliefs and the effect of social norms. For example, a group of friends may go out on a weekend, one of whom has decided not to drink alcohol. Nevertheless, because of the pressure to join in, the person may in fact drink alcohol because they do not want to be perceived as a killjoy or an outsider.

The health locus of control theory

Locus of control relates to an individual's perception of control over events (Rotter 1966). The theory suggests that those with a strong internal locus are more likely to change their behaviour than those with an external locus. Wallston and Wallston (1981) suggest that beliefs about health control fall into three categories: internal, the extent to which the individual believes that they are responsible for their health; powerful others, the extent to which the individual believes that other people such as health professionals are responsible; and chance, the extent to which individuals believe that things happen to them by fate or luck rather than because of what they choose to do.

Transtheoretical stages of change model

This model of behaviour change (Prochaska and DiClemente 1986) incorporates all of the other theories. It is used to explain how an individual moves from having no intention of making a change towards adopting behaviour that will maintain good health, and draws on different theories of health psychology around a core construct of cyclical change. Strategies based on this model can be successful for altering a range of behaviours such as alcohol and drug abuse, smoking, exercise and weight control. The key to the model is the image of a revolving door – usually the individual goes round more than once before permanent change is maintained. Prochaska and DiClemente (1986) suggest that the goal of the health professional when working with patients is not to get them through the whole change cycle, but instead to move them on from one stage to the next.

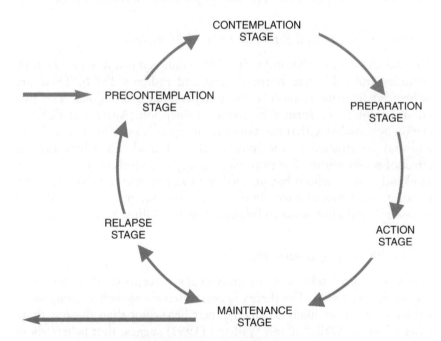

Figure 8.1 The transtheoretical stages of change model
Source: Prochaska and DiClemente (1982)

The model (see Figure 8.1) represents the stages through which people go in behaviour change. At first they may not consider changing their health behaviour (precontemplation); then they start to think about it (contemplation); the next stage is getting ready for change (preparation), followed by starting to make the change (action). The final stage is either maintenance of the change or relapse back to the precontemplation stage. At any stage within this process an individual can return to old behaviours. Stop Smoking Wales (http://stopsmokingwales.com) reports that people commonly go around this change cycle four or five times before they stop smoking. Progressing through the stages is not easy, but it is possible with motivation and help back onto the cycle after relapse.

Table 8.4 provides an outline of the process at each stage and provides the advanced nurse practitioner with methods for helping individuals move on from one stage to the next.

While behaviour change models can guide the advanced nurse practitioner through the theoretical stages of change, there are other methods that have been developed by health professionals, particularly in the mental health field.

Every Contact Counts (NHS Local 2013) provides a web-based learning resource for anyone who has contact with members of the general public. The tool gives information about how to make the most of opportunities to help people lead healthier lives. It is based around the principles of brief intervention, which relates to time available face to face with patients as opposed to any particular theory. The main aim of brief intervention is concentration on the change needed, underpinned by the following principles:

- Educating about the risks of current behaviour.
- Emphasis on patient's responsibility towards their health.
- Provision of advice about making a change.
- Exploring strategies and methods for changing.
- Action planning in collaboration with the patient.

Another method is motivational interviewing (Rollnick and Miller 1995), which draws on the principles of cognitive behavioural therapy used within mental health. This method of eliciting change is used in the NHS *Improving Health and Changing Behaviour* health trainer handbook (DoH 2008) and aims to:

- Build an empathetic relationship with the patient about the health issue and need to change.
- Discuss the advantages and disadvantages of the change for the individual.

Table 8.4 Facilitating the stages of change

Stage of Change	Process	Moving On
Precontemplation	Not aware of the need for change or has no interest in changing their health-related behaviour	Peer support/pressure Professional advice Effects on current health Role model
Contemplation	Starting to realize that there may be a need to change. Expressing some interest in change	Discussion of costs/benefits Ways of making the change discussed Assess confidence level Reflect on past experiences Others who have been successful
Preparation	Actively seeks information and support May be planning when the change will happen	Provide information such as leaflets, support groups, books, websites Set SMART goals (Specific, Measurable, Attainable, Realistic and Timely) Set a start date Discuss potential barriers and ways to overcome them Identify facilitators
Action	The change begins – this may be viewed as a trial period or may be approached with enthusiasm	Keep a diary of thoughts, feelings, barriers and facilitators Review progress regularly Praise success
Maintenance	The new health behaviour has been established – on average six months is considered the time after which the behaviour has changed with a small chance of relapse	Review coping strategies Acknowledge that everyone has setbacks and offer ways of dealing with them Review progress Rewards Ask them to help/speak with other people in their previous situation
Relapse	The patient does not like the change, lacks motivation, feels pressured Finds certain situations difficult Does not feel supported	Reinforce that relapse is not the end of the process Review the goals and adjust if needed Self-monitoring Revisit earlier stages

Source: Adapted from Prochaska and DiClemente (1984) and DoH (2008).

- See resistance to change as a normal part of the process.
- Support autonomy in changing the behaviour.

The goal of motivational interviewing is empowerment of the patient.

Conclusion

This chapter should provide the advanced nurse practitioner with an understanding of the multi-disciplinary nature of public health and health promotion, and, more importantly, of their role within the process, as well as of the theoretical underpinnings of behaviour and behaviour change. Advanced practice and public health are not seen as strongly associated, but they are linked and will develop alongside the emerging advanced nurse practitioner role. Strong recognition of health promotion, health protection and disease prevention within advanced practice nursing competencies (RCN 2012a) highlights the contribution that advanced nurse practitioners can make to improving the health of their patients. Additionally, the knowledge inherent within the role can offer much to policy makers in terms of highlighting need, providing evidence of effectiveness and advocating for individuals, families and communities.

Reflective questions
1. How would you define public health and health promotion? What influences your definitions? Are they structured around your values, beliefs, professional or private role?
2. What aspects of your role would you consider to be public health focused? What skills do you possess that help you to promote health with your patients?
3. Do you feel you possess the RCN competencies, outlined in Table 8.3? If not, why not? What can you do to develop those you are lacking?

References

Ajzen, I. and Fishbein, M. (1980) *Understanding Attitudes and Predicting Social Behavior*. Englewood Cliffs, NJ: Prentice Hall.

Ball, J. (2006) *Nurse Practitioners 2006: The Results of a Survey of Nurse Practitioners Conducted on behalf of the RCN Nurse Practitioner Association*. Hove: Employment Research.

Becker, M.H. (1974) The Health Belief Model and Personal Health Behavior. Thorofare, NJ: Slack.

Berry, J.A. (2006) Pilot study: Nurse practitioner communication and the use of recommended clinical preventative services. *Journal of the American Academy of Nurse Practitioners* 18: 277–283.

Department of Health (2008) *Improving Health and Changing Behaviour.* London: DoH.

Department of Health (2010) *Healthy Lives, Healthy People: Our Standard for Public Health in England.* London: HMSO.

Department of Health, Social Services and Public Safety (2011) *Health Survey Northern Ireland: First Results from the 2010/11 Survey.* Belfast: DHSSPS.

Douglas, J. (2010) The rise of modern multidisciplinary public health. In J. Douglas, S. Earle, S. Handsley et al. (eds), *A Reader in Promoting Public Health.* Milton Keynes: Open University.

Faculty of Public Health (2009) *Stepping Up: Using Health Standards to Improve Public Health.*

King's Fund (2011) *Transforming Our Health Care System: Ten Priorities for Service Planners and Commissioners.* London: King's Fund.

Marmot, M. (2010) *Fairer Society, Healthier Lives: Strategic Review of Health Inequalities in England post 2010.* London: The Marmot Review.

Naidoo, J. and Wills, J. (2009) *Foundations for Health Promotion*, 3rd edn. London: Bailliere Tindall.

NHS Local (2013) Every Contact Counts. http://learning.wm.hee.nhs.uk/course/every-contact-counts (ccessed 18 February 2015).

Nursing and Midwifery Council (2004) *Standards of Proficiency for Specialist Community Public Health Nurses.* London: NMC.

Nursing and Midwifery Council (2010) *Standards for Pre Registration Nurse Training.* London: NMC.

PHORCaST (2012) Practitioner registration. http://www.phorcast.org.uk/page.php?page_id=278 (accessed 22 February 2015).

Prochaska, J.O. and DiClemente, C.C. (1986) Towards a comprehensive model of change. In W.R. Miller and N. Heather (eds), *Treating Addictive Behaviors: Processes of Change.* New York: Plenum.

Prochaska, J.O. and DiClemente, C.C.D. (1982) Transtheoretical therapy: toward a more integrative model of change. *Psychotherapy: Theory Research and Practice* 19: 276–88.

Prochaska, J.O. and DiClemente, C.C. (1984) *The Transtheoretical Approach: Crossing Traditional Foundations of Change.* Homewood, IL: Dow Jones/Irwin.

Public Health Wales (2012) *Public Health Strategic Framework.* Cardiff: Welsh Assembly Government.

Rash, E. (2008) Advanced practice nursing students' perceptions of health promotion. *Southern Online Journal of Nursing Research* 8(3). http://www.resourcenter.net/images/snrs/files/sojnr_articles2/Vol08Num03Art03.pdf (accessed 18 September 2013).

Rollnick, S. and Miller, W.R. (1995) What is motivational interviewing? *Behavioural and Cognitive Psychotherapy* 23: 325–334.

Rotter, J.B. (1966) Generalised expectancies for internal versus external reinforcement. *Psychological Monographs: General and Applied* 80(1): 1–28.

Royal College of Nursing (2012a) *Advanced Nurse Practitioners: An RCN Guide to the Advanced Nurse Practitioner Role, Competences and Programme Accreditation.* London: RCN.

Royal College of Nursing (2012b) *Going Upstream: Nurses' Contribution to Public Health.* London: RCN.

Scriven, A. (2010) *Promoting Health: A Practical Guide,* 6th edn London: Baillere Tindall.

Scottish Government (2010) *Health Behaviour Change Competency Framework: Competences to Deliver Interventions to Change Lifestyle Behaviours that Affect Health.* Edinburgh: Scottish Government.

Skills for Health and Public Health Resource Unit (2008) *Multidisciplinary/ Multiagency/Multiprofessional Public Health Skills and Career Framework.* Oxford: Public Health Resource Unit.

Tannahill, A. (1985) What is health promotion? *Health Education Journal* 44(4): 167–168.

Thomson, P. and Kohli, H. (1997) Health promotion training needs analysis. *Journal of Advanced Nursing* 26: 507–514.

Tones, K. and Tilford, S. (2001) *Health Promotion: Effectiveness, Efficiency and Equity,* 3rd edn, Cheltenham: Nelson Thornes.

Upton, D. and Thirlaway, K. (2010) *Promoting Healthy Behaviour: A Practical Guide for Nursing and Healthcare Professionals.* Harlow: Pearson.

UK Public Health Workforce Advisory Group (2013) Public Health Skills and Knowledge "Refresh" – Final Report. Accessed at http://www.phorcast.org.uk/page.php?page_id=313

Wallston, K.A. and Wallston, B.S. (1981) Health locus of control scales. In H. Lefcourt (ed.), *Research with the Locus of Control Construct,* Vol. 1. New York: Academic Press.

Wanless, D. (2004) *Securing Good Health for the Whole Population.* London: HMSO.

Welsh Assembly Government (2010) *Our Healthy Future.* Cardiff: WAG.

World Health Organization (1986) The Ottawa Charter for Health Promotion. http://www.who.int/healthpromotion/conferences/previous/ottawa/en/ (accessed 30 April 2012).

World Health Organization (2011) *Noncommunicable Diseases: Country Profiles 2011.* Geneva: WHO.

CHAPTER 9

Ethics and the role of the advanced nurse practitioner

Rachel Duncan and Linda Nelson

Chapter outline

- Introduction
- Ethical principles
- The nature of contemporary healthcare
- An ethical decision-making framework
- Case study analysis
- Conclusion

Introduction

Nurses everywhere have long struggled with ethical challenges in patient care. In the late nineteenth century Florence Nightingale's *Notes on Nursing* discussed the ethical duties of confidentiality, communication and the centrality of meeting patients' needs (Nightingale 1859; Ulrich and Zeitzer 2009). An ethical issue can occur in any healthcare situation in which profound moral questions of rightness or wrongness underlie professional decision making and patient care based on optimum evidence. Patients have a right to make decisions about their own healthcare, and health professionals have a duty to support them to make these decisions by providing impartial advice and information about treatment options.

Advanced nurse practitioners (ANPs) are ideally placed to facilitate ethical decision making within healthcare teams. Enhanced knowledge and clinical skills enable them to act as experts in their own specialist field, ensuring the primacy of patient rights. Kilpatrick et al. (2011) state that the ANP contributes to care by applying an expanded scope of practice and integrating in-depth knowledge and experience in domains related to clinical practice, education, research, professional development and leadership with effective resource utilization. With an expanded scope of practice comes enhanced professional autonomy, but this is counterbalanced by additional responsibility and accountability, which all ANPs must acknowledge.

An integral part of the ANP role is the need to act as a therapeutic conduit between the healthcare team, the patient and their family. As skilled clinicians, ANPs have the confidence, skills and knowledge to communicate effectively with the multi-disciplinary team (MDT) and have the authority to facilitate ethical decision making, and to assert the needs and rights of patients and families under their care. However, in every healthcare environment there are factors that can enhance and impede optimum ethical decision making. This chapter will explore the nature of these challenges and provide thought-provoking analysis of ethical dilemmas that move beyond the routine experiences of the registered nurse. In doing so, it will highlight the role of the ANP as key to the successful achievement of individualized patient care, grounded in a comprehensive understanding of how ethical principles and theories can enhance decision making.

Ethical principles

Ethical principles are rules, standards or guidelines for action that are derived from theoretical positions about what is good for humans (Grace 2009). Throughout this chapter such principles will be applied to the presenting problem to enable the ANP to understand how this can assist in the decision-making process to achieve the best possible outcome for the patient. It is useful at this point to introduce the major ethical principles. Beauchamp and Childress (2009) provide a comprehensive analysis of competing moral perspectives and identify four major principles that have been influential in teaching and writing about biomedical ethics: respect for autonomy, beneficence, non-maleficence and justice.

Respect for autonomy

There are several definitions of autonomy in the healthcare literature, but all agree that it relates to individuals having the capacity to think and decide what is best for themselves freely and independently. Philosopher Immanuel Kant (1724–1804) believed that respect for autonomy comes from the recognition that all individuals have unconditional worth and the capacity to decide their own moral destiny. There is a general belief that people know themselves better than anybody else and consequently have the right to exercise their freedom of autonomy without interference (Grace 2009). That would include the decision to accept or refuse any treatment or intervention offered.

This may be the case for the majority of patients with whom an ANP comes into contact on a daily basis, but not all will have the mental capacity to make a free and voluntary decision. Reasons for this in the short term could be hypoxia, an impaired level of consciousness, trauma and pain. In the longer term, and on a more permanent basis, patients experiencing dementia, vegetative states and serious mental impairment lack the capacity to make informed decisions. If a voluntary choice is to be made, then the ANP must evaluate the individual's mental capacity to make that decision. The application of this and the challenges it can present are discussed in the case histories later in this chapter.

Non-maleficence

The principle of non-maleficence in medical ethics is associated with 'doing no harm' or not inflicting harm on others (Beauchamp and Childress 2009). Many nursing activities are in themselves potentially harmful and an ANP will perform them on a regular basis. Take the simple example of giving a vaccination, which all nurses will have performed on numerous occasions. How many times have you said 'just a sharp scratch' prior to inserting the needle into the patient's skin? This action will cause pain for some people, so could it be classed as harm? Beauchamp and Childress (2009: 113) recognize that 'a harmful act by one party may not be wrong'; in this situation the injection may be to prevent disease or in fact reduce pain, so there is a longer-term benefit. Harm therefore relates to any *avoidable* distress caused to the patient during care delivery or observed by a professional and experienced by a patient that is not acted on (Grace 2009).

The principle of non-maleficence has implications for many areas of biomedical ethics and in your role as an ANP you will engage with challenges related to this principle of 'doing no harm'. Examples are issues around the terminally ill and withdrawal of treatment, which are explored in detail in the case studies.

Beneficence

Morality requires not only that we treat people autonomously and refrain from harming them, but also that we contribute to their welfare. The principle of beneficence potentially demands much more than non-maleficence, as it suggests that positive steps must be taken to help others, not merely refraining from harmful acts (Beauchamp and Childress 2009). According to Beauchamp and Childress (2009) there are two principles of beneficence: positive beneficence and utility. Positive beneficence relates to ANPs providing care that will benefit others, whereas utility requires a balance of benefits, risks and cost to achieve the best possible result for the patient. We should maximize benefits and minimize harm and risks to patients in our care. Grace (2009) observes that the interventions and goals of healthcare professionals are in themselves inherently beneficent and intended for the patient's good and well-being.

Beneficence underlies all a professional's actions while working within their role and engaging with patients on a daily basis. However, Rumbold (1993: 192) raises an interesting question when he asks: Who decides what is in the best interests of the patient and on what basis? There will be occasions in your role as an ANP that ensuring beneficence seems to be in conflict with the patient's autonomy, and again this will be explored in the case histories.

Justice

Justice is commonly thought of in two ways: justice as fairness and justice as punishment. Justice as fairness is violated when people who are equal in all relevant aspects are treated unequally (Seedhouse 2009). When discussing the principle of justice in healthcare, it is often referred to in the literature as social justice. Think about the concept of a 'postcode lottery' and how this can result in varying levels of access to some treatments. This inequity is often based on issues of local policy, organizational structure and cost. An individual in one part of the country with cancer could receive a drug that may extend their life, whereas in another part this treatment would be denied. This is a good example of the principle of justice and fairness, where healthcare resources are subject to inequalities based on geography and location. As an ANP this could be a challenge and circumstance with which you are faced and it is the role of the nurse to promote justice in healthcare; without this the most vulnerable patients will remain at risk.

The nature of contemporary healthcare

The changing nature of healthcare in contemporary society has increased the complexity of ethical decision making. The development of scientific knowledge, the growth of computer-enhanced technology and the escalation of public knowledge and expectations within a limited healthcare budget have provided an increase in the scope and nature of the ethical dilemmas that healthcare professionals face. The role of an ANP requires developed skills of critical thinking, self-exploration and the ability to sift through contextually relevant elements of ethical situations (Kalb and O'Conner-Von 2007).

Within pre-registration nursing curricula, students are introduced to the primacy of patients' rights and the need for ethical thinking when caring for patients. However, this introduction to the complexity of ethical decision making cannot fully prepare them to contribute confidently to such decisions in clinical practice. It will at best provide insight into ethical dilemmas without necessarily developing the required skills to facilitate a satisfactory resolution. In contrast, Kalb and O'Conner-Von (2007) assert that ANPs are frequently at the forefront of advocating for patients and their families. As such, they require an enhanced level of ethical decision making, which integrates professional standards, encompassing diverse disciplinary perspectives and an understanding of bioethics and related philosophies. There is a need for ethics education beyond the basic graduate level to enable the ANP to engage confidently in case reviews and competently guide the healthcare team in complex ethical issues.

In order to do this, ethical decision making must be guided by a sound knowledge of ethical principles and theories. It is not enough for ANPs to be guided by their own virtues when considering ethical dilemmas. While virtue ethics has its place within personal experiences of the world, in professional ethics it must be utilized in combination with other approaches when a challenging ethical dilemma is encountered. In teaching ethics to pre-registration healthcare professionals, a common response when analysing ethical dilemmas is often: 'If it were me in that bed, I wouldn't want you to do that to me.' ANPs must progress beyond this level and be able to express a coherent, balanced moral argument, as well as confidently to challenge perspectives expressed by other members of the healthcare team, in order to achieve the best outcome for the patient and their family. The ANP must also ensure the right of all patients to participate in decision making, by familiarizing themselves with the patient's experience, their situation and the people involved (Edwards 2009). This will enable them to undertake the role of patient advocate more effectively if the need arises.

An ethical decision-making framework

There are many approaches to ethical decision making. Beauchamp and Childress (2009) provide a comprehensive analysis of competing moral perspectives, but they also acknowledge the need for a decision-making procedure. Seedhouse (2009) has developed a decision-making framework that guides the user through the main approaches in a single model. The aim of the Ethical Grid (see Figure 9.1) is to make moral decision making more comprehensive and explicit. Seedhouse is careful to point out, however, that it does not deliver the correct answer to any dilemma. Instead, it seeks to guide the healthcare worker through a practical and accessible route into moral reasoning, making the process clearer for those unfamiliar with this way of thinking. Seedhouse (2009) asserts that it is not a substitute for personal judgement; indeed, practitioners are often alerted to potential dilemmas and respond initially on a personal level. Furthermore, Steinboch et al. (2003) stress the need for practitioners to recognize the relationship between feelings and ethical decisions, suggesting: 'Our feelings may provoke us to moral inquiry, but the inquiry does not terminate there' (2003: 6).

The Ethical Grid is intended to make certain tasks easier, by ensuring clarity and a comprehensive, logical analysis of a situation. As Seedhouse (1991: 173) stresses: 'It cannot direct or prioritise the task, responsibility for this still lies with the user, not the Grid.' The tool is helpful in case conferences or team meetings to facilitate open discussion between team members (Seedhouse 2009). Using the Ethical Grid both prospectively, in everyday clinical practice, and retrospectively, following acute/emergency interventions as a method for team debriefing, will enable students and practitioners to reflect on moral dilemmas, with a view to refining and clarifying their moral reasoning when exposed to similar clinical dilemmas in the future.

The Ethical Grid consists of four layers, each illustrating the main approaches to ethical decision making at that level. Seedhouse (1991) suggests that the user can begin anywhere in the Grid, depending on the crux of the dilemma as they see it. Practitioners are encouraged to formulate a hypothesis, then try to show what is wrong with it using the Grid, rather than employing it as evidence to confirm their initial views. Not all portions of the Grid may be relevant to all dilemmas, but each should be considered prior to making a final decision. Seedhouse (2009: x) stresses that 'the Grid is not a calculating machine, it is merely a euphemism for ethical reflection'. It is through a more detailed understanding of the related moral philosophies underpinning each of the layers of the Grid and practice in using the framework that ANPs can truly maximize their ethical decision-making potential.

The innermost layer of the Grid focuses on the principle of autonomy. This is central to any attempt to clarify and find solutions to a moral dilemma. The practitioner's ability to enhance and respect autonomy for

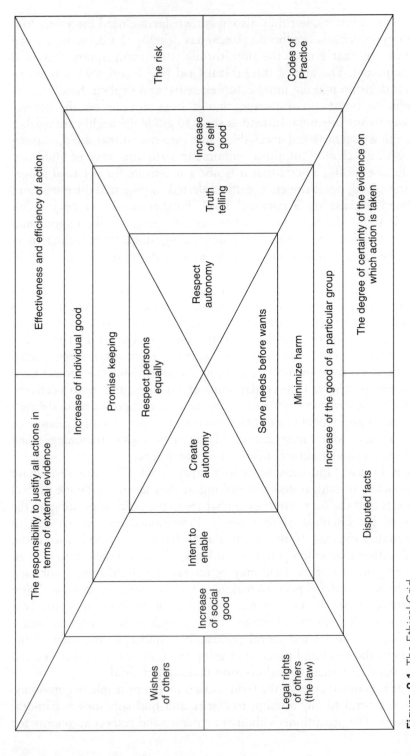

Figure 9.1 The Ethical Grid
Source: Seedhouse (1991).

each person is a fundamental moral duty. Contemporary healthcare recognizes the mentally competent patient as an essential part of clinical decision making. Thus the ANP must first ask: 'Can the patient help me to clarify or resolve this dilemma?'

The Grid then incorporates a layer that enables the user to examine a dilemma from a moral principles approach. Principles of beneficence, non-maleficence, truth telling and promise keeping are enshrined in professional practice and development. The first two layers are principles advocated by deontologists (sometimes referred to as non-consequentialists), who see people as ends in themselves, rather than as a means to an end. Deontology is an ethical theory that sees respect for the rights of the person as the ultimate standard of morality (Thiroux 2004).

The third layer of the Grid guides the user to consider the principle of the 'greatest happiness' and how this can be created and maximized within a given situation. This is the primary focus of the ethical theory of consequentialism, which looks at the end result of the actions or rules that a person follows, rather than the means to the end as with deontology. When combined with hedonism (the pleasure principle), consequentialism is referred to as utilitarianism. This ethical theory is purely concerned with maximizing happiness for the greatest number, in relation to outcomes, rather than the moral character of the agent. It encourages practitioners to look at the results of their actions, rather than ensuring that the means to the end is morally acceptable.

Seedhouse (1991) acknowledges that ethical decisions cannot be made in a moral vacuum. The outer layer of the Grid recognizes external considerations and major competing influences on moral decision making; these include the family, law, resource constraints and professional codes. Healthcare professionals cannot ignore the impact of environmental, politico-economic, cultural and legal influences on decision making. ANPs are more familiar and therefore practised in the elements of the outer layer. In combining this knowledge with increased insight into moral principles and ethical theories, they can enhance their role and status within the healthcare team, improving the quality and primacy of patient care through effective advocacy skills.

In his most recent book, Seedhouse (2009) updated the Ethical Grid to include issues of resource allocation. Use of the Grid has also been developed into an online decision support programme called the Values Exchange, in which practitioners can enter into online ethical debates. The programme, at www.values-exchange.com, may be a useful resource for you to develop your ethical decision-making skills.

Case study analysis

The case studies in this section have been selected on the basis that the issues they contain create anxiety and concern to clinical nurses. The ANP can support other practitioners in providing informed solutions to these dilemmas, enhancing the ethical climate in practice. Using an effective framework is essential to ensuring a comprehensive analysis of any situation, and Seedhouse's Ethical Grid is employed to analyse critically a number of these challenging experiences. Reflective questions are offered at the end of each practice focus to facilitate personal appraisal and multidisciplinary debate, which will hopefully lead to enhanced professional understanding and mutual respect.

DNACPR

Case scenario

Joan is a 58-year-old married woman who retired early from her job as a head teacher, due to progressive Parkinson's disease. She was diagnosed with primary lung cancer six months ago and has been receiving radiotherapy. She was admitted to the Medical Assessment Unit (MAU) with an acute urinary tract infection.

Joan appeared mentally competent on arrival to the MAU and was able to respond to the questions asked during the admissions procedure. The ANP was concerned that her condition might deteriorate due to the acute infection and potentially cause impairment in her mental capacity over the next few hours. The ANP approached the doctor to suggest that he discuss with Joan her preference for resuscitation, should the need arise. The doctor felt that this was not necessary as it was his job to stabilize her and transfer her to a medical ward, at which time this issue could be discussed with Joan and her family. The ANP thought that this might be too late, as Joan was becoming increasingly tired, affecting her ability to communicate her wishes. The ANP tried to emphasize the importance of establishing the patient's opinion on this matter while she could still express her views clearly and competently. The doctor disagreed.

Discussion

Successful end-of-life care is determined by an empathetic, compassionate response to the holistic needs of each patient. It is crucial that the healthcare team work together to ensure that each patient has the opportunity to participate in decision making, if this is their wish.

Conflict may occur between the need for individualized, holistic patient care and the potentially depersonalizing approach of the paternalistic model of healthcare, as the physical needs of the patient, as perceived by the doctor, take priority within the care setting. Eliott and Olver (2010) recognize the potential for conflict if the physician–patient relationship is not based on shared decision making, especially towards the end of life. ANPs can manage the successful integration of both perspectives to ensure that patient care is holistic and comprehensive, facilitating a smooth transition for the patient along their healthcare journey. ANPs work in a variety of healthcare settings and have a key role in facilitating care that is in the best interests of the patient and based on the patient's wishes.

In considering what is best for Joan, the ANP is recognizing the unstable nature of her health status, to ensure that Joan's expressed wishes are integrated into her care plan. The British Medical Association/Resuscitation Council/Royal College of Nursing (2007) guidelines fully endorse the need to make clinical decisions regarding the patient's resuscitation status in advance of any deterioration in their mental capacity or clinical status that may impede active participation. Crisis decision making leads to inaccurate assumptions regarding the wishes of the patient, so action in turn may be contrary to those wishes. Patients have a right to receive information in a manner they can understand in order to consider their options and express their wishes, prior to a potentially futile attempt at cardiopulmonary resuscitation (CPR). The General Medical Council end-of-life care strategy (GMC 2010) recognizes that patients with terminal illness are denied informed choices regarding the remainder of their life and the manner in which they die. The GMC states that those patients who are likely to die within the next 12 months can be defined as 'approaching the end of life', thus due consideration is required regarding their right to participate in end-of-life decisions. It supports the view that a patient who has a condition that will impair capacity as it progresses must be given every opportunity to express their wishes. Inappropriate resuscitation of terminally ill patients may prolong the dying process, cause loss of patient dignity, dissonance within the healthcare team and distress for the patient's family, and is potentially a waste of healthcare resources. This view is reinforced in a report by the National Confidential Enquiry into Patient Outcome and Death (2012), which stresses that it is not good medical practice to fail to anticipate the needs of the patient before an emergency arises. The report claims that in a number of cases CPR was attempted when the researchers thought that an earlier DNACPR (do not attempt resuscitation) decision should have been made. In 47% of cases there was a deficiency in patient assessment, which led to the failure to formulate an appropriate plan (NCEPOD 2012: 6).

In the UK it is the responsibility of the senior clinician to discuss end-of-life issues with the patient; this can be a suitably experienced nurse (BMA/RC/RCN 2007), although in reality the task is infrequently undertaken by nurses. A number of authors have commented that nurses may be in good position to approach the patient to discuss end-of-life issues. Loertscher et al. (2010), in a small study of two hospitals in the USA, remarked on the lack of training in communication skills and of doctors' confidence when discussing DNACPR status with patients. A situation highlighted at Addenbrooke's Hospital, Cambridge whereby a patient had a DNACPR order applied without her consent resulted in the Court of Appeal declaring that this was unlawful. Medical staff are now required to consult with all patients before applying such a notice to their medical records (Saul 2014).

Developing the role of the ANP to include strategies to achieve more individualized, compassionate end-of-life decisions may be one such improvement. However, despite nurses' attempts to influence care, a study by Sulmasy et al. (2008: 1817) reported that nurses referred to themselves as 'the responsible powerless'. They provide the majority of care, but are frequently excluded from DNACPR decisions. The GMC encourages medical staff to consult the healthcare team, patients and their families prior to end-of-life decision making, although it has defended the doctor's right to decide whether to inform the patient and their family. Current guidance on who is responsible for decision making regarding CPR states that a 'suitably qualified nurse' could make such decisions following appropriate training and education (BMA/RC/RCN 2007: 19). However, the NCEPOD report (2012) states that of 62 DNACPR decisions made over a 14-day audit period in November 2010, no decisions regarding CPR status were made by nurses. In addition, none of the patients who had the opportunity to discuss their status with a healthcare practitioner did so with a nurse. There is clearly a role for the ANP in such decision making, due to their expert knowledge and more cogent therapeutic relationship with the patient, although a change of culture is required.

In this case scenario, using the Ethical Grid the ANP can confidently challenge the doctor's decision regarding Joan's care. Initial assessment of the patient's needs has alerted the ANP to the volatile, terminal nature of her illness and the potential need for future resuscitation in the event of a cardiac arrest. Legally, if the patient's views regarding their resuscitation status are unknown and a DNACPR order has not been written, the healthcare team has a duty to resuscitate. A decision not to resuscitate should only take place if a mentally competent patient has refused CPR, a valid advance refusal has been made regarding CPR, or resuscitation is unlikely to be successful or, if successful, would lead to a length and quality of life that would not be in the best interests of the patient (Dimond 2011).

During the initial assessment of Joan's needs, the ANP recognizes that she is currently mentally competent, as she fulfils the criteria outlined in the Mental Capacity Act (DoH 2005). Joan is able to understand and retain the information given to her regarding aspects of her care, weigh it up and communicate her wishes. In light of Joan's understanding of her current health status, the ANP is confident that she would be able to participate in end-of-life decision making. The ANP wishes to respect Joan's right to autonomous choice regarding her future care. The Human Rights Act 1998 supports this right, as Joan has the right not to be subjected to inhumane or degrading treatment (Article 3), which may be a consequence of the doctor's reluctance to discuss resuscitation status with her if she is later resuscitated. NCEPOD (2012: 60) recognizes that appreciation of urgency, supervision of junior doctors and seeking advice from senior doctors regarding DNACPR decisions were all poor. It further emphasized the necessity to refer to a consultant in the event that the patient continues to deteriorate. This report supports the duty of ANPs to refer to senior colleagues in the event of disagreement with junior medical staff, thus safeguarding their advocacy role.

During the admissions process it is important that the nurse enquires whether Joan has an Advanced Directive to Refuse Treatment (ADRT) outlining her future wishes regarding care and treatment, or whether she has signed a lasting power of attorney. ADRTs are covered by the Mental Capacity Act 2005. If an ADRT exists, it is crucial that the ANP checks that it is in writing, signed and dated by Joan and also signed by a competent witness. The ADRT will state that she is 'refusing the treatment identified even if her life is in danger' (DoH 2012a). However, an ADRT or lasting power of attorney would not be applicable while Joan is mentally competent, as she can instruct the healthcare team regarding her own wishes; they will only become legally enforceable if her mental capacity deteriorates. If an ADRT exists, the ANP must make this known to the team and make a note in the patient's records. If Joan has appointed someone with a legal power of attorney who is registered with the Office of Public Guardians, they must be consulted in all matters concerning her in the event of her losing capacity. Nevertheless, while guidelines encourage the team to work closely with family members (GMC 2010; NMC 2008), as long as Joan remains competent she should be consulted prior to sharing any sensitive information with family members.

The Ethical Grid encourages the ANP to recognize the delicate balance between beneficence (doing good) and non-maleficence (doing no harm) in this situation. Respecting Joan's right to participate in decision making may lead to her refusing a potentially life-saving treatment. However, resuscitating a patient who is approaching the end of life may lead to a greater balance of harm over benefit, as it may in fact prolong the dying process and cause unnecessary distress. While it is important to recognize a patient's right to refuse life-sustaining treatment, Joan cannot insist that she is resuscitated if the doctor believes this clinical intervention to be futile (GMC 2010). In order to reduce the potential for harm occurring, the clinician must explain the treatment options to Joan, what her goals are regarding care and the risks, benefits and burdens of CPR. Many people have an unrealistic expectation of success following CPR due to television dramas that portray unrealistically high positive outcomes (GMC 2010). Although the decision to withhold CPR may be the rational option in Joan's case, it is essential to recognize that other treatments will be provided for her. For instance, the urinary tract infection is potentially treatable with low-cost antibiotics and good nursing care.

The distinction between ordinary and extraordinary treatments has been used to support the rights of patients to certain interventions, while refraining from administering others. The criteria often stipulated a focus on 'ordinary means' of care/treatment as 'all medicines and treatments which offer a reasonable hope of benefit, are without excessive expense, pain or inconvenience', and 'extraordinary means' as 'all medicines and treatments that cannot be obtained without excessive expense, pain or other inconvenience, or which if used would not offer a reasonable hope of benefit' (Beauchamp and Childress 2009). In Joan's case CPR can be considered to be an extraordinary intervention, while antibiotics for her urinary tract infection are ordinary. However, Beauchamp and Childress (2009) have criticized the ordinary/extraordinary distinction for having a confusing array of meanings and thus being open to interpretation. Many of the concepts used in this distinction are ambiguous and abstract, therefore careful team discussion is required to determine a consensus regarding the limits of 'excess', 'benefit' and 'inconvenience'. The ANP must be clear that the ordinary/extraordinary distinction does not apply to specific interventions, but only to the intervention as it relates to the needs of each individual patient, in this case Joan. Treatment considered as 'extraordinary' for one patient may in fact be 'ordinary' for another, depending on their health status.

Specific strategies can improve the quality of decision making towards the end of life. The principle of veracity or truth telling is central to the promotion of autonomous decision making. In order for Joan to participate in decision making, it is essential that she is informed of her health status and that it is openly acknowledged that she has a right to refuse life-sustaining treatment. The ANP can try to establish the reason for the doctor's reluctance to discuss Joan's resuscitation status with her. Time constraints and pressure of work are not suitable explanations and should be challenged. If poor communication skills and lack of confidence are issues (Lachman 2010), a well-trained ANP can take on the responsibility of approaching and discussing end-of-life issues with the patient. Palliative care nurses have developed a wealth of knowledge and skills regarding how to facilitate such discussions. Various authors, including Jepson (2003) and Lachman (2010), maintain that nurses are the least likely to find talking about DNACPR decisions with patients or surrogates difficult. Unlike the house officers, the nurses viewed these conversations as a gratifying experience and part of their role as patient advocate. The researchers concluded that nurses were ready to take a more active role in initiating end-of-life discussions.

Poor communication is often to blame for inappropriate end-of-life interventions (GMC 2010). The role of the ANP extends beyond the acute setting into the community and patients are likely to meet ANPs anywhere along their healthcare journey. It is the ANP's responsibility to ensure that end-of-life decisions are formalized and transferred along with the patient throughout this journey, to ensure that the patient's rights are not infringed. The role of the ANP within primary care should thus be developed to include the opportunity to review the end-of-life wishes of patients with chronic long-term conditions. These patients should be given the opportunity to attend their GP practice to discuss issues openly and compassionately with an expert practitioner. ANPs working in GP surgeries can be attached to residential and nursing homes so that they visit the residents and develop a therapeutic relationship with them. A study by Lawrence (2009) found that ANPs were well prepared to help facilitate advanced decision making towards the end of life, and reported an increase in the number of advanced decisions being written if ANPs were placed in nursing homes to perform early identification, diagnosis and end-of-life care planning for residents with significant changes in health status. Early communication with patients and families is essential for effective end-of-life decision making.

> ### Reflective questions
>
> 1. What are the rights and duties of each member of the healthcare team and how can the ANP manage conflict within the team?
> 2. How can you enhance your practice to ensure that the rights of the patient are central to your considerations?
> 3. How can you develop your communication/interpersonal skills to ensure the seamless transition of care along the patient journey?
> 4. What are the rights of family members to information regarding the patient and how can the ANP manage any conflict within the healthcare team regarding consulting the family first?

Deactivation of cardiac device

Case scenario

Peter is 74 years old and a retired engineer. He is married with two grown-up children. Three years ago he had an implantable cardioverter defibrillator (ICD) inserted due to malignant cardiac arrhythmias. He has lived successfully with the ICD despite initial anxieties. He returned to see his GP as he was feeling tired and had seen blood in his urine. Following referral to a urologist, Peter was diagnosed with prostate cancer, with metastatic spread to his liver. He discussed his treatment options with a physician and was left feeling concerned regarding the likely success of radiotherapy and chemotherapy. He comes to see you, the advanced nurse practitioner in the cardiac outpatient clinic, the following week for his routine heart check-up. He presents as confused and concerned about the implications of this new diagnosis and suggested treatment. He asks about the possibility of his ICD being deactivated before the cancer destroys what little quality of life he may have left. You recognize the need to discuss Peter's options with him, but feel uncomfortable that deactivating his ICD may shorten his life prematurely.

Discussion

The use of sophisticated technology in the care of patients with malignant cardiac conditions has developed rapidly in the last 50 years. In our enthusiasm to achieve the optimum physiological conditions for patient survival, the moral implications of advanced practice tend to get left behind, as the ability to predict moral dilemmas is not an exact science. There is absolutely no doubt that the use of ICDs has enhanced the lives of thousands of cardiac patients who would otherwise have died. Sudden cardiac death occurs in approximately 50,000–70,000 people annually in the UK, and ICDs can be used for the primary prevention of life-threatening arrhythmias in individuals at risk of sudden cardiac death, as a secondary measure post-cardiac event, to stabilize patients with unstable heart rhythms or for treating those patients presenting with certain types of congenital heart disease (NICE 2006).

Due to the increasing number of patients presenting with cardiac disease, the likelihood of a nurse encountering a case like Peter's is increasing. ANPs working in cardiology will be part of the multi-disciplinary team that prepares patients for device insertion and immediate aftercare. Other ANPs working within medicine and palliative care are likely to meet a patient with an ICD as they present with end-of-life issues not related to their primary cardiac condition.

The Ethical Grid can provide an effective decision-making platform for multi-disciplinary bioethical discourse regarding this moral dilemma. Petrucci et al. (2011) also assert the need for an organized, ethically sensitive approach that begins at the initial stage of consent for implantation of the ICD and suggest a three-phase approach: initial information (understanding consent); pre-implant preparation (future directions); and specific end-of-life issues (withdrawing care). A working knowledge of both the Ethical Grid and Petrucci et al.'s 10-point model will provide a comprehensive opportunity for the analysis of the issues by clinical teams.

Petrucci et al.'s 10-point model:

Phase 1 Initial information (understanding consent)

Point 1. Surgical intervention
Point 2. Device technology
Point 3. Expected recovery
Point 4. Changing plans

Phase 2 Pre-implant preparation (future directions)

Point 5. Care planning
Point 6. Appointing a decision maker
Point 7. Cultural preference
Point 8. Conflict resolution

Phase 3 End-of-life care

Point 9. Palliative plan
Point 10. Acceptable withdrawal

Source: Petrucci et al. (2011).

Phase 1 of Petrucci et al.'s model includes the need to gain informed consent from Peter for implanting the ICD. The doctrine of informed consent is now legally, morally and professionally enshrined within all aspects of patient care in the UK. Every mentally competent adult has the right to accept or decline any or all treatments if they are mentally competent and do not wish treatment to commence or be continued. This is based on the principle of respect for autonomy and a person's right to bodily integrity. If a clinician continues to administer treatment to which the patient has not consented (unless in an emergency situation where consent is not possible, or the person lacks mental capacity and the clinician proceeds using the 'best interests' principle), or the person has refused consent to a proposed treatment, the clinician can be open to accusations of battery (Dimond 2011).

Effective informed consent should include the facts regarding the risks, benefits, side effects, alternative interventions and the consequences of having/not having the ICD implanted. This discussion should take place with Peter and his family, a cardiologist and an ANP who has specialist cardiology knowledge, to ensure comprehensive, consistent and continued holistic support throughout the process. Within this first phase Peter would have been prepared for the possible effects of ICD implantation, which include stroke, infection and multi-organ failure (NICE 2006). Dunbar (2005) also reports pain, sleep disturbance and multiple ICD activity 'storms', which are very distressing to patients. Nurses also cannot under-estimate the significance of psychosocial issues related to ICD implantation, which include anxiety, depression, anger and fear (Dunbar 2005). Device failure and re-implantation must also be discussed pre-operatively. It is within this first phase that Petrucci et al. (2011) include the need to begin to prepare Peter and his immediate family for end-of-life issues. The patient's values, beliefs and preferences are discussed and the importance of advance planning and the need for an advocate in the event of future incapacity are introduced, to ensure adherence to Peter's choices. Lachman (2011) stresses the need to create a 'preparedness plan', as many patients still do not have an advanced directive or engage in discussions regarding device deactivation towards the end of life. She asserts:

> The decision to begin is at least as important as the decision to stop; it is important to elicit the patient's values and views on quality of life and end of life, when they are still capable of reflection. (Lachman 2011: 99)

Phase 2 of Petrucci et al.'s model develops the initial discussion into active care planning pre-operatively. Lachman (2011) recommends referral to a palliative care specialist to ensure that the patient has an opportunity to discuss deactivation of the device and to seek reassurances of effective symptom management once deactivated. Opportunities for 'what if' questions need to be provided and responses should be open, honest and sensitive. An ADRT needs to be completed prior to the insertion of the device. A study by Mueller et al. (2010) suggested that only 50% of ICD patients had advanced directives and out of this number none mentioned deactivation. Goldstein et al. (2004) found that decisions to deactivate were not well planned in advance of the patient's death, but were a reaction to distress in the days, hours and minutes before that. They explain that even among patients with DNACPR orders, discussions about deactivating the ICD occurred in fewer than 45% of cases. This creates another dilemma for the healthcare team, as some members may see the ICD as a means of resuscitation, while others view it as a way of managing cardiac arrhythmias (Mueller et al. 2010). Either way, in Peter's case death is likely to be due to metastatic spread and associated symptoms, rather than cardiac failure, as the ICD will remain active until deactivated. Goldstein et al. (2004) emphasize the need to ensure that DNACPR documentation instructs clinicians to address the issue of deactivating ICDs where appropriate.

Peter must be informed of the process for deactivating the ICD to reassure him that it is not an open, invasive procedure. The procedure is practically quite simple considering the profound outcome. It consists of a magnet being placed over the skin above the ICD, which disables the defibrillator activity while maintaining pacing mode only (Nambisan 2004).

Peter also needs to select a decision maker to advocate for his wishes in the event that he becomes incapacitated. This will ensure that the healthcare team adheres to his final wishes. The Mental Capacity Act (DoH 2005) supports the appointment of a lasting power of attorney even if the patient has made an ADRT. Information regarding both the ADRT and the lasting power of attorney must be readily available to the clinical team and documentation provided to prevent confusion and delays. In the case of family conflict or when a person has no known family or friends, an independent mental capacity advocate or court-appointed deputy would be appointed to act on the patient's behalf. Petrucci et al. (2011) recommend the involvement of the institution's ethics committee when conflict exists. However, in the UK the role of ethics committees is for research review. Multi-disciplinary case reviews tend to be the preferred option for ethical analysis and related clinical decision making.

It is during the final Phase 3 that the decision to deactivate the ICD comes into effect and determines the validity of the two earlier phases.

Peter has approached the ANP in the clinic to discuss his options, one of which is deactivation at a time of his choosing. The ANP must remain non-judgemental and listen as Peter expresses his values, beliefs and preferences regarding his future choices and quality of life. Mueller et al. (2010) assert that patients have more authority to make decisions than clinicians and that their decisions have priority over clinical decision making. Berger (2005) believes that patients' decisions relating to quality of life are often based on their predicted levels of cognition or physical function. They determine what medical intrusions would diminish their quality of life sufficiently to render it no longer of value, making the decision 'exquisitely personal'. If the ANP is unable or unwilling to discuss deactivation due to personal, cultural or religious beliefs, they must refer Peter to another clinician. Healthcare professionals have a right to conscientiously object to certain issues, but must make their views knows to their manager (NMC 2008).

A patient's request to deactivate an ICD may create a moral dilemma for which the ANP is ill prepared. Some nurses may see deactivation of the ICD as assisted suicide or active euthanasia, as they judge it to be a constitutive therapy because it 'takes over the function that the body can no longer provide for itself' (Lachman 2011: 99), and thus will be unwilling to support the patient's request. Other nurses will recognize the primacy of respect for individual autonomy while appreciating the potential conflict between beneficence and non-maleficence, since the ICD actively impedes the dying process by inappropriately triggering cardiac defibrillation towards the end of life. The distinction lies with the intention of the healthcare professional performing the act of withdrawal. The doctrine of double effect attempts to differentiate between those acts that are intended to cause harm and those where harm is a reasonably foreseeable effect. Sometimes in trying to act beneficently the nurse can foresee two distinct outcomes to the proposed intervention, one good and the other potentially harmful. Administration of morphine towards the end of life is an example, where the intended effect is to ease pain and promote patient comfort, but the nurse recognises that a foreseeable side effect is respiratory depression. If the intention is beneficent rather than malevolent, the action is morally supported.

Beauchamp and Childress (2009: 162) identify four criteria that must be satisfied for an act with a double effect to be justified:

- The act must be good, or at least morally neutral, independent of its consequences.
- The agent intends only the good effect, not the bad effect. The bad effect can be foreseen, tolerated and permitted, but it must not be intended.

- The bad effect must not be a means to the good effect. If the good effect were the causal result of the bad effect, the agent would intend the bad effect in pursuit of the good effect.
- The good effect must outweigh the bad effect. The bad effect is permissible only if a proportionate reason compensates for permitting the foreseen bad effect.

The doctrine of double effect examines the intention of the person performing the act, by asserting that if the intention is to remove a treatment that is not beneficial or is burdensome, to terminate the treatment rather than the patient, then the act is morally justifiable. Indeed, precedent already exists to withdraw other treatments like ventilatory support and haemodialysis towards the end of life. However, Beauchamp and Childress (2009) suggest that the concept of intention is ambiguous, as it says nothing about a person's motivation and character, which can make a difference to the moral assessment of the action. The continued defibrillation of a patient via an ICD at the end of life violates the right of the patient to a good death and is therefore futile. The term futile refers to a situation in which irreversibly dying patients have reached a point at which further treatment provides no physiological benefit or is hopeless and becomes optional (Beauchamp and Childress 2009). If it were not for the ICD, the patient at the end of life may already be dead. The motivation to deactivate the ICD is to terminate a treatment that inhibits the natural progression of a lethal pathology (Mueller et al. 2010). Death will be due to cardiac arrest, not medical intervention, and is therefore not considered as assisted suicide or euthanasia and can be considered as justifiable according to the doctrine of double effect. Deactivation of the ICD allows a randomly assigned disease to progress, whereas suicide and euthanasia cause death irrespective of disease (Berger 2005). If the procedure is being carried out at home, as per the patient's request, a clinician/nurse practitioner should be present when deactivation is attempted to support all those involved.

Every person is entitled to a good and dignified death, but defining exactly what a good death is remains elusive. Perceptions of a good death vary, depending on the individual and their personal needs and wishes at the end of life. Staff's perceptions of a good death may differ from those of the individual and the family, resulting in confusion and distress at the end of life. In her study of death and dying in the intensive care unit, Seymour (2001: 129) suggests that a good death involves maintaining the integrity of the natural order and the dying individual's personhood. This, combined with trust between healthcare staff and patients' companions, leads to the core elements attributed to a good death. From the patient's perspective, freedom from inhumane and degrading practice (DoH 2008) is enshrined in the Human Rights Act, Article 3. This right affirms the importance of being treated as an individual, with dignity and respect, without pain and other symptoms, in familiar surroundings and in the company of close family and/or friends. These principles are identified as key to a good death in the Department of Health's end-of-life care strategy (2008).

Nurses must ensure that they uphold their duty to the patient and the family in respect of these principles. The provision of effective support, comfort and symptom control is essential towards the end of life and following deactivation of the device. Patients and their families will be scared and hesitant when the decision to deactivate the ICD is put into action. The development of Locality Registers (GMC 2010) for all patients receiving end-of-life care will help to ensure that they are not readmitted to hospital when death is imminent, thus preventing further inappropriate treatment and suffering. A report published by the Department of Health's End of Life Care Programme (2012b) emphasizes the need to develop policies that alert all members of the healthcare team to situations where patients have refused further clinical interventions. This includes ambulance staff, who are often faced with difficult decisions if called to a person's home. It recommends robust information systems to ensure that the person's wishes are communicated in a timely manner to the ambulance service and staff. In Peter's case the ANP could ensure that his GP has left a 'statement of intent' in the event that relatives are alone at home with Peter when his ICD is discontinued. This will prevent unnecessary intervention by ambulance staff in the event that they are called to assist, which would override Peter's wishes.

Until access to good-quality palliative care is provided as an absolute right within all healthcare environments and resources are sufficient to enable a good death, Mueller et al. (2010) assert that nurses can take courage from the belief that death from a cardiac arrhythmia may be a better mode of death than that from terminal cancer. An ICD impedes the dying process and maintains a moribund or permanent state of unconsciousness, a condition referred to as 'destination nowhere' (Bramstedt 2008: 1).

Reflective questions

1. Does the doctrine of double effect support the right of healthcare practitioners to perform immoral actions if the intention is good?
2. Consider how a consequentialist and a deontologist might view the doctrine of double effect. How can the potential conflict be managed in practice?

3. Try to think of other examples from your practice in which the doctrine of double effect can be applied to help explain the actions of a healthcare practitioner.

Respect and dignity in death

Case scenario

Following a failed resuscitation attempt in Accident and Emergency (A&E), the consultant invites the junior doctor to practise his defibrillation technique on a patient, prior to certifying the patient dead. All attempts at resuscitation have failed and the team decides to discontinue active measures; the patient subsequently dies. The junior doctor has no experience of defibrillating a real patient and is keen to practise the skill while under the supervision of the consultant. The ANP is not comfortable with this request, but is unsure of where she stands legally, morally and professionally.

Discussion

This is an extremely controversial issue that challenges the realms of possibility in contemporary healthcare, and we make no apologies for including it. Since the implementation of the Human Tissue Act 2004, healthcare professionals are unable to perform ad hoc teaching on the imminently or newly deceased without adhering to strict legal guidelines. However, despite legislation and moral concern being attached to such practices, they still occur, albeit on very rare occasions, a view supported by anecdotal evidence from clinical colleagues. The right of the medical staff to perfect their clinical skills is in direct conflict with the right of the patient to a dignified death. ANPs must not circumvent issues of such a contentious nature, but embrace them as they strive to provide holistic quality care.

The key elements of this dilemma focus on the status of the patient and their right to consent, dignity and respect, while acknowledging the greater need of society to have confidence in the competence of doctors, especially in an acute situation. Previous literature (Berger et al. 2002; Denny and Kollek 1999; Ardagh et al. 1997) concentrates on the distinction between therapeutic interventions aimed to benefit the patient, which occur prior to death, and training or practice, which occurs post mortem. This is an important distinction, although crucially it rests on the time at which the emergency consultant decides that continued resuscitation is futile and that death is irreversible. Berger et al. (2002) recognize that there is significant disagreement between practitioners about when this occurs during the resuscitation process.

The consultant's intention when inviting the junior doctor to defibrillate the patient is critical to the debate. In this scenario the request to defibrillate occurs prior to the declaration of death, so as such the issues involved are different from those manifesting post mortem. As death has not been declared, the suggested intervention remains within the remit of therapeutic treatment. It is evident that the patient, having failed to be resuscitated, is clinically if not legally dead when the consultant asks his junior doctor to perform additional defibrillation. Only when the patient is verified dead by the consultant and time of death is recorded is the patient legally recognized as deceased. Until verification has been made the patient remains open to further therapeutic interventions. Following verification of death, any procedure the junior doctor performs is not for therapeutic purposes, but specifically for training. The British Medical Association's consent guidelines state that 'the use of human tissue used after death for educational purposes requires consent from the donor, a person with parental responsibility (in the case of a child) or a qualifying relative' (BMA 2009: 26). In the case study the patient has not yet been verified as dead, therefore remains within the law governing informed consent. Seedhouse (2009) stresses the importance of ensuring that all the facts in a dilemma are determined prior to taking any action. The consultant must be able to justify all actions with a sound evidence-based rationale.

There has been much debate in the medical literature over the last 25 years regarding the appropriate use of nearly dead and recently dead bodies for education and training. Iserson (1993) is the main proponent of using dead bodies for training junior doctors in critical care areas. More recent analysis by Van Bogaert and Ogunbanjo (2008) recommends that institutions consider their position regarding this issue and develop stringent guidelines to limit the procedure to only those staff who can truly benefit from it. It supports the right of doctors to practise certain techniques on the nearly and recently deceased, particularly in emergency situations. The rationale for this is the utilitarian principle of 'increasing the greater good for the greatest number', which allows the interests of society to override those of the individual (Beauchamp and Childress 2009: 198). Allowing doctors to practise clinical techniques on the recently deceased will improve their clinical competence, thus benefiting future patients and society.

Beneficence is a fundamental moral principle in healthcare. Healthcare professionals must respect the autonomous choices of patients and contribute positively to their welfare. Beauchamp and Childress (2009) assert that the principle of beneficence demands much more than that of non-maleficence, because agents must take positive steps to help others, not merely refrain from harming them. Seedhouse (2009) prompts the decision maker to consider these principles within his Ethical Grid.

Central to the Grid is respect for patient autonomy, a fundamental moral principle that underpins all aspects of contemporary healthcare. To ensure that this principle is upheld, it is essential that ANPs recognize the need to assess the mental capacity of all their patients prior to determining the extent to which they can contribute to the decision-making process. Due to the critical nature of the patient in this case study, mental capacity and thus autonomy are absent; therefore, the patient is unable to participate in decision making. It is essential that as nurses we protect the rights of the patient. ANPs must be 'aware of the legislation regarding mental capacity, ensuring that people who lack capacity remain at the centre of decision making and are fully safe-guarded' (NMC 2008). It is crucial that ANPs recognize the essential nature of their role as patient advocates in this situation. A sound knowledge of the Human Tissue Act (DoH 2004) is required, as this stipulates in Schedule 1: Part 2 that consent is required to undertake any education or training relating to human health. Whether the patient is alive or dead, the principle of informed consent will still override any use of the body for training purposes.

The Human Tissue Act (Part 1, Section 1:10) stipulates that 'appropriate consent must be given voluntarily by an appropriately informed person, who has the capacity to agree to the activity in question'. It is clear that the wish of the patient is indeterminable during such a critical event. The patient may have previously donated their body to a university for the purpose of training and education, but this is not usually known in A&E unless relatives provide the information. The patient may also have an organ donation card, but this does not presume consent to training on an ad hoc basis in A&E. However, the Guttman scale (Trochim 2002) suggests that if an extreme procedure is accepted, then less extreme procedures on a given scale will also be accepted. If we apply this principle to consent, Ardagh (1997) believes that it may support the assumption that if a patient consents to something more extreme, like organ donation, it makes it potentially acceptable for doctors to practise their skills, as this is less burdensome than organ donation. However, in the scenario here, the patient has not yet been verified dead and his status regarding organ donation is unknown, which challenges this presumption.

Since the patient in this scenario has failed to respond to resuscitation and is mentally incapacitated, doctors must work in his best interests. They have a duty of care to take life-saving action, unless they are aware of any advanced decision to refuse such intervention. This is based on the statutory powers of the Mental Capacity Act (DoH 2005), which stipulates that 'An act done or decision made, for or on behalf of a person who lacks capacity must be done, or made, in his best interests'. The Act requires the healthcare professional to take into consideration any of the person's known views and to consult relatives and friends. If the patient's views are unknown or the relatives inaccessible, the doctor must consult an independent mental capacity advocate to report on the person's best interests (Dimond 2011). Consultation regarding consent to teach a junior doctor defibrillation prior to verifying death is impractical, inappropriate and also immoral.

Despite the moral and legal arguments against the use of a nearly dead body for practice and training, it remains a concern to some nurses. Inviting a junior doctor to practise defibrillation (or indeed any other clinical procedure) prior to verifying death cannot be in the patient's best interests. It is therefore unethical, which supports the need for the ANP to intervene and challenge the right of the healthcare professional to undertake the procedure. To do this, the ANP must take their role as patient advocate seriously and develop the assertiveness skills required to perform this role confidently. That requires close partnership working with colleagues to ensure that clear policies are in place within the department to identify training needs and ensure that ethical practices are followed. The ANP has an opportunity to become an effective role model for others and develop knowledge and skills in ethical matters in order to present a valid rationale for action. The use of a decision-making framework will enhance their ability to present a coherent justification for action. It also enables the ANP to appreciate the views of others when trying to reach a consensus. The development and use of ethics consultation teams and multi-disciplinary case reviews within departments can help to determine a morally acceptable approach to difficult cases, either prospectively or retrospectively. One way forward is for ANPs to instigate the development of case reviews whenever they believe that the rights of the patients are being infringed. This is part of their key role in facilitating effective solutions to moral dilemmas in clinical practice.

Reflective questions

1. Do the rights of the individual outweigh the rights of the general public to competent practitioners?
2. Many practitioners can see the overall utility of practising complex skills on dead bodies, especially infants, due to the complex nature of the

procedures and the ultimate consequence of failure. How can this be balanced with the right of the person to a dignified death?
3. What are the implications of the Guttman scale in other areas of your clinical decision making?
4. Is it appropriate to seek the views of relatives in an acute situation or should the team be left to work in the best interests of the patient?
5. What skills do you require to be an effective patient advocate? How would you apply them in this case scenario?

Conclusion

Healthcare practitioners frequently encounter moral dilemmas. Reality is morally complex and ethical theories are not mutually exclusive, but serve to provide a plethora of philosophical beliefs, a toolkit for the ANP to master their art. It is not a question of determining which moral theory is correct, since all of them contribute in some way to the complex clinical reality. Add to this non-moral dimensions such as economics and the law and we soon have a recipe for conflict. Having advanced technical competencies is only one dimension of ANPs' multi-faceted responsibility. Practitioners must endeavour to explore and understand the complex nature of human behaviour and to integrate the rights of patients and their carers into the web of clinical decision making. ANPs are not expected to be supererogatory when going about their daily encounters, but they are expected to ensure that patients are not harmed by any acts or omissions by them or their colleagues. Seedhouse's Ethical Grid decision-making framework helps in providing workable solutions to difficult moral problems. As Paniagua (2010) states, advanced nursing practice is not a role, but a way of thinking. ANPs must embrace the additional responsibilities of their role and take active steps to develop knowledge and competence in ethical decision making.

References

Ardagh, M. (1997) May we practise endotracheal intubation on the newly dead? *Journal of Medical Ethics* 23: 289–294.

Beauchamp, T.L. and Childress, J.F. (2009) *Principles of Biomedical Ethics*, 6th edn. Oxford: Oxford University Press.

Berger, J.T. (2005) The ethics of deactivating implanted cardioverter defibrillators. *Annals of Internal Medicine* 142: 631–634.

Berger, J.T., Rosner, F. and Cassell M.D. (2002) Ethics of practicing medical procedures on newly dead and nearly dead patients. *Journal of General Internal Medicine* 17: 774–778.

Bramstedt, K.A. (2004) Elective inactivation of total artificial heart technology in non-futile situations: Inpatients, outpatients and research participants. *Death Studies* 28: 423–433.

Bramstedt, K.A. (2008) Destination nowhere: A potential dilemma with ventricular assist devices. *American Journal of Artificial Internal Organs* 54: 1–2.

British Medical Association (2009) *Consent Toolkit*, 5th edn. London: BMA.

British Medical Association, Resuscitation Council (UK) and Royal College of Nursing (2007) *Decisions Relating to Cardio-pulmonary Resuscitation*. London: BMA/RC/RCN.

Denny, C.J. and Kollek, D. (1999) Practicing procedures on the recently dead. *Journal of Emergency Medicine* 17(6): 949–952.

Department of Health (1998) *The Human Rights Act*. http://www.legislation.gov.uk/ukpga/1998/42/schedule/1 (accessed 15 June 2012).

Department of Health (2004) *The Human Tissue Act*. London: HMSO.

Department of Health (2005) *The Mental Capacity Act*. London: HMSO.

Department of Health (2012a) Your Right to Refuse Future Medical Treatment. http://webarchive.nationalarchives.gov.uk/20121015000000/http://www.direct.gov.uk/en/governmentcitizensandrights/death/preparation/dg_10029429 (accessed 22 February 2015).

Department of Health (2012b) *National End of Life Care Programme: The Route to Success in End of Life Care – Achieving Quality in Ambulance Services*. London: End of Life Care Programme.

Dimond, B. (2011) *Legal Aspects of Nursing*, 6th edn. London: Pearson.

Dunbar, S.B. (2005) Psychosocial issues of patients with implantable cardioverter defibrillators. *American Journal of Critical Care* 14(4): 294–303.

Edwards, S.D. (2009) *Nursing Ethics; A Principled-Based Approach*. London: Macmillan.

Eliott, J. and Olver I. (2010) Dying cancer patients talk about physician and patient roles in DNR decision making. *Health Expectations* 14: 147–158.

General Medical Council (2010) *Treatment and Care towards the End of Life: Good Practice in Decision Making*. London: GMC.

Goldstein, N.E., Lampert, R., Bradley, E., Lynn, J. and Krumholz, H.M. (2004) Management of implantable cardioverter defibrillators in end of life care. *Annals of Internal Medicine* 141: 835–838.

Grace, P.J. (2009) *Nursing Ethics and Professional Responsibility*. London: Jones and Bartlett.

Guardian (2011) NHS hospitals warned over 'Do not resuscitate orders'. 5 November. http://www.guardian.co.uk/society/2011/dec/05/nhs-hospitals-warned-resuscitate-orders (accessed 22 February 2015).

Iserson, K.V. (1993) Postmortem procedures in the Emergency Department: Using the recently dead to practise and teach. *Journal of Medical Ethics* 19: 92–98.

Jepson, J. (2003) Do not attempt resuscitation decisions: The nursing role. *British Journal of Nursing* 12(7): 1038–1042.

Kalb, K. and O'Conner-Von, S. (2007) Ethics education in advanced practice nursing: Respect for human dignity. *Nursing Education Perspectives* 28(4): 196–202.

Kant, L. (1967) Foundations of the metaphysics of morals. In P.J. Grace (ed.), *Nursing Ethics and Professional Responsibility*. London: Jones and Bartlett.

Kilpatrick, K., Lavoie-Tremblay, M., Ritchie, J.A. and Lamothe, L. (2011) Advanced practice nursing, health care teams and perceptions of team effectiveness. *The Healthcare Manager* 30(3): 215–226.

Lachman, V. (2010) Do not resuscitate orders: Nurses' role requires moral courage. *Journal of Medical Surgical Nursing* 19(4): 249–251.

Lachman, V. (2011) Left ventricular assisted device deactivation: Ethical issues. *Journal of Medical and Surgical Nursing* 20(2): 98–100.

Lawrence, J.F. (2009) The Advanced Directive prevalence in long-term care: A comparison of relationships between a nurse practitioner healthcare model and a traditional healthcare model. *Journal of the American Academy of Nurse Practitioners* 21: 179–185.

Loertscher, L., Reed, D.A., Bannon, M.P. and Mueller, P.S. (2010) Cardiopulmonary resuscitation and do not resuscitate orders: A guide for clinicians. *American Journal of Medicine* 23(1): 4–9.

Mueller, P.S., Swetz, K.M., Freeman, M.R. et al. (2010) Ethical analysis of withdrawing ventricular assist device support. *Mayo Clinic Proceedings* 85(9): 791–797.

Nambisan, V. (2004) Dying and defibrillation: A shocking experience. *Palliative Medicine* 18: 482–483.

National Confidential Enquiry into Patient Outcome and Death (2012) *Time to Intervene?* London: NCEPOD.

National Institute of Health and Clinical Excellence (2006) Guidance on the use of implantable cardioverter defibrillators for arrhythmias. *Technology Appraisal* 95. London: NICE.

Nightingale, F. (1859) *Notes on Nursing: What It Is and What It Is Not*. London: Harrison.

Nursing and Midwifery Council (2008) *The Code: Standards of Conduct, Performance and Ethics for Nurses and Midwives*. London: NMC.

Paniagua, H. (2010) Reviewing the concept of advanced nurse practice. *Practice Nursing* 21(7): 371–375.

Petrucci, R.J., Benish, L.A. and Carrow, B.L. (2011) Ethical considerations for ventricular assisted device support: A 10 point model. *American Society for Artificial Internal Organs* 57: 268–273.

Rumbold, G. (1993) *Ethics in Nursing Practice*, 2nd edn. London: Balliere Tindall.

Saul, H. (2014) Do Not Resuscitate orders: Doctors must consult patients before putting notice on medical records, Court of Appeal rules. *Independent*, 17 June. http://www.independent.co.uk/news/uk/home-news/do-not-resuscitate-orders-doctors-have-legal-duty-to-consult-rules-court-of-appeal-9542969.html (accessed 1 March 2015).

Seedhouse, D. (1991) *Ethics: The Heart of Healthcare*. Chichester: John Wiley and Sons.

Seedhouse, D. (2009) *Ethics: The Heart of Healthcare*, 3rd edn. Chichester: Wiley-Blackwell.

Seymour, J.E. (2001) *Critical Moments: Death and Dying in Intensive Care*. Milton Keynes: Open University Press.

Steinboch, B., Arras, J.D. and London, A.J. (2003) *Ethical Issues in Modern Medicine*, 6th edn. New York: McGraw-Hill.

Sulmasy, D.P., Kai He, M., McAuley, R. and Ury, W.A. (2008) Beliefs and attitudes of nurses and physicians about do not resuscitate orders and who should speak to patients and families about them. *Critical Care Medicine* 36(6): 1817–1822.

Thiroux, J. (2004) *Ethics: Theory and Practice*, 8th edn. Upper Saddle River, NJ: Pearson/Prentice Hall.

Trochim, W.M.K. (2002) General Issues of Scaling. http://www.indiana.edu/~educy520/sec5982/week_3/scaling_trochim.pdf (accessed 5 July 2012).

Ulrich, C. and Zeitzer, M. (2009) Ethical issues in nursing practice. In V. Ravitsky, A. Fiester and A. Caplan (eds), *The Penn Center Guide to Bioethics*. New York: Springer.

Van Bogaert, K. and Ogunbanjo G.A. (2008) 'Don't ask, don't tell'. Ethical issues concerning learning and maintaining life-saving skills. *South African Family Practise* 50(4): 52–54.

CHAPTER 10

Careers and career development for advanced practice

Hilary Walsgrove and Heather Griffith

Chapter outline

- Introduction
- Advanced practice role development
- Career planning and development for advanced practice
- Advanced practitioner interviews
- A picture of advanced practice

Introduction

This chapter considers career development for advanced practice. A series of advanced practice career profiles illustrate how individuals develop from experienced, competent practitioner to advanced practitioner, along a number of different, sometimes challenging pathways. The practitioners who have shared their profiles were drawn from a purposive, convenience sample of individuals (Holloway and Wheeler 2010; Robson 2011) known to the authors through clinical practice and educational arenas within the UK. They encompass roles from both primary and secondary care settings. Some of their journeys have been straightforward and structured around specific areas of practice or roles already established, but for others the picture has been quite different.

Advanced practice role development

Advanced practice roles in the UK are a relatively new concept, when compared with the experience of the USA, where advanced nurses have been practising for decades. Advanced nursing practice in the USA emerged as a result of increases in medical specialization and the inaccessibility of medical care (Marsden et al. 2003; Pearson and Peels 2002; Schober and Affara 2006; Sheer and Wong 2008). The UK's experience dates back to around the 1980s when nurses looked to the experience of other nations (Sheer and Wong 2008) in their quest to improve care for patients and to fill gaps in an ever-changing Health Service (Stilwell 1984; Marsden et al. 2003). Australia and New Zealand appeared to take a similar path from the 1990s onwards (Nurse Practitioner Taskforce 2000; Gardner et al. 2010). More recently, Ireland, the Netherlands, Switzerland and Scandinavia have reported on the emergence of advanced practice roles in their healthcare services (Lindpaintner 2004; Roodbol et al. 2007; Callaghan 2008; Fagerstrom and Glasberg 2011).

The concept and definition of advanced practice

As a result of the emergent nature of advanced practice, numerous different roles, with a plethora of titles and profiles, have developed with little in the way of structure or coherence (Furlong and Smith 2005; Currie 2010). What is clear is that a concept of advanced practice, particularly related to nursing but also as a feature within other healthcare professions, is a global trend. It is growing and developing as a support and sometimes an alternative to traditional medical treatment and as an enhancement of established patient care. A body of knowledge of advanced practice has emerged and continues to develop, shaping and reshaping itself alongside constantly changing healthcare services and patient needs and demands. This is strengthened and supported by evidence indicating that advanced practice brings about improvements in patient outcomes and plays a valuable role 'in providing a beneficial contribution and filling a gap in healthcare services' (Callaghan 2008: 205).

Recently, advanced practice has reached a point in its evolution where a globally agreed definition can be proposed. Although this mainly concentrates on nursing, it is the generic skills and knowledge of the practitioner, rather than the professional background per se, that are key to the advanced practice role. Thus, the core principles that have predominantly been applied to nursing (NES 2008; DoH 2010; NLIAH 2010) are also being adopted by other healthcare professionals. It is widely acknowledged that advanced practice nurses are nurses practising at a higher level than traditional nurses (Sheer and Wong 2008). The identification of an overarching term for advanced practice was also facilitated through the International Council of Nurses (ICN), which launched the International Nurse Practitioner/Advanced Practice

Network (INP/APNN) in 2000. The global membership of this network acknowledges that, despite some international differences, there is sufficient similarity between nations to enable a generic definition. The INP/APNN definition states that advanced practice nurses are:

registered nurses who have acquired the expert knowledge base, complex decision-making skills, and clinical competencies for expanded practice, the characteristics of which are shaped by the context or country in which they are credentialed to practice. (ICN 2001)

The early stages of development

During the evolutionary phases of advanced practice, individuals and the organizations within which they were employed had little on which to base their role development. Thus, these roles emerged in an ad hoc, unstructured manner, in response to what was required for the service, in accordance with patients' needs and with reliance on the experience, skills and knowledge of the individual practitioners (Sheer and Wong 2008). Studies of some of the early examples of advanced roles reported that the drive for their development tended to fit into one of three categories: enthusiastic individuals developing roles when money was not available; replacement of doctors; and nurse-led initiatives (Scholes et al. 1999).

Without a solid background of advanced practice being available, these practitioners and their managers/employers needed to consider what education and professional development needs were required to facilitate the advancement of a role that would fit the purpose required. As a result, the numerous roles that developed featured an array of different levels and parameters (Furlong and Smith 2005; Pulcini et al. 2010; Currie 2010).

Developing frameworks for advanced practice roles

It is only in the last few years that frameworks have started to be developed that provide organizations and aspiring advanced practice nurses with more clarity on the domains of practice and competencies of advanced practice. These have the potential to guide and structure roles and career development (Bryant-Lukosius and DiCenso 2004; Gardner and Gardner 2005; NES 2008; NLIAH 2010; DoH 2010), as well as avoiding barriers to the successful introduction of advanced practice roles (Griffin and Melby 2006; RCN 2012; Barton et al. 2012). Such a proactive and systematic approach has only become possible since the body of advanced practice knowledge, and evidence to support it, has gradually grown, been reported on and disseminated widely. Without the early years of innovation, creativity, trial and error, pioneering spirit and risk taking, there would have been little in the way of advanced practice development.

A small selection of these frameworks for advanced practice development are explored in this chapter to provide a flavour of what is emerging as a repertoire of development and evalution tools.

The 'Strong model' is a conceptual framework designed by Ackerman et al. (1996) consisting of five domains of practice: direct comprehensive care, education, research, support of systems, and publication and professional leadership. Ackerman et al. (1996) focused on the development from novice to expert advanced practice nurses, looking at the expectations of individuals as leaders in the professional practice of nursing.

The 'PEPPA' framework was developed for the introduction, development, implementation and evaluation of advanced practice nursing roles in Canada. It focuses on a 'participatory, evidence-based, patient-focused process' (Bryant-Lukosius and Di Censo 2004: 530) that is goal directed and outcomes based. One of its key aims is to enable the development of roles that are instrumental in addressing patients' health needs by providing coordinated care systems and ensuring collaborative working relationships with healthcare providers.

From the 1990s inwards, the Departments of Health for the four countries of the UK (NLIAH 2010; NES 2008; DoH 2010), as well as other influencing organizations such as the Nursing and Midwifery Council (NMC 2005) and the Royal College of Nursing (RCN 2002), have started to build frameworks for advanced practice roles, focused on the delivery of quality services for patients across the whole healthcare arena (Laurant et al. 2005; Callaghan 2008; Carryer et al. 2007; Pulcini et al. 2010). Part of this has involved the definition of competencies for advanced practice.

Competencies for advanced nursing practice

During the 1990s the National Organization of Nurse Practitioner Faculties (NONPF) in the USA developed and released advanced practice nursing competencies within seven domains of practice (NONPF 2002):

- Management of patient health/illness status
- Nurse practitioner–patient relationship
- Teaching/coaching function

- Professional role
- Managing and negotiating healthcare delivery systems
- Monitoring and ensuring quality of healthcare practice
- Cultural competence

This has provided an international advanced nursing practice model and has guided national and international curriculum development in a number of countries, most notably the UK (RCN 2002, 2012).

The RCN used the NONPF competencies as a baseline on which to develop a set of competencies for advanced nurse practitioners in the UK (RCN 2002). The vast majority of these competencies were then adopted by the NMC as it embarked on a plan to regulate and/or register advanced nurses (NMC 2005). Work has continued to develop a framework for advanced practice. Although the Scottish, Welsh and English Departments of Health have issued individual documents, the frameworks considered as a whole provide a consensus for advanced practice in the UK (NLIAH 2010; NES 2008; DoH 2010).

In Ireland, the National Council for the Professional Development of Nursing and Midwifery established a framework for advanced nursing practice roles (NCNM 2001), followed by accreditation procedures for the first advanced nurse practitioners (NCNM 2006). This framework identified leadership, autonomy, expertise and research as some of the essential components of the role. In addition, Callaghan (2008) cites other pertinent aspects as including evidence-based practice, consultancy, collaboration and clinical decision making. These components are equally identified within other international frameworks and models of advanced practice (Daly and Carnwell 2003; Furlong and Smith 2005; Hampel et al. 2010; Gardner et al. 2010; Lowe et al. 2012).

The various pieces that have been built and refined over decades of development are now beginning to knit together into a complete patchwork quilt that represents a sound base and a clear framework for advanced practice. On this solid base, individuals and organizations can develop appropriate roles and services, while maintaining a flexible, innovative and creative approach that meets patient and service needs effectively and efficiently.

A local framework

Within the UK there are local examples of advanced practice strategies and frameworks. A recent framework for advanced nurses in an acute hospital in the South of England provides an illustration of how an organization can develop its own workforce. An organization-wide review was undertaken of all nurses working in posts that were identified as fitting

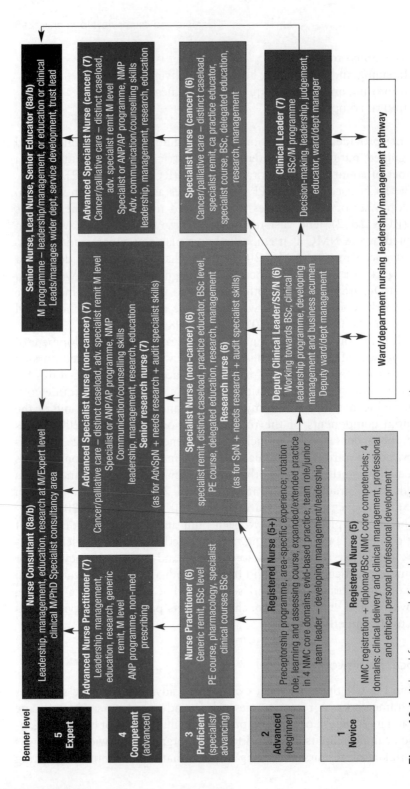

Figure 10.1 A local framework for advanced practice career progression
Source: The Royal Bournemouth and Christchurch Hospitals NHS Foundation Trust (2012)

into the local context of advancing and advanced practice. As a result, a number of tools were developed to help in career progression and to provide consistency and parity across the organization.

This included a framework within which the nurses work, with a career progression pathway that provides clear but flexible routes for individual nurses and succession planning for the organization (see Figure 10.1). Relevant professional development and education and training requirements are identified for individuals to develop and maintain competence, and to progress in advanced practice nursing careers that are fit for purpose and in line with the requirements of the organization and within the context of the definition of advanced practice that is recognized globally (ICN/APNN 2000), nationally (DH 2010; RCN 2012) and locally at the hospital in question.

As can be seen in Figure 10.1, the roles identified fall into seven categories, ranging from Band 6 to Band 8b on the Agenda for Change scale (DoH 2004): nurse consultant, advanced nurse practitioner, nurse practitioner, advanced specialist nurse, specialist nurse, senior research nurse and research nurse. A series of template job descriptions have been developed for the various levels and categories of posts. Development work has continued and there is now an ongoing commitment across the organization to consider the introduction and development of advancing and advanced roles in a more structured and cohesive manner, representing a hospital-wide strategy.

Career planning and development for advanced practice

It is widely acknowledged that nurses in advanced roles can make a significant, positive contribution to healthcare delivery (Horrocks et al. 2002; Furlong and Smith 2005; Laurant et al. 2005; Ball 2006) and that developments in advanced nursing practice have taken place in response to changes to contemporary heathcare delivery (Gibson and Hooker 2004; Callaghan 2008; Lowe et al. 2012). This has provided an impetus for nurses who wish to remain in clinical practice, as they are able to consider how they can utilize their expertise as the cornerstone for planning and developing their careers. Advanced nurse practitioner roles provide an innovative, exciting and yet challenging opportunity to work at an advanced level of clinical practice (Carlisle 2004; Walsgrove and Fulbrook 2005), offering promotional prospects and acknowledgement of a clinical career pathway from intial registration through to expert practice level (Benner 1984; Daly and Carnwell 2003; Griffith 2004).

The ever-changing environment of healthcare practice requires its workforce to take control of their own careers and futures. Healthcare

> **Box 10.1 Career planning and development: reflective questions**
>
> - What have I been doing?
> - How have I got where I am today?
> - Where am I now and why?
> - Where would I like to be and why?
> - What is stopping me get there and what am I doing about it?
> - How will I get to where I want to be?

practitioners need to be career resilient, which involves a high degree of flexibility and adaptability, the hallmarks of a profession. Such career resilience is in line with definitions of professional practice as including autonomy, self-direction and continuous professional development (ICN 2002). Continuous career planning needs to be integral to the development of individuals within or considering advanced roles, and is a means of responding to both short-term and long-term healthcare changes (Carlisle 2004; NCNM 2005; Livesley et al. 2009; Currie 2010). Such a planning process requires individuals to understand their work and the environment within which they are working, to have the ability to identify both their strengths and limitations and to articulate their personal vision within a realistic plan for the future, and then to realize their career goals through marketing and collaborative strategies that meet the requirements of their organizations as well as the patients they serve.

The use of reflective skills to answer the questions in Box 10.1 can act as a starting point for individual practitioners as they embark on career planning (Moon 2006; Casey and Egan 2010).

Once the practitioner has reflected on their current situation and started on the road to career development, it is worth focusing on elements relating more specifically to developing as an advanced practitioner. Barker (2009: 50) draws on a four-step career development planning model, devised by Donner and Wheeler (2001), as a tool for helping practitioners to understand their development needs in this context.

1. *Scan the environment* to understand the local and wider context, to identify the needs of the healthcare environment, and to be aware of the organization's vision and shared values and how you can contribute to moving these forward as an advanced practitioner.
2. *Complete a self-assessment*, asking yourself about your own values and beliefs about your profession and healthcare more generally;

identifying the strengths and knowledge, skills and experience you have to build on and what you require for the future; and acknowledging your personal limitations and how these might be overcome within the context of an advancing role.

3. *Create a career vision,* using the reflective questions detailed in Box 10.1, but with a focus on your overall career goal as an advanced practitioner.
4. *Create a career development plan,* identifying goals, plans, timelines and resources, in conjunction with a suitable mentor (Anderson et al. 2002; Girot and Rickaby 2008).

While considering an advancing role and how you are going to realize your career aspirations at the same time as improving and enhancing patient care, it is useful to refer to the ever-growing body of advanced practice knowledge (Bryant-Lukosius et al. 2004; Barker 2009; Lowe et al. 2012) and to look at the reality of advanced practice roles within your own area as well as more widely. The next section provides an overview of eight roles based on a snapshot of points emerging from interviews with practitioners.

Advanced practitioner interviews

We carried out interviews with advanced nurses and practitioners from different clinical and geographical areas across England and Wales. From the data gathered during the interviews, we created brief career development profiles to illustrate a selection of real-life examples of advanced practice roles. Some emergent characteristics appeared to be shared by all the interviewees, such as autonomous practice, critical thinking, a high level of decision making and problem solving, improving practice, risk taking, innovation and leadership. While these will be discussed in more detail later in the chapter, here we should say that they are very similar to the categories outlined in the work undertaken by NHS Scotland to developed its advanced practice toolkit (NES 2008). What also came to the fore was the diversity of the roles, all of which fit within the context of advanced practice (NES 2008; DoH 2010; NLIAH 2010).

To help in understanding advanced practice careers and their development, we used the reflective questions in Box 10.1 as a starting point for the interviews. Participants were asked to discuss their roles and to explore the journey they had taken to become an advanced nurse practitioner, focusing on their career development. Box 10.2 describes the interview format that we employed to guide the dialogue and create the

> ## Box 10.2 Advanced practice careers and career development interview format
>
> - Their current post
> - The population they serve
> - What 'unique' contribution they make to delivery of patient care
> - The journey the individual took from their decision as an experienced, competent nurse to where they are now
> - The education and professional development they undertook
> - Some of the celebrations, influences along the way, who and what helped them during their progress, how and why
> - Challenges they faced on the way
> - Changes of direction required, why their quest failed
> - Where they see themselves in the future
> - Where they see advanced practice in the future
> - What advice they have for aspiring advanced practitioners

profiles. Once the interviews had been transcribed, the interviewees checked the contents for accuracy. All were keen to share their stories and gave their consent for their profiles to be included in this book. To maintain confidentiality, we have used pseudonyms.

Profile 1: Advanced nurse practitioner (gynaecology), acute hospital trust

Pam is an advanced nurse practitioner (ANP) for a team of six consultant gynaecologists. Her work is mainly based around elective and emergency surgical patients in an outpatient and operating theatre capacity, with continuity along the patient's pathway provided through the inpatient ward. She leads the gynaecology pre-operative assessment service, working clinically, assessing patients prior to surgery using advanced nursing skills, obtaining patients' consent for their procedures, taking detailed drug histories and transcribing patients' own drugs. She also identifies any patients with potential problems that may compromise their surgical journey and refers on to relevant healthcare professionals, following the issues up as required in order to ensure the smooth running of the patient's journey through the service. She is a resource for and provides training and support to junior doctors and nurses, acts as an advanced scrub practitioner in the operating theatre and follows patients up in her ANP-led outpatient clinic after surgery. She acts as a point of contact for patients throughout their surgical journey, providing support, information and advice. Despite being a member of the gynaecology team, Pam identifies that she has a great deal of autonomy within her role, and the main focus of all the aspects of her role is that they are within the context of ANP-led services that she has developed, leads and manages, using a high level of clinical judgement and decision making, only seeking advice and guidance from the team when required. Her role is one that dovetails with and supports both nursing and medicine. With the advanced scrub practitioner role, Pam has replaced a senior house officer, as there was not enough medical cover.

Pam has a wealth of nursing experience in a variety of specialties within acute hospital settings dating back 30 years. She spent 22 years in medicine working up to a ward sister's post and then a hospital site manager's role, where she was responsible for the management and leadership of the hospital as a whole. A shift in roles and a desire to do something different took Pam down a surgical career route. She worked on an orthopaedic ward and then specialized within orthopaedic pre-assessment.

It was within this environment that she started to develop advanced assessment skills, through a physical examination module, leading to completion of an advanced nurse practitioner course. This course as well as the advanced scrub practitioner programme enabled her to develop the required generic clinical skills at an advanced level. She also needed to build up knowledge and skills within the specialty, as this was fairly new to her. Pam took on a gynaecology ANP role partway through her ANP course. Although she had very little experience of gynaecology, it was identified that she had a high level of generic advanced nursing skills and knowledge that would form the backbone of the work she would be doing. She also had demonstrable leadership and management skills and service and practice development abilities, and is able to work independently but always within her scope of practice (NMC 2008). Completion of the advanced scrub practitioner (ASP) course gave her the required complement of competencies, knowledge and skills to function in the role. As it was a new role, Pam was instrumental in developing the role and gaining the requisite knowledge and skills herself to ensure that patient needs and service requirements were met, meeting gaps she saw in the service, such as lack of ownership of pre-assessment and a need to lead on the follow-up of patients being assessed. She uses innovative and creative approaches, along with tireless energy, commitment and motivation, as the drivers for success.

Key points about the role

It has been a very individual journey. I haven't followed anybody else ... One thing leads to another. One of the keys to my post was to be able to take ownership of ... the pre-assessment service.'

(Interviewer) 'With the ASP role, if they didn't have you doing it they would have to employ a medical practitioner, wouldn't they? Essentially you've replaced an SHO.' (Pam's response) 'Yes, yes.'

'The ANP and scrub practitioner, some would argue are not related, but I would disagree with that, they are interlinked in my role.'

'It's the generic skills that make the ANP role transferable into any specialty. The core skills are transferable over any area. I could transfer the skills into a primary care setting, but then you would need new skills relevant to that area of practice.'

'Moving from a management role managing people to managing yourself as an autonomous practitioner requires a high level of leadership and management skills.'

'I had experience in other areas.'

Challenges

Pam had reached a senior level as a nurse manager and had experienced some upheaval due to service changes and ward closures, requiring her to think about a change in career direction. She then found herself going back to a junior staff nurse position in a different specialist area and then a 'novice' as she embarked on her ANP and ASP training, which was not always easy. However, she maintained a very positive approach throughout this period and felt that as one door closed another opened. Pam remarked: 'The opportunities are always there. If you turn the clock back, no way would I have expected to be where I am today. Nothing is ever lost, you gain something from everything you do.'

Role transition is often described as being difficult and Pam experienced some hurdles along the way: 'Coming into the gynae job halfway through doing the ANP course wasn't an easy transition in having a brand new job with not taking over from someone. It was a development job.'

Although Pam had successfully completed her ANP degree programme, her training and education for the role were not complete. 'I work as an advanced scrub practitioner ... It was part of my job description ... so not really having a background in theatre, it was something that when I did I felt quite uncomfortable doing it at that stage. Very embarrassing at first, everybody in theatre seemed to know what they were doing. I required formal training.'

She now finds herself in a position where the job has grown beyond expectations and as the only ANP in the team she is struggling with the expanded workload: 'The job is growing all the time. To develop the role further I would need pressures taken off ... you just manage the work ... which is quite frustrating, you don't want the high standards you've built to drop.'

Celebrations

Pam has achieved a great deal in a sort space of time, but now has no plans to go anywhere else, just to grow within the role she is in.

She talked enthusiastically about her role: 'It's probably the best job I've ever had. Yes it's very exciting.' She added: 'I actually see patients in pre-assessment, assist at their operation and see them and discharge them, which is fantastic.'

However, one of her celebrations, knowing she had achieved competence as an advanced scrub practitioner, is to 'actually be requested by consultants on a regular basis, going in to assist them'.

Advice for others

'The opportunities are always there.'

Profile 2: Colorectal advanced specialist nurse, acute hospital trust

Debra has been in post as a colorectal advanced specialist nurse for seven years. She works in a multi-disciplinary team, with patients who have colorectal cancer. She sees them in endoscopy or outpatient department, when a cancer is first suspected, explains any concerns to them and the investigations that need to be done. She takes patients through the journey from suspicion to diagnosis and pre-operatively if surgery is the first line of treatment. She does surveillance for patients who have been treated and their follow-up for up to five years. She sees all the post-surgery patients in a nurse-led clinic. Debra's remit as a key worker is multi-functional, dealing with the psychological as well as the physical care and treatment of patients, using advanced communication and advanced assessment skills. The specialist skills relevant to this patient case load, as well as the more generic advanced skills, are utilized within her role.

Debra had been a surgical ward sister for 16 years, 14 years on a colorectal ward. She loved the job but wanted a change and took a job in the community, but missed the hospital life and the relationships she formed with patients. She was offered the advanced specialist nurse job on condition that she undertook an advanced nurse practitioner course of study. This was to enable her to autonomously run her own nurse-led clinics, which was what was required of the post. The model for this role was different from the traditional cancer nurse specialist (CNS) role, which is usually much more focused on the psychological support of patients; what was wanted was a role that merged the ANP with a CNS, creating a joined-up role that encompasses both psychological as well as physical skills at an advanced level of practice.

Key points about the role

Debra believes that for this role, she needed to be a good communicator who is open and honest and able to communicate with the patient on their own level. She had to have a caring approach, some life experience and maturity, which she believes is at the heart of functioning effectively in her role. Debra commented: 'I'm not sure I could have done this as a young nurse.' The specialty-specific experience and community experience were valuable to the development of her role. In relation to the surgical knowledge and skills, Debra commented: 'we're talking major surgery that these people are having and you need to know your anatomy, because if you don't how can you explain to a patient why they are having the symptoms and what to expect once we've altered their plumbing.'

Debra believes that being an advanced nurse enables her to deal with the unpredictable work pattern. She thinks that 'you have to have a good sense of priority because what was your priority five minutes ago is suddenly not! You have to be able to explain to patients why you are leaving them to go elsewhere, which does cause problems.'

Challenges

Debra talked about the responsibility inherent in the role, particularly as the majority of her patients have cancer: 'particularly with the bowel screening patients who come along having no symptoms whatsoever, think they're just coming for a quick test and hey presto they've got a cancer'. She also described how 'I think uniquely we are telling patients that they may have cancer and that's something that lots of people will shy away from doing ... often it is us telling them what they've got.'

Debra's role is very unpredictable and she never knows from one day to the next how the day is going to go, even if she has set clinic patterns and so on, so this requires her to work very reactively. 'You never know who is going to contact you, when new patients are going to be discovered ... no way of knowing which patients are going to have a cancer.' She added: 'It moves all the time, and we have to take into account patients' health generally, their mental state and we may have to move goal posts.'

Lack of communication has been a barrier at times from an organizational point of view, 'when people are taking things forward and kind of leave us out'. This also occurs when things are not considered priority.

The whole service is only covered by Debra and one other colleague, so it is hard to keep the service going and ensure it is effective when one of them is away, and they have to be very organized.

Celebrations

Debra has merged the nurse practitioner role with the more 'classical' cancer nurse specialist role to create a joined-up, psychological and physical, integrated role. She said: 'It's a nice role to have because you get the whole patient, whereas in oncology you don't always get the opportunity to do the physical side of it ... hands-on to be done and it's a nice combination.'

Debra discussed what a 'huge difference' the Nurse Practitioner course made to her role: 'It was great to be amongst other specialities and to hear how they managed. It gave me confidence to know that what I was doing was OK.' She explained: 'From a knowledge point of view it enhanced what I already knew, and knowing I had passed this or that part of the course meant that I was safe to practise. Just gaining that confidence.' Also she achieved the same experience and confidence building by attending an advanced communications skills course.

Debra felt she had a lot of highlights to share from the last six years: 'just when patients say, "we're so glad you're here or you're there at the end of a phone, we know we can call you if we need to."' Also 'discharging someone when they've reached five years, it's great.' She went on to say that 'a big sense of achievement with me was finally getting the degree ... Because I never thought it was going to happen.'

Debra commented on the fact that she felt they were very lucky as they had 'a very progressive thinking multi-disciplinary team: 'If we had wanted to take things forward, they have pretty much allowed us to.'

One of her highlights was a successful survivorship project, for which a presentation was given at a local conference 'to see the benefits the patient gets from it'.

Advice for others

'I think they need to work within the specialty and have a good, sound knowledge and to have worked with patients with stomas, have had to go through bowel preparation and have been through major surgery and you have to understand how that part of the body works and the effect it has on the rest of the body.' They need 'a solid foundation over a number of years'.

They should be prepared to take things forward and be part of service development.

Debra felt that it was important to have good leadership skills, as you need to be able to influence people, often your superiors, senior managers and so on: 'You would need to be confident and be able to stand your ground if you come up against dissidence.'

Debra summed up by saying: 'I think it's a valuable role and I think for the right person it is very satisfying, very satisfying.'

Profile 3: Ophthalmology nurse consultant, acute hospital trust

Jane is a nurse consultant within the ophthalmology outpatient service, focusing mainly on emergency care, and leading from a clinical aspect rather than a managerial one. She works closely with the clinical leader, particularly from a service development perspective for the department, as well as having a wider remit outside of the hospital, locally and nationally. The clinical aspect is key, as she sees, diagnoses and treats patients within her own daily clinics and also gives expert practice advice and education to both junior nurses and doctors, and she acts as a resource for the department. Staff have said of her that 'if Jane doesn't know, then who does know?' The triage nurse decides if something is appropriate to be seen by Jane, the doctor or one of the nurses, based on protocols, with Jane tending to see the more complex presentations.

Jane was a pioneer in the role within the department and therefore the role was set up from scratch. She is a qualified advanced nurse practitioner and a non-medical prescriber. Her role has a high level of autonomy and she makes her own decisions about what patients need, whereas the nurses work to protocols and patient group directives. Once a week, Jane runs a follow-up clinic for patients who have been seen in the acute referral clinic. A significant part of her time is spent supporting, developing and teaching junior nurses, so that the department had now built up a career structure for its nursing staff, allowing for clear career progression from staff nurse, nurse practitioner, advanced nurse practitioner up to nurse consultant.

Key points about the role

Jane had always wanted to be an ophthalmic nurse. Her aim was to become a general nurse, obtain a bit of experience, then get specialist training in a specialist unit. She eventually became a manager, but this had never been her plan, and although she was good in the role, she missed the clinical side of things and she was 'starting to get frustrated with that … there's no job satisfaction in it.' She added: 'And I hadn't been happy for a while.' This led her to consider what she could do. Although she had done an ophthalmic course, she wanted to get a degree: 'I thought the Nurse Practitioner degree for me seemed the perfect thing as I could make it specific to ophthalmology.' She saw this as her opportunity to get back into the clinical practice side of things.

Jane was proactive in developing a role within the department and was responsible for putting together a business case for an advanced nurse practitioner. She could see a need for something like this as 'we weren't meeting targets of assessing patients within the time as walk-ins and it was just a bit chaotic. So I thought there is a role there.' The two aspects with regard to this development were changing the service and developing her role. At the same time as undertaking the course, she was also developing the clinical practice side of things, supported by the medical staff. What Jane found was that 'there is quite a gap between working within protocols at a certain level and actually advancing your role … being autonomous'.

Jane commented: 'I am a role model for the department and for that reason I do feel it is important to be professional, knowledgeable, cheerful and to treat your patients properly.' As 'an advanced nurse you know people do look to you'. She also felt that 'clinical credibility (and a reputation) for listening to new ideas and getting things done' were important.

Jane talked about the leadership aspects of her role and the importance of maintaining standards of practice as key.

Challenges

When Jane's role as an advanced nurse practitioner was reviewed and the decision made that she should progress to that of a consultant nurse, this was challenged by the medical staff, who weren't happy with it: 'I think it was the concern that no, I wasn't a consultant, I was a *nurse* consultant.'

There is also an ongoing issue with Jane taking on some of the follow-up clinic patients, which she feels she could grade appropriately: 'They seem to have this idea that if someone else grades their clinics then they will be inundated with patients and they feel they are losing control.'

She remarked: 'Having to go through so many hoops is very frustrating because you can't just get on with it. That's a hindrance.'

Celebrations

Jane commented on some main achievements: 'turning the department around into an efficient service, an appointment-based service where people are assessed immediately and given an appointment, which means generally they don't wait around'.

She developed an electronic patient pathway with an external company, which she felt had been a great achievement, particularly as this has now been rolled out to other departments in the region.

Jane has published three books on ophthalmic nursing. She was also pleased to talk about the success of her team: 'We got to the final of the *Nursing Times* Team of the Year award several years ago, so that was good.'

'I have always been very supported by management,' she stressed.

Advice to others

Jane felt that her own personal eye problems were an asset, as she is able to reassure patients by saying: 'I know what you are talking about and it will be OK.'

She considered that doing the Nurse Practitioner course made her think much more objectively about what she wanted to do, 'rather than thinking the department needed this or that. It made me think where I was now and where I wanted to be and where I wanted the department to be in the future. It made you think more widely, in a more analytical way.'

She also felt she came out of it as 'a much more rounded person ... able to justify my actions, more confident'.

Jane was keen to discuss that she felt that it was important not to advance your role and become a 'mini doctor', but that working in partnership with the patient is the most important thing, as this helps to foster trust and to ensure patients cooperate and comply with treatment and care, 'empowering patients'. She also talked about the different approach that an advanced nurse has that supports this way of working through problems with the patient.

'My own management experience has helped because I know who to go to ... I'm a reasonable negotiator.'

'Getting yourself known in the community, in your organization. Widen your knowledge, broaden your horizons.'

Jane summed up by saying: 'I really enjoy what I do. When I look at an eye and I don't know what's going on and I've got to use my brain and my differential diagnosis skills and think ways through things, and also I think it is the interactions with the patients.' She added: 'I love the team. We've got a really nice team here.'

Profile 4: Advanced paramedic practitioner, GP out-of-hours service, acute hospital trust

Ann is an advanced paramedic practitioner, who has been working since 2004 as a member of an urgent care out-of-hours team within a hospital-based treatment centre in a geographically remote and rural area. The team consists of GPs and two non-medical practitioners (Ann and an advanced nurse practitioner), who cover the north and south of the county, alongside appropriately trained nurses who triage the patients using an electronic triage protocol. The team work from treatment centre bases, either advising patients, seeing them in the centre or in their own homes, depending on acuity. The more complex and often sicker patients are referred to the GP or advanced practitioner, who makes decisions about their management, as the triage nurses only work at a certain level, not at that of an advanced practitioner or GP. There is usually a GP on at the same time as Ann when she is working from the base, with both of them seeing any patients who come through the door, or if a patient needs to be seen in their home, whoever has been allocated to be 'mobile' will go out and leave the other person to cover the patients in the base or arrange appointments for patients to be seen when they return from home visits.

Although Ann manages patients independently and uses patient group directives for most medicines, she does access the GPs if prescriptions are required and if she wants to discuss or check anything. She also gets involved in triaging if the nurses are busy. As the service is hospital based, there is a certain amount of cross-cover between the service and the Accident and Emergency (A&E) Department, with patients moving between the two areas if needs be. Ann also works in A&E seeing some of the minor injuries or in the majors area or clerking patients for admission, if it is particularly busy. 'I work, I guess similar to a middle grade [doctor]', she explains. There are emergency nurse practitioners who work in A&E, but Ann feels she has a wider scope of practice, due to her primary care and pre-hospital care experience and expertise. She also teaches one day a week on master's-level advanced practice modules at the local university.

Key points about the role

Ann had worked in the health service in a nuclear medicine department before becoming a paramedic. She had been a paramedic for six years before she undertook one of the first pre-hospital care degree courses, followed by a full-time, fully funded master's programme in advanced practice, on which five paramedics were enrolled as part of a pilot project, funded by the government health department, aimed at 'treating more people in the community and therefore not transferring and admitting patients that could be treated elsewhere. This was a very good success.' The programme involved working in a variety of practice placements, supported and guided by a senior medical mentor in each placement.

Ann sees her role as one that has developed and continues to develop as an unscheduled care role, characterized by advanced practice. The aim is to meet whatever the patient's needs are rather than being restricted by who provides the treatment, such as the doctor, nurse, paramedic, and where the treatment is carried out (A&E, treatment centre, patient's home). All of this has to be fitted within a service that is compromised by difficulty recruiting staff, particularly medical staff, and in an area that attracts visitors in the summer, thus there is an unpredictable case load of patients at certain times. This is well summed up when Ann says: 'sometimes with advanced practice we learn to navigate the best we can'.

Ann believes that advanced practice is a set of core skills, which are transferable, rather than being profession specific. This was confirmed through her multi-professional course: 'it beautifully showed for me that it's not about the profession, it is about the person with these generic set of skills. It doesn't really matter what label you stick on them.' She also talked about the holistic aspects of advanced practice, discussing how the four pillars of advanced practice (clinical, leadership/management, education and research) are intertwined and are all integrated with master's-level study. She strongly advocates that the hallmark of all advanced roles needs to be the clinical aspect: 'the clinical practice, if you don't practise every day then I think you get skill erosion'.

When asked about what unique contribution Ann felt she had on patient care as an advanced practitioner, she responded by saying: 'I think that patients are more satisfied with care, there is more holistic care. I feel that they [patients] are better communicated with … and I think that is vital and it is all about holistic communication as well as clinical care.'

Challenges

Ann talked about developing an advanced practice role and undertaking the course of study linked to it: 'I guess the actual amount of work, study time and everything, I think it is about finding your own temporary boundaries for acquiring knoweldge at a particular time and because obviously you can just dive off. It's a bit like an amoeba. I think it's like jumping in the sea and wherever you are there's just more sea! You can forever go on to seek out new knowledge, new skills, and it's about finding that balance and having the maturity to say, well I need to know this and this. It's like doing a list of this is essential, this is desirable, this is luxury. You have to get the essentials done before you move on, before you then go off and do something that's, you know, to learn about more specifics.'

She also talked about transition into an advanced practice role: 'I think everyone finds it difficult to make that transition. I think it's easier for paramedics. They always work unsupervised, they always work in the community, and therefore there is always an inherent core about the clinical risks, about not having to be supervised. So I think that in my experience a lot of nursing colleagues found that more difficult because they have generally been brought up in an environment where they have always had someone next door, looking over their shoulder or working with them. It almost seems like the drop is bigger.'

Although Ann has not been restricted in her role by being unable to prescribe, she has found it frustrating at times, as she has undertaken the prescribing course. However, 'because my base qualification is paramedic not nurse, I'm currently not legally allowed to do that.'

Once she had completed the advanced practice programme and the pilot project, Ann became frustrated that her role was not being utilized appropriately, particularly as the pilot project had been so successful and had generated a high level of patient satisfaction. An example of the project's success was in terms of 60% of the chest pain patients who were kept at home who would have been admitted. Ann said she 'personally felt discouraged, and I was aware I wasn't using the skills I had acquired'. This was the impetus she needed to do something about the situation and so she looked around at different areas and wrote to several organizations about what she could offer. This led to her current role as an advanced paramedic practitioner.

Although Ann did not experience any particular difficulties, she does feel that challenges for advancing roles can come from a few members of the medical profession who think that advanced practitioners are taking over their roles and that certain activities do not belong outside medicine. She also considers that there is a lack of understanding of the importance of education for advanced roles, and that some people are quite negative about the links between education and advancing practice. However, she thinks these negative elements are a lot to do with people's perceptions, which can be altered: 'I believe that as soon as you've engaged with them, work alongside them and when those insecurities are put to rest ... for every one that you get that is quite negative, then time will change that, or happily you get other people who are more than happy for you to work with them, very interactive, very much mutual respect both ways, and understand what you can do and what you can't do and what you need in terms of support.'

Celebrations

Ann does not believe there are many paramedics who work in the same way as she does and thinks she is probably 'a bit of an anomaly'. Although the advanced nurse practitioner in the team works within the treatment centre, she does not go out on home visits as Ann does. Ann's advanced role enables her to work alongside GPs providing an effective and efficient urgent care service within the most appropriate environment, depending on the patient's condition. Her paramedic background in pre-hospital care, with her emergency assessment and treatment skills, means that she is very proficient at recognizing and deciding if patients need to be brought into hospital, particularly with the more acutely ill patients. She is able to give patients medications that fit into the paramedic's 'exemption drugs' category, such as morphine. Her contribution to the team is complementary to that of the GPs, as she has the emergency skill base to deal with immediate emergency conditions. Ann illustrates this point with an example: 'If somebody did have a respiratory arrest then I can intubate. Most GPs wouldn't want to touch that with a barge pole!'

Advice for others

Ann believes that 'it doesn't matter what your profession is, it's about what you provide as an advanced practitioner'. She talked about being a pioneer of advanced paramedic practice roles: 'My dissertation was called "Walking in the snow" and the reason for that was because it felt that I was the first one walking through with no one in front of me.'

Ann considers that 'there are enormous opportunities for advanced practice in the future and not just because of the poor medical recruitment, you know, all the health care professionals developing'.

'My ambition would be to incorporate a role that's leading an advanced practice team in whatever profession it's possible, in primary or secondary care, to include those skills and possibly a rotation so that people are becoming more generic. I think there's not enough generalists around. Potentially I could set up a unit that would rotate people in hospital, to the emergency deparment, to the clinical assessment units etc. That would increase their skills, keep everybody on board, it would be able to have incredible flexibility in terms of care.'

Ann believes that advanced practice should be on a separate part of the register, 'because that would be a way of bringing professions from different areas into a core area to demonstrate advanced practice'.

Profile 5: Advanced occupational therapy practitioner, community services

Ellen is an advanced occupational therapy (OT) practitioner. Her current job title is Community Liaison OT Specialist (Long-Term Conditions). She has been in her current post since 2010, as part of the community matron service. She is employed as the link in the hospital for the long-term conditions service and her role is to try to keep patients out of hospital, but if they do need to be admitted she is a communication link between hospital and community, and plays a key role in discharge planning, educating staff and keeping everyone informed of new services and processes that are constantly changing and developing. She deals with any incidents involving problematic hospital discharges and sees patients who have been readmitted, as well as doing community follow-up visits. Although Ellen feels she does not use the advanced clinical skills she learnt during her advanced practice course as much as she would like to, she does carry a small case load of patients and she is involved in a new pilot project called virtual ward. The ward was set up by the hospital, but is staffed by community staff. The team follow up patients who have been discharged from hospital to the community, assess, identify any issues, make sure they understand their medications, their diagnoses, what advice they have been given and that all the follow-ups have been arranged. As Ellen explained: 'Keeping them out of hospital again, that's the main part of it.' She also described the contribution of her role: 'I'm definitely a figure within the hospital that people know to ring me if they've got anyone that they don't know what to do with and I'll do my best to find out or work out what the answer might be.'

Key points about the role

When Ellen applied to do the advanced practitioner course, she was working as a senior OT in a community-based crisis intervention team, trying to get patients out of A&E more quickly. The multi-disciplinary team all worked together, and had done standard training across professions so they could all do the same generic assessment, although they utilized their specialist skills as well. It was while Ellen was doing this job that that she started to think she wanted to do more, but was not exactly sure what that would lead to. The course seemed to fit with her job as well as her ideas for the future. She had good support from her manager and a GP mentor to guide and support her. When she started the course she did not realize how focused it was on advanced nursing and had to keep this in mind throughout. Any assessments or essays she did, she made sure she reflected at the end how it fitted with OT, 'because the course wasn't at all geared to OT'. She was the first OT to undertake the course and was the only non-nurse in her group, which was quite difficult at times.

Ellen was in the second year of the advanced practitioner course when she started working in her current role. The course helped her to gain a much better understanding of many different conditions, signs and symptoms. However, it was the critical thinking skills rather than the hands-on clinical skills that she found most valuable: 'I didn't just do the course to do skills, it's the whole advanced-level thinking. I saw it as adding to the OT skills that I've already got. To do the best OT assessment that I can.' She continued, in reference to herself: 'I always wanted to be an OT. It was never anything about becoming anything else. I want to be the best I can be at that.' Ellen went on to talk about what she gained from undertaking the course: 'with any condition, it's just having the confidence, that even if I don't know about it I know that I am capable of looking up about it, knowing what my competencies are, who to ask and that it's OK to ask. It's about safe practice at the end of the day.' And when discussing the clinical focus of the course she said: 'The course really stressed that so much of your examination is about taking a history and getting that right and the exam is almost concerning what you're half expecting anyway. I'm sure if I think about it I'm using those clinical history taking skills all the time, but you just don't think that you're doing it.' Ellen was keen to stress: 'I don't think I would ever want to not spend at least some of my time clinical, because it would be a waste, as I am good with patients and work well with patients.'

Challenges

'I think OTs who would consider themselves as working as advanced practitioners within OT would be quite condition specialized, an orthopaedic or mental health specialist OT … whereas I see myself as an advanced practitioner in primary care working as an OT.' Ellen viewed her advanced practitioner role as more of a generic role: 'a general practitioner OT, a primary care OT, because that's just how my career path ended up and where my skills have led me, that's what I do. That really isn't a formalized role.'

Celebrations

'It's a culmination of all my years of experience working in the community as an OT, together with the added critical thinking skills and the added medical model knowledge that I gained from doing the course. All put together plus my personality, which I think does play a part, means that when I assess a patient they get as holistic an assessment as I possibly could give. I'm not just thinking about what brought you into hospital, you understand your medical condition, medications, I also am thinking about how this is this affecting your life. Is there anything we could do to make any of this any better. So I think the patient feels that they have understood why they've been in hospital and what they need to think about, when, where they could go and if they've got any problems, any concerns. Also that their social and home life has been considered, things that they didn't know that anyone would care to ask them about or they haven't thought about.'

Ellen recalled a patient she had seen that day, which is a good illustration of her input based on her assessment of the whole situation: '[The patient's] main thing was that she had been told that she wasn't allowed to get up and go to the kitchen and make herself a cup of tea, so the carers were getting her tea in a mug and she couldn't get at it herself and really she likes her tea in a pot. I got her up and she seemed to do quite well on her feet, but she couldn't lift the kettle. So I went back and got her a kettle tipper and she made herself a pot of tea and took it back into the lounge. The carer was there and was quite shocked that she was even out of the chair. And basically the OT who brought her on the home visit told her that she wasn't safe to walk with the trolley, so the carers had been telling her that she wasn't allowed to. So I said, well, so at the time she'd been poorly and she obviously wasn't as strong as she is now and you look at her now and you can see how well she's walking, and she'd never seen her walking so well. Had I not been there and done that follow-up visit, she'd still now be sitting in the chair having everything brought to her without any control over it. I don't think anyone would have tried to see if she could do it because everyone's scared of her falling over. But to her the most important thing is to be able to get that little pot of tea.' Ellen talked about 'negotiating with patients and not dictating to them. You understand there are risks with boiling water and walking, but she understands that she's got to be careful. She's got a seat and she can sit down.'

This is a powerful illustration of what Ellen feels she can offer patients and how satisfying it can be: 'That's why I wouldn't not want to be clinical, the little things that make the job worthwhile. It's not about the money, it's about knowing that you've gone and done a visit and made someone's life a bit better, not a huge amount better but that's made a difference.'

Advice for others

Ellen talked about how much hard work undertaking an advanced practice course is and stressed the time it takes and the dedication it requires. She continued by saying: 'there's no point putting yourself through that unless you truly believe that doing it is going to benefit your patient care. If you think you're doing it because it's going to get you more money or you're doing it for prestige, I really don't think it's worth the amount of effort and thought. You need to be doing it because you want to be a better practitioner and then that makes the hard work worth it. You can see the reasons behind what you know and why you're doing it. So I think you need to be doing it for the right reasons.'

'I think being an ambassador ... what I already said about having the wisdom to know, to accept that the more you know the more you don't know, but working within your competencies, striving to learn more all the time, being able to demonstrate advanced clinical skills, critical thinking in your field and being a role model.'

Profile 6: Advanced paediatric nurse practitioner, acute general hospital

Gill has worked as a paediatric advanced nurse practitioner in an acute general hospital since completing her nurse practitioner degree five years ago. She is a dual trained Registered General Nurse and Registered Sick Children's Nurse and previously worked as a ward sister on the acute admissions unit.

Currently she is specializing in the assessment of children with allergies and has commenced a master's programme in the management of allergic diseases. Many of her referrals come directly from GPs or from other consultants, some of whom work outside the paediatric team. An example is the ENT consultants, who may request an allergy 'work-up' in a child with severe rhinitis that has proven unresponsive to conventional treatment. Her assessment includes a detailed review that investigates any indication of the 'allergic march', which may have commenced at the time of weaning.

This is a very different role from the one she had envisaged, and the one she commenced after completing her nurse practitioner training. But her adaptability to service demands and financial constraints has led to unexpected rewards, and she finds herself now in a fulfilling role providing valuable care for anxious families.

In addition to her specialist role she also works regular sessions in an out-of-hours GP service located within the hospital. Audit shows that more than half of the patients who seek care are children and Gill reports that GP and NP colleagues are very supportive of her input. This enables her to maintain her skills, while providing specialist support and teaching to generalist colleagues. She also perceives that she has intercepted inappropriate referrals to the ward and has empowered families to care for their children appropriately in their own homes.

Key points about the role

When Gill first did her nurse practitioner degree, her vision for future practice was focused on how she was going to evolve as a nurse practitioner in the acute paediatric assessment unit. As a ward sister she had responsibility for managing a team of nurses and overseeing the clinical care of all admissions, from acute paediatric medical emergencies through to daycare patients and those attending outpatients. Although she enjoyed this role, she felt her passion lay with the clinical aspects and supporting junior nurses rather than the managerial and administrative responsibilities. She had also been influenced by colleagues who worked in other wards within the hospital, who warned of the complexity of trying to combine the ward sister and nurse practitioner roles. This prompted her to visit paediatric hospitals in London and various other places to explore how advanced practitioners had been integrated into the ward environment. This was beneficial from two perspectives: not only did she initiate contact with knowledgeable and enthusiastic peers, but she also discovered that some units had developed very specific, specialist roles, which was precisely what she wanted to avoid. However, in one hospital she observed an advanced nurse working on an inpatient assessment unit undertaking ward rounds alongside medical colleagues in a model that she aspired to. On return, she completed a mapping exercise that examined her skills at that point and all the advanced aspects of care she anticipated being able to undertake on completion of her training. This appealed to her medical colleagues, some of whom proved to be important advocates, and she was inspired to produce a presentation in which she clearly articulated her proposal.

Gill recalled frustration during times of slow progress, particularly when she eventually finished her nurse practitioner degree and there was no money for project development. She was anxious that people would lose sight of the fact that she was a potential asset, so she negotiated working one day a week as a nurse practitioner and undertaking her sister role on the remaining four days. This enabled her to demonstrate her clinical skills, seeing patients and assessing them in exactly the same way as the medical staff. Her needs analysis had identified a short-age of experienced doctors on the wards during the mornings, as the single registrar was often busy on the high-dependency unit. Therefore she undertook the registrar reviews, which involved the assessment of children who had recently been discharged home but who required a 'safety net' check on the ward a few days later. This proved extremely valuable, as patients and their families were seen promptly, had any outstanding results explained to them and, importantly, had the oppor-tunity to share concerns and ongoing issues. Medical staff were appre-ciative and even on her 'sister' days Gill would help with the registrar reviews if the opportunity arose.

At around this time scrutiny of the senior nursing staff occurred when financial constraints became apparent. The necessity of having three ward sisters within the 26-bed unit was questioned and clinicians became vulnerable in a climate of cost cutting. Gill viewed this as an opportunity for change and volunteered to amend her position from that of ward sister to nurse practitioner within the month. This was accepted and she was able to devote her time completely to her advanced practice role.

However, within six months, as financial constraints gripped, a further review by the clinical director hinted that a full-time position on the wards may be unsustainable. It also transpired that the director, a medic, felt that the nurse practitioner role was encroaching on the junior doctors' learning experience. Suspecting that her position had once again become vulnerable, when the opportunity within the allergy team became available, Gill took the initiative.

Challenges

One of the main challenges that Gill encountered was disseminating her vision for practice in a meaningful way to varied audiences. She was inspired by one of her university lecturers, who encouraged 'entrepre-neurial thinking' by 'knowing your audience'. By anticipating what would appeal to their specific needs, Gill was able to adapt her generic presentation on the nurse practitioner role for each audience. For exam-ple, when presenting to nurses on the wards, who at that time were often having to deal with frustrated patients kept waiting when medical staff were delayed or busy, her emphasis would be on the nurse practi-tioner's potential to expedite patient care. When presenting to the matrons within the hospital, her emphasis would be on the development of innovative nursing roles that made the unit look 'dynamic'. And for managers her emphasis would be on the potential cost effectiveness of appointing a nurse practitioner to undertake aspects of care such as the registrar reviews.

An additional challenge for Gill was undertaking a nurse practitioner degree programme that focused on the adult patient. However, she reported being able to adapt everything she learned and she welcomed the broad curriculum. This may have been due to her being dual RGN and RSCN trained, although she conceded that some elements of the pharmacology unit may not have been as relevant. Her recommendation is to be determined and focused on achieving your desired goal. She continues to seek out learning opportunities and has recently visited a regional specialist centre to observe immune challenges.

Celebrations

Gill has benefited from the support and camaraderie of both nursing and medical colleagues. She credits her nursing team as being key to the successful implementation of her novice nurse practitioner role while she was combining the responsibilities of ward management. Her medical colleagues also acted as advocates and her mentor supported her with regular clinical supervision and case reviews. She, too, made an effort to collaborate with colleagues and would recommend 'keeping involved' by attending team meetings to raise awareness of your vision.

'I love the fact that I have a really good working relationship with both nurses and medical staff, and although I feel I don't belong in any team, I'm not the sort of person who's going to sit in a corner being quiet.'

Advice for others

Gill recommends developing your self-identity, taking the initiative and keeping focused on your personal goal: 'It's about knowing yourself. If, like me, you're not a completer-finisher you may need somebody else to be your inspiration – to push you along a bit.'

'Know what you want ... find out what's out there, because although you think you know what you want, you have to really make sure it's what you want.'

'Know your audience when you're presenting – and know what you want to get ... and have an idea of what is going to tick their boxes ... It's about trying to sell yourself and focus on that when you're doing any sort of presentations ... and stick with it!'

Profile 7: Advanced nurse practitioner, general practice

Mandy is an advanced nurse practitioner in a large general practice on the south coast of England. She has been in post for ten years and undertakes home visits in addition to 'on the day' assessments.

Mandy had an established career as a district nurse and team leader for almost 10 years before she decided it was time to 'do something different' and applied to undertake a nurse practitioner degree in her early 50s. She had been based at a general practice that had participated in a pilot study to integrate an experienced nurse practitioner in the late 1990s, and admits that this insight into 'the potential' of advanced nursing practice encouraged her to seek out development opportunities. Throughout her degree programme she continued to manage the team of community nurses, although she found the demands of university combined with both clinical responsibilities and a leadership role quite challenging at the time. But she was 'determined' to succeed and reflects that the 'hard work' has reaped rewards, as she is now in a role that she finds immensely satisfying, and one that is appreciated by her patients and her employers.

Key points about the role

Mandy's extensive experience working in the community enabled her to share the home visits with GPs soon after completing her nurse practitioner degree. At first she personally selected these according to her confidence and previous knowledge, but quickly developed her competence and now reviews two or three patients from the visit list in their homes after each morning surgery. She was originally employed to assist GPs with their unmet demand for 'on the day' appointments and this has proved beneficial in reducing waiting times for patients in addition to relieving the GPs' workload. A 'pivotal' development for Mandy was completing non-medical prescribing, as this has facilitated her autonomy and she is no longer dependent on medical colleagues to write prescriptions for her patients. She has also developed specific skills in dermatology and has now replaced one of the GPs running the weekly cryotherapy clinic.

Challenges

One of the greatest challenges for Mandy was changing her professional identity from an established district nurse to that of a nurse practitioner based in a general practice. She explained that this persists today with some older patients making assumptions about her role: 'I think some patients found that quite difficult. And even now, for example this week, I've had a gentlemen come to see me with a problem – well, it looks like a leg ulcer, and he said to me, "Oh, this is fine because you know all about leg ulcers, don't you? You know all about dressings?" and I said to him, "Do you how long ago that was? That was 10 or 12 years ago!"'

From a personal perspective she recommends having a clear vision for your future role at an early stage in career development. For Mandy, however, there was no clear route for advanced practice development as a district nurse and she thinks this led to personal uncertainty at first. She reflected that this may have been different if the community matron role had been established at the time of her training. However, without a clear strategy for role development within the district nurse team, when she was approached by one of the GPs looking to employ a nurse practitioner, she took up the invitation to apply for the post and was successful. Mandy took 'the risk' as she perceived it, particularly as employment was on a three-month trial basis only.

Mandy also recalled that nursing colleagues, medical practitioners and the practice staff were initially unsure of what an advanced nursing role would involve (she was the first nurse practitioner employed at the surgery). Her strategy was to patiently explain, repeatedly when necessary, precisely what her goal was: 'I think you have to work at it, don't you? To explain to the GPs your capabilities and what you can bring to the surgery. It takes effort.' She also understood that reception staff would be central to marketing her role to patients, although this too required determined intervention: 'Nobody had a clear idea of what I could do ... I would hear receptionists sometimes say, "Well, she's like a doctor but she can't prescribe" [at that time], but I had to say to the practice manager, "they mustn't say she's like a doctor – I'm a nurse practitioner". And in end they had a list of things that I could see and sent a newsletter out to patients.'

Mandy benefited from regular clinical support from her medical mentor, which took the form of weekly random case reviews and analysis of 'challenging cases'. She stresses that all of the GPs were supportive of her developing role, but that it took at least 12 months to become established and comfortable with the 'unpredictability' of general practice.

Celebrations

The ability to demonstrate her personal competence has been central to Mandy's professional development, and this has often required her to seek out learning opportunities in addition to collating evidence within a personal portfolio. A GP with a 'special interest' in dermatology mentored Mandy in clinical practice and she now sees 15–20 patients each week (all of whom have been previously assessed either by her or their GP) for treatment for varied conditions such as verrucae, warts, seborrhoeic warts, skin tags and actinic keratosis.

Advice for others

Mandy recommended being mindful that the journey into advanced practice will involve stepping into unfamiliar territory, and that this may be unsettling at first. She perceived that she has taken 'personal risks' in terms of her professional development by leaving the 'comfort' of her team-leader role for a position that was unsecure and unknown at the time. But she clarified that 'personal risk' is quite distinct to 'professional risk' and that having insight into your personal competence and professional accountability is imperative. Mandy illustrated that some nurses may not want to 'look outside the box' and say 'that's not my job ... that's not my responsibility', but stressed that advanced practitioners require a willingness to extend their 'level of responsibility'.

She also recommended identifying your personal learning needs and taking any opportunity for further education. In addition to regularly attending a local nurse practitioner group for professional support, she meets regularly for educational evenings with GP colleagues.

Profile 8: Advanced practitioner, drug intervention programme

Steve is a registered mental health nurse (RMN) specializing in substance misuse. He is currently employed as a drug intervention programme (DIP) nurse and primarily treats ex-custodial clients with complex needs. He completed a postgraduate Advanced Nurse Practitioner programme two years ago and is a registered non-medical prescriber. His role, which is unique in the region, was originally commissioned through a drug and alcohol addiction team and is now funded through the local Primary Care Trust (PCT). He is the only clinician in the county who is specifically employed to prescribe immediately for clients with significant alcohol and/or drug dependence. Although there is good evidence that early intervention with these clients has a positive outcome, there are very few DIP advanced practice nurses employed in the UK.

Steve is based in a small coastal town in a county that has a distinctive profile, with a higher number of heroin addicts per capita than anywhere else in the country. As he explained: 'They call it "end of the line" syndrome – literally it's at the end of the line from London – and it's a seaside town ... and a lot of drugs come through Bristol, which is reasonably close. And we have a significant number of PPOs [Priority Prolific Offenders] that we have to deal with.'

There are also five prisons in the region, which has an impact on Steve's case load. Statistics show a high rate of reoffending in people who are released from prison with addictions, and therefore his role involves early intervention – often on the same day as someone is released. His referrals come direct from either the prison drug treatment system or the police (if an offender identified as having an addiction has been arrested). Their details are passed on to him when they leave custody and he makes contact immediately after their release. The success of this model of early intervention is revealed in the continued funding and support from the PCT.

Key points about the role

Steve always had an interest in substance misuse and tailored many of his placements to further his learning during his RMN training. Following his qualification in 2004, he worked as a 'detox nurse' in both acute and community settings before completing a BSc in addictions. He then qualified as a non-medical prescriber and become involved in the DIP. The increased responsibilities associated with this unique role led him to investigate advanced practice programmes and he commenced a postgraduate Advanced Nurse Practitioner diploma at a local university in 2008. This course was generic and most of his peers on the programme were registered general nurses. Steve recalled a 'steep learning curve', notably in the development of his physical examination skills and study of pathophysiology. He reflected that, although this was one of the most demanding elements of his course, it had proved a key attribute of his advanced practice role: 'As an RMN in Substance Misuse I think the hardest thing has been developing the physical examination aspect of healthcare. However, things have developed as a direct response to my training and I am now doing physical health assessments that are tailored to my clients.'

There is a high rate of respiratory problems, including TB, in the 'complex' substance misuse clients that Steve treats, in addition to an increased risk of DVTs, infected skin wounds and abscesses. Inevitably his caseload has reduced as his management responsibilities have increased, but the clinical focus of his work remains central to his advanced practice role: 'I'm still prescribing methadone for about 15 patients each week – occasionally this can be quite a high dose, for someone who has just left prison, for example. These are the more complex patients who I monitor until they're stable enough to move into the Drug Advisory Service.' Early notification from prison staff allows Steve to visit and assess clients while they are still in custody, resulting in timely and prompt treatment when they are released.

Steve's involvement in service development and leadership has expanded considerably since he completed his diploma. This was illustrated recently in a project he initiated that resulted in an improved referral process to the Drug Advisory Team following admission of clients to hospital. His suspicion was raised some months ago when he realized that clients with addictions had been known to secondary care services (antenatal, medical or surgical clinicians) for some time prior to their referral for help. Following negotiation with the medical directorate at the local hospital, he conducted an audit that clearly demonstrated that the low numbers of referrals were not a true representation of the actual need: 'We arranged to meet a group of consultants from the wards where our clients had been inpatients – at my request – and I led a meeting on how we might capture these clients, how we might audit this ... it showed the numbers were between 7–10 times higher than we were getting referrals. And there was a very variable service from different ward areas.' Through teamwork and negotiation, Steve conducted a series of teaching sessions for ward staff, although he admitted he felt daunted by the prospect at first. He addressed nursing, midwifery and medical teams in addition to managers and clinical leads with positive results. He gained confidence with repeated sessions and realized that raising awareness in colleagues had a direct impact on patient care: 'It actually surprises me sometimes how little knowledge some of the senior, experienced medical clinicians have about our clients. So a bit of training can go a long way.'

Challenges

Steve experienced a degree of isolation in his practice development, in that his role is unique. There are few 'substance misuse advanced nurse practitioners' in the UK, and there were none in the locality when he commenced his training: 'I couldn't find one when I started the course – you know, someone I could pick up the phone to and say, "How did you incorporate this into your role?"' This remained a challenge, but he stayed confident that what he was learning was valuable and would have the potential to enhance client care. He described an 'inner conviction' that 'kept him going', while also being mindful that he would have to continuously convince those around him of the benefits that he envisaged.

To some extent he did not have a clear vision at the outset of training, and his personal experience of role development was more spontaneous advancement as opportunities arose. His advanced nurse practitioner course was generic in that he could 'tailor' his assignments, wherever possible, to focus on his role in substance misuse and he built a portfolio of evidence based on his client group. Despite the majority of his peers being registered general nurses rather than mental health specialists, he described an enhanced learning experience in which knowledge and expertise were shared reciprocally.

Steve provides physical health assessments to a client group who are at serious risk of developing problems because of their alcohol consumption. He delivers this care in the community and there remains one aspect of his role development that has been a continued source of frustration – that is, the ability to administer Pabrinex injections when necessary. As he explained: 'It's Thiamin – B complex vitamins –which can be given IV or IM. What it does in alcoholics is give their immune system a complete boost and if it's caught early enough it can actually stop people developing Wernicke–Korsakoff syndrome and prevent their memory from deteriorating rapidly.' Due to the risk of anaphylaxis when given IV, the drug is usually administered during inpatient treatment. However, Steve has argued that his 'extreme' client group would benefit if the injection was given IM in the community (this carries a lower risk of anaphylaxis). He has support from the regional Addictions Medical Consultant and has drafted guidelines for administration, but has met resistance from the local medicines management team: 'We would like to able to give this in the community, however, we're finding the negotiations with the MHRA and our local Medicines Management Team challenging. We've researched this considerably and are fully aware of the potential risks [of allergic response] and, you know, taking adrenaline with us to a client's home and an AED if necessary. But sometimes the client is so physically unwell – perhaps in a bedsit in the far end of town – they can't get here. And we just want to be able to give them the three to five days of Pabrinex ... These are the kind of things that we come up against – you know, when we're considering what would be really good for the patients. Because this drug could really help – really prevent someone's life deteriorating very rapidly. And yes, there is a risk they could still be drinking – but this drug could sustain them over decades. I feel I am always having to convince people!'

Steve perceives that, in this case, the system intended to support service development has been obstructive rather than facilitative, but he is determined to succeed and 'won't give up'. The Addictions Consultant, an advocate, is assisting him in a further 'redraft' of the proposal.

Celebrations

The ability to utilize audit strategies with a demonstrable impact on client care has been rewarding for Steve and something he had not anticipated. He conceded that in previous roles he had very little involvement in audit evaluation, but now has insight into the potential it has for identifying gaps in service provision. As a direct result of the study, funding was secured for a Band 7, non-medical prescriber who works full time in the hospital with the new detox team.

Advice for others

Steve recommended resilience in your advanced practice development. Sometimes the transition can be isolating, particularly when trying to establish a pioneering role that inevitably comes under greater scrutiny. Having support from peers is beneficial, but this may not be consistent. Steve encountered disparity within the regional Drug Advisory Team; although his local colleagues were supportive, he met negativity in others and recalled being in meetings that felt 'confrontational and intimidating'. He recommended being prepared to encounter resistance: 'I think my way of dealing with that is to be really inclusive, to be understanding, to look at the reasons why they may be being resistant. You know, conventional management skills.' He also made an effort to persuade peers and superiors about the value of the role.

He cautioned that promotion to a 'clinical leadership' role does not always equate to 'advanced practice' and, in his experience, completion of an advanced nurse practitioner course was key to his success. He had recommended the programme to other nurses because 'it gives a much more "overall" picture of a client's health – including physical rather than just mental health'.

Steve's personal confidence has grown with the challenges he has encountered and he suggested that this resulted from being clinically focused. Although as clinical lead he has management responsibilities, he successfully balances these with his personal case load. He recommended sharing your personal knowledge with colleagues, even when, at first, the prospect seems daunting. Steve now speaks on substance misuse to advanced practice students at university in addition to non-medical prescribers, doctors and other healthcare practitioners.

A picture of advanced practice

The advanced practitioners' profiles detailed in this chapter provide a rich and insightful view of their roles and some of the challenges faced and achievements realized while advancing their practice. Although the roles are diverse, their backgrounds varied and the journeys taken are different, some themes emerge that would appear to identify the shared characteristics of these advanced practitioners (Shearer and Adams 2012; Lowe et al. 2012). This develops a picture of eight different roles, all exhibiting elements that fit into the four identifed pillars of advanced practice: clinical, education, management/leadership and research (NES 2010; DoH 2010; NLIAH 2010) within an integrated advanced professional role. At a more specific level, it can be seen that these practitioners meet the criteria for advanced practice such as those detailed by the Department of Health for England (DoH 2010). What is demonstrated through all the profiles is the uniqueness of these practitioners' role development, which has on occasions made them feel isolated. However, they do appear to have gained in strength from this.

So what is it that brings these practitioners together under the umbrella of advanced practice? Drawing on the dialogue from the interviews and analysing and synthesizing what the individuals were describing, an overall profile of an advanced practitioner emerges. They all fit with Davies and Hughes's (2002: 147) interpretation of advanced practice role characteristics as a 'constellation of competencies embedded in a variety of roles, rather than in terms of particular roles'. There are various sub-roles, including clinician, educator, researcher and consultant. Reflecting back on the interviews, both interviewers got a sense that it was not what they knew that made the participants advanced practitioners, but rather how they used what they knew.

Starting out as experienced practitioners

All eight interviewees had strong, well-established clinical backgrounds and were experienced healthcare professionals who had been qualified for 5–25 years. In addition, they had been working in a variety of different roles across a number of specialist areas. It takes a considerable time to develop an advanced practice role and this is reliant on a sound background of relevant practice experience, with the right knowledge and skills, abilities, attitudes and values (Currie and Grundy 2011), which appear to be evident in the interviewees' profiles.

Education and development needs

All of the interviewees identified that, although expert in their field of practice, they had reached a point at which further education and training as advanced practitioners was required, in order to support them in meeting their visions for improving patient care through the development of their advancing roles. They clearly articulated in each of the interviews that they have a strong desire to learn. They had sought out courses and embraced opportunities to help support their role progression. They drew on the expertise of others to enhance their own learning and development, such as through the identification of appropriate mentors (Anderson et al. 2002; Girot and Rickaby 2008), who were able to provide the specific input they required. It was not solely the identification of suitable mentors for their educational requirements that was important, but also the identification of advocates, often medics, as well as alliances with nursing or other healthcare peers. These practitioners consciously sought out the support and camaraderie of professional groups, peers and medics as they advanced their practice and roles.

They had all undertaken an academic, clinically focused educational programme, which included a significant amount of application into practice of the knowledge and skills that they were developing (NES 2007; RCN 2012). Additionally, they adapted their learning experiences to ensure that these were tailored to the needs of their practice and the service they were providing. Gill highlighted this when she commented on the fact that she adapted the generic advanced nurse practitioner programme that she undertook to suit her specific needs as a paediatric nurse. Steve took the same course, but was able to keep his primary focus on mental health, and Ellen and Ann both took advanced practice courses that were predominantly nursing orientated.

The educational programmes and developments within their practice settings supported the interviewees, who felt that they were able to apply a greater depth and breadth of knowledge and complexity of decision making to their practice. Currie and Grundy (2011) list some of the underpinning principles of advanced practice as autonomous practice, critical thinking, a high level of decision making, problem solving, values-based care and improving practice, concepts echoed widely in the literature (Hanson and Hamric 2003; Bryant Lukosius et al. 2004; Mantzoukas and Watkinson 2006; Pulcini et al. 2010). It is exactly these characteristics that the interviewees identifed as being key elements of their developing roles, which required a high level of education and training with a strong practice application, supported by their managers and other members of the multi-disciplinary team (Currie and Grundy 2011).

Delivering quality patient-centred care

The interviewees exhibited a passion for their profession and dedication to maintaining high standards of quality care for patients. They are committed to improving patient journeys and could see that developing their roles as advanced practitioners was a way to help make a real difference at both practice and service levels. At the heart of their practice is a strong values-driven, patient-centred approach (Kitson et al. 2013), which mirrors the dimensions of patient-centred care defined in the work of Gereteis et al. (1993), with a focus on the centrality of patient experience and care that is adapted according to patient needs and values within an integrated management approach (McCormack and McCance 2006; Tutton et al. 2007).

Box 10.3 Drivers for improving patient care and advanced practice career development

- Visionary – innovative, creative ways to improve practice, 'anything is possible'
- Drive and determination – believing in patient benefit
- Articulating an 'early' vision for their professional future
- Ambition/personal motivation
- Tenacious, sticking with it. 'I was like a bee in their bonnet really ...'
- Motivated, dedicated, conscientious healthcare professional
- Committed to developing and promoting holistic healthcare within a multi-disciplinary team
- Values driven – compassionate and caring, passionate about quality care
- Pioneering spirit – able to see beyond current practices, seize opportunities
- Desire to make a difference for their patients by being proactive and an advocate
- Courageous – prepared to take risks, challenge practice, trial and error
- Developing professional confidence – strong belief in self (and personal knowledge/competence) and being assertive with strong sense of self-identity

Some of the drivers for improving patient care and advanced practice career development that these interviews revealed are captured in Box 10.3.

Clinical practice

All the interviewees viewed the nature of their roles as providing holistic healthcare, emphasizing the well-being of every aspect of what makes a person whole and complete and treating the individual as a whole and individual person (Barker 2009). They described a holistic approach to each healthcare episode, enabled by a combination of their advanced clinical practice built on the fundamentals of their base professional practice, rather than either in isolation (Lowe et al. 2012). They made a conscious decision to maintain the clinical practice element of their role, utilizing advanced skills regularly and dealing with complexity in their patient consultations.

The way the practitioners described their roles is that they are characterized by an extension of their professional practice, be it nursing, occupational therapy or paramedic, rather than a substitution of identified tasks (Hanson and Hamric 2003). For each of the practitioners, one of the reasons for embracing an advanced practice role was to reduce the fragmentation of care and treatment inherent in healthcare in the UK, and to move towards the delivery of an enhanced, more complete and integrated package of care for the patient (Kilpatrick 2008).

It was apparent that the interviewees exercise a significant degree of autonomy in their practice and function independently within their roles, at the same time as working alongside the multi-disciplinary team, with the patient at the heart of this joined-up approach to treatment and care (Mantzoukas and Watkinson 2006; Wong and Chung 2006). All were able to identify a distinct case load of patients whose care and treatment they manage, regardless of what type of service they work in, with most of them running their own 'clinic' and consulting with patients within a therapeutic encounter (DoH 2010). They all use a high level of critical thinking, problem-solving and decision-making skills, despite each role being quite different with regard to the specific areas of expertise and the knowledge on which they draw (Barker 2009; RCN 2012). They are very aware of their own accountability and the increased level of responsibility that comes with working as advanced practitioners, and they strive to keep their competencies up to date and at a safe level.

These are self-perpetuating, unique, challenging and pioneering roles, that require creative thinking, flexibility and adaptability, invariably involving a certain amount of risk taking, while at the same time still ensuring safe and effective practice delivery. Key to all is that they work across traditional professional boundaries, particularly medicine, while maintaining a philosophical underpinning based soundly within their own identified profession (Running et al. 2006; Gould et al. 2007).

Education

The nature of their roles and the expert knowledge, skills and experience they have, along with their ability to develop therapeutic relationships with their patients, enables these practitioners to incorporate a high level of health education and health promotion into their consultations, whether as a snapshot, in an emergency or acute episode or as a more comprehensive, sometimes ongoing health education or information-giving activity (Chen et al. 2009; Jennings et al. 2009). Linked to this is their knowledge of supporting services and other health and social care professionals, and thus the ability to enhance patient care further through appropriate referral mechanisms when required.

Staff education, training and professional development support are key elements of all the practitioners' roles. They act as role models for advanced practice, sharing knowledge and skills with colleagues, taking on both formal and informal education and training roles within their own practice areas and providing support to ensure that practice is of a high quality across the workforce, not merely in relation to their own professional practice.

Management/leadership

All the interviewees talked about their clinical leadership roles in managing care (DoH 2010; NLIAH 2010). Other people look to them to provide expert advice, vision and commitment to quality care. They hold credibility within their organizations for the advanced practice role and the services they provide, and they all have reputations for getting things done and being tenacious. One talked about part of her leadership role as having 'ownership of the care and service I provide'. Ann focused on how she influenced the developing service in which she worked: 'Sometimes with advanced practice we learn to navigate the best we can.' Negotiating and influencing skills in relation to directing, leading and managing patient care were highlighted, and the interviewees felt these were facilitated by their experience at a senior level within their organization. All the practitioners discussed their roles in terms of leading service and practice development in proactive ways, as a means of facilitating improvements to patient care. They had often been instrumental in identifying gaps in service and had adopted creative and innovative ways of meeting deficits in care, invariably through use of the advanced practice elements of their roles. This is all in line with the work of Gerrish et al. (2011), who explore how advanced practitioners lead developments and support the maintenance of standards of practice.

As clinical leaders, the practitioners are key players, guiding and directing their patients' care. They act as the link between health care professionals at the centre of the patient journey. Each works within a cohesive and cooperative team (Goodrich 2009), within which they assume a leadership role, maintaining the patient as the central element of the process.

Research

These experienced practitioners dedicate time to considering and reflecting on their own and others' practice and how this can be enhanced to improve services and better meet the needs of their patients. They are involved in formal research and audit activities, often in a leadership capacity, as well as in less formal practice and service evaluation, learning from patient experiences and sharing best practice with local and wider networks. The patient is always at the heart of their enquiries.

In a wider definition of research, they are committed to knowledge management and promoting the uptake of knowledge in relation to their own practice and that of the colleagues around them. Dobbins et al. (2009) refer to this as 'knowledge brokering' in the promotion of evidence-based practice, with interpretation and application of knowledge, and the ability to synthesize knowledge and incorporate key elements from research into the local context. This is managed through role modelling, problem solving and decision making, facilitating change and teaching (Gerrish et al. 2011).

This chapter has considered career development for advanced practice by reviewing the career profiles of advanced practitioners. As advanced practice is still at a relatively early stage in its evolution in the UK, this approach was felt to be the most appropriate to illustrate the varied pathways that practitioners experience in following their career trajectory.

References

Ackerman, M., Norsen, L., Martin, B., Wiedrich, J. and Kitzman, H. (1996) Development of a model of advanced practice. *American Journal of Critical Care* 5: 68–73.

Anderson, M., Kroll, B., Luoma, J. et al. (2002) Mentoring relationships. *Minnesota Nursing Accent* 74: 24–29.

Ball, J. (2006) *Nurse Practitioners 2006: The Results of a Survey of Nurse Practitioners Conducted on Behalf of the RCN NP Association.* London: RCN.

Barker, A.M. (2009) *Advanced Practice Nursing: Essential Knowledge for the Profession.* Burlington, MA: Jones and Bartlett.

Barton, T.D., Bevan, L. and Mooney, G. (2012) Advanced Nursing 2: A governance framework for advanced nursing. *Nursing Times* 108(25): 22–24.

Benner, P. (1984) *From Novice to Expert: Excellence and Power in Clinical Nursing Practice.* Menlo Park, CA: Addison-Wesley.

Bryant-Lukosius, D. and Dicenso, A. (2004) A framework for the introduction and evaluation of advanced practice nurse roles. *Journal of Advanced Nursing* 48: 530–540.

Bryant-Lukosius, D., Dicenso, A., Browne, G. and Pinelli, J. (2004) Advanced practice nursing roles: Development, implementation and evaluation. *Journal of Advanced Nursing* 48(5): 519–529.

Callaghan, L. (2008) Advanced nursing practice: An idea whose time has come. *Journal of Clinical Nursing* 17(2): 205–213.

Carlisle, C. (2004) *New Nursing Roles: Deciding the Future for Scotland.* http://www.gov.scot/Publications/2004/04/19201/35584 (accessed 22 February 2015).

Carryer, J., Gardner, G., Dunn, S. and Gardner, A. (2007) The core role of the nurse practitioner: Practice, professionalism and clinical leadership. *Journal of Clinical Nursing* 16(10): 1818–1825.

Casey, D.C. and Egan, D. (2010) The use of professional portfolios and profiles for career enhancement. *British Journal of Community Nursing* 15(11): 547–552.

Chen, C., McNeese-Smith, D., Cowan, M., Upenieks, V. and Affifi, A. (2009) Evaluation of a nurse practitioner-led care management model in reducing in-patient drug utilization and cost. *Nurse Economist* 27(3): 1680–1688.

Currie, K. (2010) Succession planning for advanced nursing practice: Contingency or continuity? The Scottish experience. *Journal of Healthcare Leadership* 2: 17–24.

Currie, K. and Grundy, M. (2011) Building foundations for the future: The NHS Scotland advanced practice succession planning development pathway. *Journal of Nursing Management* 19(7): 933–942.

Daly, W.M. and Carnwell, R. (2003) Nursing roles and levels of practice: A framework for differentiating between elementary, specialist and advancing nursing practice. *Journal of Clinical Nursing* 12: 158–167.

Davies, B. and Hughes, A.M. (2002) Clarification of advanced nursing practice: Characteristics and competencies. *Clinical Nurse Specialist* 16(3): 147–152.

Department of Health (2004) *The NHS Knowledge and Skills Framework.* London: HMSO.

Department of Health (2010) *Advanced Level Nursing: A Position Statement.* Leeds: DoH.

Dobbins, M., Robeson, P., Ciliska, D. et al. (2009) A description of a knowledge broker role implemented as part of a randomized controlled trial evaluating three knowledge translation strategies. *Implementation Science* 4(23): 1–9.

Donner, G.J. Wheeler, M.M. (2001) Career planning and development for nurses: The time has come. *International Nursing Review* 48(2): 79–85.

Fagerstrom, L. and Glasberg, A.L. (2011) The first evaluation of the advanced practice nurse role in Finland: The perspective of nurse leaders. *Journal of Nursing Management* 19(7): 925–932.

Furlong, E. and Smith, R. (2005) Advanced nursing practice: Policy, education and role development. *Journal of Clinical Nursing* 14(9): 1059–1066.

Gardner, A. and Gardner, G. (2005) A trial of nurse practitioner scope of practice. *Journal of Advanced Nursing* 49(2): 135–145.

Gardner, G., Gardner, A., Middleton, S. et al. (2010) The work of nurse practitioners. *Journal of Advanced Nursing* 66(10): 2160–2169.

Gereteis, M., Edgman-Levitan, S., Daley, J. and Delbanco, T. (1993) *Through the Patient's Eyes: Understanding and Promoting Patient-Centred Care.* San Fransisco, CA: Jossey-Bass.

Gerrish, K., McDonnell, A., Nolan, M. et al. (2011) The role of advanced practice nurses in knowledge brokering as a means of promoting evidence-based practice among clinical nurses. *Journal of Advanced Nursing* 67(9): 2004–2014.

Gibson, F. and Hooker, L. (2004) Defining a framework for advanced nursing practice. In F. Gibson, L. Soanes and B. Sepion (eds), *Perspectives in Paediatric Oncology Nursing.* London: Whurr.

Girot, E.A. and Rickaby, C.E. (2008) Evaluating the role of mentors for advanced practitioners: An example from community matrons in England. *Learning in Health and Social Care* 8(1): 1–12.

Goodrich, J. (2009) Exploring the wide range of terminology used to describe care that is patient-centred. *Nursing Times* 105(20): 14–17.

Gould, O., Johnstone, D. and Wasyikiln, L. (2007) Nurse practitioners in Canada: Beginnings, benefits and barriers. *Journal of the American Academy of Nurse Practitioners* 19: 165–171.

Griffin, M. and Melby, V. (2006) Developing an advanced nurse practitioner service in emergency care: Attitudes of nurses and doctors. *Journal of Advanced Nursing* 56(3): 292–301.

Griffith, H. (2004) Nurse practitioner education: Learning from students. *Nursing Standard* 18: 33–41.

Hampel, S., Procter, N. and Deuter, K. (2010) A model of succession planning for mental health nurse practitioners. *International Journal of Mental Health Nursing* 19: 278–286.

Hanson, C.M. and Hamric, A.B. (2003) Reflections on the continuing evolution of advanced practice nursing. *Nursing Outlook* 51(5): 203–211.

Holloway, I. and Wheeler, S. (2010) *Qualitative Research in Healthcare*, 3rd edn. Oxford: Blackwell.

Horrocks, S., Anderson, E. and Salisbury, C. (2002) Systematic review of whether nurse practitioners working in primary care can provide equivalent care to doctors. *British Medical Journal* 324: 819–823.

International Council of Nurses (2001) *Definition and Clarification of the Role.* Geneva: ICN Advanced Practice Network.

International Council of Nurses (2002) *Definition and Characteristics of the Role.* Geneva: International Council of Nurses.

Jennings, N., Lee, G., Chao, K. and Keating, S. (2009) A survey of patient satisfaction in a metropolitan emergency department comparing nurse practitioners and emergency physicians. *International Journal of Nursing Practice* 15(3): 213–218.

Kilpatrick, K. (2008) Praxis and the role development of the acute care nurse practitioner. *Nursing Inquiry* 15(2): 116–126.

Kitson, A., Marshall, A., Bassett, K. and Zeitz, K. (2013) What are the core elements of patient-centred care? A narrative review and synthesis of the literature from health policy, medicine and nursing. *Journal of Advanced Nursing* 69(1): 4–15.

Laurant, M., Reeves, D., Hermens, R. et al. (2005) Substitution of doctors by nurses in primary care. *Cochrane Database Systematic Review:* CD001271.

Lindpainter, L. (2004) Teaching clinical assessment skills: The Basel curriculum. 3rd ICN/APNN Conference, June 29–July 2, Groningen, Netherlands.

Livesley, J., Waters, K. and Tarbuck, P. (2009) The management of advanced practitioner preparation: A work-based challenge. *Journal of Nursing Management* 17(5): 584–593.

Lowe, G., Plummer, V., O'Brien, A.P. and Boyd, L. (2012) Time to clarify – the value of advanced practice nursing roles in healthcare. *Journal of Advanced Nursing* 68(3): 677–685.

Mantzoukas, S. and Watkinson, S. (2006) Review of advanced nursing practice: The international literature and developing the generic features. *Journal of Clinical Nursing* 16: 28–37.

Marsden, J., Dolan, B. and Holt, L. (2003) Nurse practitioner practice and deployment: Electronic mail Delphi study. *Journal of Advanced Nursing* 43: 595–605.

McCormack, B. and McCance, T.V. (2006) Development of a framework for person-centred nursing. *Journal of Advanced Nursing* 56(5): 472–479.

Moon, J. (2006) *Learning Journals: A Handbook for Reflective Practice and Professional Development*, 2nd edn. London: Routledge.

National Leadership and Innovation Agency for Healthcare (2010) *Framework for Advanced Nursing, Midwifery and Allied Health Professional Practice in Wales*. Llanharan: NLIAH.

National Organization of Nurse Practitioner Faculties (2002) *Domains and Core Competencies of Nurse Practitioner Practice*. Washington, DC: NONPF.

National Council for the Professional Development of Nursing and Midwifery (2001) *Framework for the Establishment of Advanced Nurse Practitioner and Advanced Midwife Practitioner Posts*. Dublin: NCNM.

National Council for the Professional Development of Nursing and Midwifery (2005) *A Preliminary Evaluation of the Role of the Advanced Nurse Practitioner*. Dublin: NCNM.

National Council for the Professional Development of Nursing and Midwifery (2006) Advanced nurse practitioners accredited. *National Council for the*

Professional Development of Nursing and Midwifery Quarterly Review 23: 20.

NHS Education for Scotland (2007) *Background Information for Participants and Sponsors: Advanced Practice Succession Planning Development Pathway.* Edinburgh: NES.

NHS Education for Scotland (2010) Advanced Practice Toolkit. http://www.advancedpractice.scot.nhs.uk (accessed 21 January 2013).

Nurse Practitioner Taskforce (2000) *The Victorian Nurse Practitioner Report: Final Report of the Taskforce.* Melbourne: Department of Human Services. https://acnp.org.au/sites/default/files/docs/nurse_practitioner_taskforce_ report_0.pdf (accessed 22 February 2015).

Nursing and Midwifery Council (2005) *The Proposed Framework for the Standard of Post-registration Nursing.* London: NMC.

Nursing and Midwifery Council (2008) *Standards of Conduct, Performance and Ethics for Nurses and Midwives.* London: NMC.

Pearson, A. and Peels, S. (2002) Advanced practice in nursing: International perspective. *International Journal of Nursing Practice* 8(2): S1–S4.

Pulcini, J., Jelic, M., Gul, R. and Loke, A.Y. (2010) An international survey on advanced practice nursing education, practice and regulation. *Journal of Nursing Scholarship* 42(1): 31–39.

Robson, C. (2011) *Real World Research*, 3rd edn, Chichester: John Wiley.

Roodbol, P., Sheer, B., Wong-Ru, T., Loke, A. and Usami, S. (2007) Policy in action: A comparison of the development of regulation for advanced practice nurses in several countries. ICN conference, Yokohama, Japan.

Royal College of Nursing (2002) *Nurse Practitioners: An RCN Guide to the Nurse Practitioner Role, Competencies and Programme Accreditation.* Lonon: RCN.

Royal College of Nursing (2010) *Advanced Nurse Practitioners: An RCN Guide to the Advanced Nurse Practitioner Role, Competencies and Programme Accreditation.* London: RCN.

Royal College of Nursing (2012) *Advanced Nurse Practitioners: An RCN Guide to Advanced Nursing Practice and Programme Accreditation.* London, RCN.

Running, A., Kipp, C. and Mercer, V. (2006) Prescriptive patterns of nurse practitioners and physicians. *Journal of the American Academy of Nurse Practitioners* 18(5): 228–233.

Schober, M. and Affara, F. (2006) *Advanced Nursing Practice.* Oxford; Blackwell.

Scholes, J., Furlong, S. and Vaughan, B. (1999) New roles in practice: Charting three typologies of role innovation. *Nursing in Critical Care* 4(6): 268–275.

Shearer, D. and Adams, J. (2012) Evaluating an Advanced Nurse Practitioner course: Student perceptions. *Nursing Standard* 26(21): 35–41.

Sheer, B. and Wong, F.K.Y. (2008) The development of advanced nursing practice globally. *Journal of Nursing Scholarship* 40(3): 204–211.

Stilwell, B. (1984) The nurse in practice. *Nursing Mirror* 158: 17–22.

Tutton, E., Seers, K. and Langstaff, D. (2007) Professional nursing culture on a trauma unit: Experiences of patients and staff. *Journal of Advanced Nursing* 61(2): 145–153.

Walsgrove, H. and Fulbrook, P. (2005) Advancing the clinical perspective: A practice development project to develop the nurse practitioner role in an acute hospital trust. *Journal of Clinical Nursing* 14: 444–455.

Wong, F.K.Y. and Chung, L. (2006) Establishing a model for nurse-led clinic: Structure, process and outcome. *Journal of Advanced Nursing* 53(3): 358–369.

CHAPTER 11

The impact of new information and communication technologies on the development of advanced practice

Anne Cooper, Dawn Dowding and David Barrett

Chapter outline

- Introduction
- Political drivers for change
- Technological advances in healthcare
- Potential issues with the use of technology
- Conclusion

Introduction

The impact of technology can be experienced in many aspects of our lives: we use handheld devices to access information from almost anywhere; we can talk to these devices and pose questions – and they answer; and we no longer use paper maps but rely on satellite navigation to help us find our way around. The previously limiting factor of remote geography has been shifted by the ease and low cost of tools like Skype, allowing us to see as well as hear each other when we are not in the same location. Many commentators argue that technology is only available for the better off in society and that access is restricted as a consequence of location, for instance there may be limited broadband availability in some areas. However, a report from the UK Office of National Statistics (ONS 2012) indicated that access to the internet and internet use are continuing to rise, with 85% of the UK population having used the internet at some point. The way we access the internet is also changing: an earlier ONS report suggested that in 2011 45% of households had mobile devices that allowed them to do so, and this number is likely to have increased.

These changes in society and the availability of technology inevitably have an effect on healthcare and nursing practice. Nurses are no strangers to the use of technology in supporting their work, not only in areas such as critical care, which are traditionally high users of technology. Many nurses have adopted technical solutions such as medical devices that record observations, basic electronic patient records and the use of the telephone to provide remote support and advice. Technology is also leading us to new types of nursing practice, moving some nursing away from direct care by employing technology to provide supportive monitoring or interventions that allow patients to remain more independent and well in their own home; these approaches are often known as telecare, telehealth and telemonitoring. All represent a shift away from what people perceive to be the role of the nurse, to the extent that many commentators see technology as providing a potential barrier to relationships with patients.

In this chapter we discuss the possible impacts of the increasing use of technology on the role and practice of advanced nurse practitioners. We suggest that nurses taking on advanced roles need to have an understanding of how technological innovations can support their role, as well as being aware of some of the issues involved in implementing such systems in clinical practice. We also reflect on how the use of technology (including innovations such as social media) can change the way in which patients interact with healthcare professionals, and the implications this has for nurses in advanced practice roles.

Political drivers for change

Reflecting changes in society in general, there is increasing political emphasis in the UK and internationally for healthcare systems to use technology to make care delivery more effective, safer and potentially lower cost (PWC 2013). The adoption of technology has been supported by substantial government funding. For instance, the UK government provided an £11.4 billion investment in the NHS via the National Programme for IT; and the HITECH act in the US provided $19 billion over six years to healthcare organizations that show they are investing in health information technology that has 'meaningful use'. The UK government has also produced an updated information strategy suggesting that healthcare should be 'digital first' (Young and Wilkins 2012). Patients should be given access to their electronic records, and there should be a culture of transparency where information about performance is made available not only to patients but also in the public domain. There should be better recording, sharing and use of information at the point of care to improve safety, efficiency, patient outcomes and quality of care. Furthermore, technology is also being employed to reduce the amount of paper used in NHS settings with a move towards, as a minimum, a 'paper-light' working environment.

What is key is what this means for nursing practice. If patients have access to their own records and information is shared across providers, then those records need to be clear and accurate. This has implications for all nurses, including advanced nurse practitioners. There will need to be more emphasis on record keeping. Patients will rightly expect to receive high-quality, understandable information and all nurses will need to develop more sophisticated skills in the navigation, assessment and selection of information resources to support patients in understanding their health and well-being requirements.

The challenge for nurses working as advanced practitioners is to harness this technology as a way of supporting practice, improving the quality of patient care and demonstrating improvement through the provision of high-quality nursing metrics. In the rest of this chapter we focus on technologies that either currently exist or are likely to be introduced into healthcare settings over the next few years and explore how they can be used to support advanced practice. We outline two areas where technology is likely to be most useful: as a way of supporting nursing practice generally; and as a way of supporting individuals who are carrying out advanced roles, including activities such as diagnosis and prescribing. Finally, we consider the implications of the wider impact of information availability on patients and their families, and how this may affect their relationship with healthcare professionals.

Technological advances in healthcare

It is useful to define exactly what we mean by technology in relation to nursing. Black et al. (2011) categorize eHealth technologies according to their function: data storage, management and retrieval; and supporting decision making. The types of system listed in Table 11.1 are independent of the ways in which individuals may access such systems; we anticipate that in the future nurses (and patients) may be able to access EPR, CDSS and other systems via mobile platforms such as tablets and smartphones, as well as via traditional computer workstations. It is the *functions* of the systems and how they are used that is of issue here, rather than the precise technology that enables them.

Table 11.1 eHealth technologies

Function	Types of technology
Data storage, management and retrieval	Electronic patient record (EPR) or electronic health record (EHR) Picture archiving and communication systems (PACS) Electronic transfer of prescriptions (ETP) Electronic appointment booking
Supporting decision making	Computerized physician order entry (CPOE) Electronic prescribing system (EPS) Computerized decision support systems (CDSS) Telehealth systems

Source: Black et al. (2011).

journals.plos.org/pols medicine/article?id=10.1371/journal.pmed.1000387

Using technology to support nursing practice

The vision of 'digital first' healthcare means that in the future all healthcare professionals will be utilizing technology such as electronic patient records (EPR) or electronic health records (EHR) to both inform and keep a record of their practice. An EHR can be defined as follows:

> a longitudinal electronic record of patient health information generated by one or more encounters in any care delivery setting. Included in this information are patient demographics, progress notes, problems, medications, vital signs, past medical history, immunizations, laboratory data and radiology reports. The EHR automates and streamlines the clinician's workflow. The EHR has the ability to generate a complete record of a clinical patient encounter – as well as supporting other care-related activities directly or indirectly via interface – including evidence-based decision support, quality management, and outcomes reporting. (HIMMS n.d.)

Integrated EHR systems will therefore have the ability to interface with the types of system that are used to support decision making. They may include access to picture archiving and communication systems (PACS) and other information systems across and between healthcare organizations. Increasingly technology is also being introduced such as smart pumps and vital signs monitors that communicate with broader data management, storage and retrieval systems such as an EHR, so that information about patients is communicated instantaneously.

The key for advanced practitioners is understanding the potential implications for practice of the introduction of such systems, and the impact they may have on the quality and efficiency of care. The potential benefits relate to the 'increased accessibility, legibility, "search-ability," manipulation, transportation, sharing, and preservation of electronic data' (Black et al. 2011). There is some evidence to suggest that nurses value the ability to read and access patient information easily in an EHR system, as well as that this may save nurses time when documenting patient care, although the evidence for this is more mixed. What is often not recognized is that EHRs enable healthcare professionals to document large amounts of information about patients easily, often at the point of care. It could be that nurses will be documenting more information, in a different way to when they used paper-based systems. It may not therefore be appropriate to use time as a metric for effects of EHRs on practice, but rather to focus on the potential effects of improved communication between members of the healthcare team and easier access to information to support patient care.

Many of the technological advances relate to sophisticated systems designed to help support decision making in practice. Advanced nurse practitioners often take on roles that include advanced assessment and diagnosis, non-medical prescribing and advancing practice through innovation and service redesign. It is in these areas that technological advances have the most potential to help.

Computerized physician order entry (CPOE) systems enable practitioners to order laboratory tests and receive the results electronically, as well as organizing referrals, and they often interface with ePrescribing systems and computerized decision support. ePrescribing systems assist with the ordering or prescribing of medications (which may include electronic prescription transfer and the use of scanning and bar coding technology to assist with the administration of medications). Computerized decision support systems (CDSS) cover a broad range of functionality ranging from passive systems that provide information when requested, through to active systems that provide patient-specific guidance at the point of decision making. CDSS often link with CPOE and ePrescribing systems to provide guidance and advice to practitioners across a range of decision situations, including assisting with diagnosis, recommendations for treatment interventions, alerts related to safe prescribing and support for long-term condition management.

Telehealth is a broad term that describes the use of information technologies to support the provision of healthcare or promotion of well-being remotely (Barrett 2012). Within this broad approach are a series of specific applications that nurses and other practitioners can use to enhance care. Pressures on healthcare delivery have catalysed the drive to embed telehealth as a modality of care. This is manifested in the UK in public strategy documents outlining the importance of telehealth (Scottish Government 2012) and specific initiatives such as England's '3 Million Lives', which aims to give 3 million people in England access to telehealth and telecare by 2017 (DoH 2012a). Here we will focus on two particular applications of telehealth: telemonitoring and teleconsultation.

Telemonitoring allows the provision of information such as vital signs and feedback on signs and symptoms from patients to practitioners. For example, someone living at home with chronic obstructive pulmonary disease (COPD) may record daily information on oxygen saturation levels, blood pressure and pulse, in addition to answering questions about levels of breathlessness. This data is sent via a broadband connection to a central server, where it can be viewed by a practitioner (often a senior nurse), who can use it to plan care or identify the need for intervention.

At a superficial level, telemonitoring may allow practitioners to gain an 'early warning' of deterioration; this then provides the cue for early intervention that can, in turn, reduce the likelihood of hospital admission. To go back to the example of our patient with COPD, a practitioner may notice, via the telemonitoring system, a decrease in oxygen saturation and reports of increased breathlessness. This might prompt a phone call from the practitioner to the patient, culminating in a recommendation to use their 'rescue pack' containing antibiotics and corticosteroids, thereby mitigating any exacerbation and preventing a hospital admission.

The interest in telemonitoring stems largely from some evidence that the service can provide clinical benefits for patients with long-term conditions. Notably, Cochrane systematic reviews indicate that telemonitoring can reduce mortality and/or hospital admissions in patients with heart failure (Inglis et al. 2010) and COPD (McClean et al. 2011). A large-scale randomized controlled trial (RCT) of telemonitoring – the Whole System Demonstrator (WSD) – in patients with long-term conditions (either COPD, CHF or diabetes) found 12-month mortality rates 45% lower in the intervention group when compared to control (Steventon et al. 2012).

Despite its promise, the evidence base for telemonitoring is not clear cut. For example, there have been some RCTs of telemonitoring that show no significant benefit (Chaudhry et al. 2011; Koehler et al. 2011).

Even the WSD, despite the encouraging clinical outcomes, showed no benefits in terms of quality of life (Cartwright et al. 2013) or cost (Henderson et al. 2013). Some of the inconsistencies and uncertainties in the evidence have led to doubts about the benefit of telemonitoring, of which practitioners should be aware when attempting to develop or deliver such a service.

Although the broad principles of telemonitoring are straightforward, there are important nuances. First, its role in empowering and educating patients should not be underestimated. Access to vital sign and symptom information can help patients understand their condition and recognize the impact of lifestyle, behaviour and medication. Advanced practitioners therefore need to engage with users of telemonitoring to ensure that they utilize the information constructively and proactively.

Practitioners must also recognize that the availability of telemonitoring data may alter the way they themselves work and require the development of new skill sets. Visits to patients in the community may, where appropriate, be replaced with remote monitoring of vital signs and symptoms, supplemented by telephone consultations. This can have an impact on all areas of the practitioner's role, from early detection of deterioration, to education and support, through to medication titration. One of the challenges for practitioners is to develop the skills necessary to contextualize telemonitoring data so that it can inform decision making. Most telemonitoring systems are relatively 'dumb'. They can record and transmit data, and raise 'alerts' if data is missing or if signs or symptoms are outside practitioner-set limits. For example, if a patient has systolic blood pressure limits of between 100 mmHg and 160 mmHg, then an alert will be raised if the recording on a particular day is outside these. However, these systems do not provide the practitioner with sophisticated decision support software. Nor in many cases do they provide information on clinically significant issues such as recent changes in medication. Practitioners using telemonitoring systems therefore need to view data as just one piece of a clinical jigsaw and make decisions based on a more holistic picture of patient need.

Technology can facilitate other modalities of remote care above and beyond telemonitoring. Teleconsultation – the use of real-time video-conferencing to facilitate clinical communication between practitioners and patients – has been used for many years. However, improvements in technology and communication speeds have allowed services to become more sophisticated and effective.

Teleconsultation can be utilized to overcome geographical distance: examples include the use of video to facilitate consultation between patients and their GPs in the Scottish Islands (Audit Scotland 2011).

Even where distance is not the primary problem, teleconsultation can help address logistical issues associated with face-to-face care. The most obvious example is its use to assess prisoners who may need medical attention. This has been shown to be an effective approach to delivering care that can in some cases avert the need for hospital admission (Cruikshank and Paxman 2013).

Finally, teleconsultation can help practitioners overcome the challenges raised by the centralization of acute services and lack of onsite specialist knowledge and expertise. Examples usually require a specialist centre ('hub') providing video-based support to hospitals without onsite specialists ('spokes'). There are many potential clinical applications for services such as this, but some of the best documented and tested relate to trauma management (Latifi et al. 2009) and acute stroke care (Demaerschalk et al. 2012).

Again, the adoption of teleconsultation as a method of delivering care has substantial implications for advanced nurse practitioners. Undoubtedly, video offers the potential to provide care to a wider range of patients in a manner that reduces inconvenience and travel. However, it does – by definition – involve functions such as assessment and advice giving to be provided without being physically 'in the room' with a patient. Certain elements of the nursing role, such as therapeutic touch, are lost, as is specific assessment information such as the smell of a wound. Utilizing teleconsultation therefore requires skills to be adapted to compensate for the lack of 'hands-on' interaction. This has parallels with the experience of nurses who took on roles with the UK telephone triage service NHS Direct, launched in 1998. Studies of nurses who provided assessment and triage based only on telephone consultation demonstrated how the development of a new skill set allowed for the necessary information to be gathered through enhanced questioning and listening skills (Purc-Stephenson and Thrasher 2010). Use of teleconsultation requires similar adaptation, albeit with the technology allowing the added value of visual assessment of the patient and their environment.

Benefits of using technology for practice

So what does this mean for advanced nurse practitioners? Technology such as CDSS has the potential to provide support to decision making across professional boundaries, and to ensure that nurses' decisions are evidence based. Organizations can also use the power of the information stored in their integrated eHealth systems to provide instant reporting to nurses at both an individual clinician level and at managerial or organizational level, on a variety of metrics related to patient safety and care quality; these are known as clinical or quality dashboards or performance scorecards. This access to up-to-date and relevant patient information has the potential to help transform the way in which care is provided and monitored, with advanced practitioners gaining the ability to monitor directly the effects that changes in care and innovation in practice have on patient outcomes.

There are a number of potential benefits related to the use of CPOE, ePrescribing and related CDSS systems. For instance, improvements in systems for ordering and reporting tests and medication prescribing should lead to greater efficiency, and the introduction of CDSS to an increase in evidence-based care and improved patient safety. Recent systematic reviews indicate that using CDSS is likely to improve healthcare practitioners' performance (Jaspers et al. 2011; Garg et al. 2005). This is particularly true for systems that are designed to assist with drug ordering and dosing and preventive care such as the management of blood pressure, diabetes and asthma (Jaspers et al. 2011). Clinicians who use such systems to support their practice are less likely to make prescribing errors, and more likely to provide care according to evidence-based guidance.

There is less evidence that the use of such systems also leads to improved outcomes for patients; however, this could be due to the size limitations of the studies that have so far been carried out. A large-scale evaluation of telehealth systems has indicated that patients who use them are less likely to be admitted to hospital and less likely to die over a 12-month period than patients who receive normal care (Steventon et al. 2012). Therefore, the evidence does suggest that when clinicians use technology to support their practice, the quality of the care patients receive is likely to improve.

Potential issues with the use of technology

Nevertheless, there are issues and problems with the introduction of technology of which advanced nurse practitioners need to be aware. By their nature, technological solutions tend to be complex, and when they are introduced they may often change the way in which people work, either intentionally or unintentionally. This can lead to changes to work processes or to how the technology is used to fit better with local practices (this is known as a 'workaround'). In turn, this can result in outcomes that in themselves could be harmful to patients, known as unintended consequences. A large body of work has considered the characteristics of the unintended consequences of introducing technology into healthcare settings (Bloomrosen et al. 2011). It suggests that often this increases rather than decreases workload, due to the additional demands of logging into computer systems, having to fill out required information and responding to alerts built into the system. Introducing technology may also change communication patterns between healthcare professionals, which leads to the 'illusion of communication' – just because something has been recorded in an information system, individuals assume that it has been read and acted on by someone else. Furthremore, technology may alter the power structure in healthcare organizations, as its use often forces clinicians to systematize they way they practise. Bloomrosen et al. (2011) suggest that this may result in an increase in the power and autonomy of nursing staff and a reduction in the power of physicians.

Changing the way individuals work can compromise the safety or quality of care that patients receive. For example, Koppel et al. (2008), in a study of an electronic bar code administration system, observed nurses reproducing patients' wristband ID barcodes and fixing them to a variety of different items (such as the patient's door, their clipboard, putting them in their pocket) so that they could easily scan them when administering medications. However, this introduces a greater risk of the wrong patient being given the wrong drug, whereas bar code medication administration is often introduced to try to reduce this happening.

As an advanced practitioner you will need to stay abreast of technical advancements and make sure that their integration into patient care avoids increasing the potential for harm. This means being aware not only of the potential benefits of technological systems, but also being mindful of the implications of individuals using systems in ways that were perhaps not anticipated.

The role of nurses in technology development

For technological systems to be successful, nurses need to be involved in the design and implementation of the specific elements of systems such as EHR, CPOE and CDSS that are related to nursing practice (such as nursing assessment, interventions and care planning). Nurses have often been reluctant to engage with the designers of technological systems, with the result that they are then left to work with a system that has either not considered the nursing input into care processes, or operates in a dual documentation system where doctors' activities are electronic and nurses are still reliant on paper.

Technology can help nurses through the provision of information at the point of care. However, if this potential is to be realized, it requires advanced practitioners who are able to produce and manage the clinical content, defined as the forms, pathways and decision trees embedded in systems and the codes and terminology that underpin these. This is a new set of skills that requires the evaluation of evidence, the assessment of risk and the translation of information into usable systems that support and direct staff to the best course of action. Governance of content will also be key, with an understanding of information standards and how and where these apply.

The wider impact of information availability

It is not only information systems that are likely to change the way nurses practise, but also the availability of information to patients and citizens. There is a move in both the US and the UK to make electronic records more available and visible to patients. In the US the Department of Veterans' Affairs uses a system called 'Health Vault', which allows patients to have access to their personal online health record; the record, depending on the type of account, can potentially allow patients to have access to the entirety of their medical record. In England the government's strategy 'The Power of Information' (DoH 2012b) clearly states an intention to make electronic records increasingly available to citizens. This means that some patients are likely to become more knowledgeable about their condition, which may change the relationship between nurse and patient. Advanced nursing practice using this transparent and open approach is likely to lead to improved shared decision making with patients and carers, and may result in patients improving their self-care if they have a better understanding of their condition.

Transparent and open records that are visible to patients also require sophisticated record-keeping practices. Good practice already includes making clear records and not using jargon. However, if patients are to read records, nurses will need to think carefully about the content of what they record and how it is expressed. The level of general literacy across a population is a key issue: in areas of cultural and linguistic diversity, nurses need to be aware of what patients can understand, but also what is acceptable in terms of technical record keeping. Recording complex information that can be understood by patients but does not lose technical meaning, and therefore reduce safety, will be an increasingly important area of nursing practice and advanced practitioners will need to evolve expert skills.

As a result of the increase in technology available, there is also a more general movement towards citizens collecting information about their health and well-being. Apps on smartphones and on websites such as 'Patients Like Me' (www.patientslikeme.com) hold information that may be useful when someone is unwell and being cared for by a healthcare team. Advanced practitioners will need to have the skills to add this information into the care process and critically appraise its relevance for safe practice.

There is more and more information online about health, access to which is becoming easier even for the poorer members of society. Timmins (2006) explored the concept of 'information need', an individual's expressed needs, which are personal and unique. Once an information need has been met, it has the potential to become enhanced knowledge. Advanced practitioners need to be able to respond to these needs using the many information resources available, but also to be able to distinguish good information from poor and use new skills to support patients in navigating the information resources available. An understanding of general and health literacy coupled with the ability to find and analyse information, working in partnership with a patient, is likely increasingly to be part of advanced practice.

Furthermore, social media has an impact on nursing practice and citizens expect to be able to interact with practitioners online. The ability to work with patients in remote digital spaces uses similar skills to those of telephone triage and telehealth, but can be played out in public spaces, as opposed to in private, one-on-one interactions. Advanced practitioners will need to pay attention to digital professionalism; that is, the ability to practise in these new and emerging digital spaces while maintaining due regard for privacy and confidentiality.

Conclusion

Technology is increasingly pervasive across all areas of life, including healthcare practice. The availability of easily accessible information to both patients and healthcare staff, together with an emphasis on transparency of information in healthcare settings, means that relationships between nurses and their patients are likely to change considerably. As advanced practitioners, nurses need to understand how technological innovations can support them in delivering effective, safe, high-quality care, as well as how to interact with patients who have access to their own records and information about care delivery services. This requires skills in information management and communication alike.

References

Audit Scotland (2011) *A Review of Telehealth in Scotland.* www.audit-scotland. gov.uk/docs/health/2011/nr_111013_telehealth.pdf (accessed 10 April 2013).

Barrett, D. (2012) The role of telemonitoring in caring for people with long-term conditions. *Nursing Older People* 24(7): 21–25.

Black, A.D., Car, J., Pagliari, C. et al. (2011) The impact of eHealth on the quality and safety of health care: A systematic overview. *PLOS Medicine* 8(1): e1000387.

Bloomrosen, M. Starren, J., Lorenzi, N.M., Ash, J.S., Patel, V.L., Shortliffe, E.H. (2011) Anticipating and addressing the unintended consequences of health IT and policy: A report from the AMIA 2009 Health Meeting. *Journal of the American Medical Informatics Association* 18: 1, 82–90.

Cartwright, M., Hirani, S., Rixon, L. et al. (2013) Effect of telehealth on quality of life and psychological outcomes over 12 months (Whole Systems Demonstrator telehealth questionnaire study): Nested study of patient reported outcomes in a pragmatic, cluster randomised controlled trial. *British Medical Journal* 346: f653.

Chaudhry, S., Mattera, J., Curtis, J.P. et al. (2011) Telemonitoring in patients with heart failure. *New England Journal of Medicine* 363: 2301–2309.

Cruikshank, J. and Paxman, J. (2013) Yorkshire and the Humber Telehealth Hub: Project Evaluation. 2020health. http://www.2020health.org/2020health/Publications/Publications-2013/Yorkshire-Telehealth.html (accessed 22 February 2015).

Demaerschalk, B., Raman, R. and Meyer, B. (2012) Efficacy of telemedicine for stroke: Pooled analysis of the Stroke Team Remote Evaluation Using a Digital Observation Camera (STRokE DOC) and STRokE DOC Arizona telestroke trials. *Telemedicine and eHealth* 18(3): 230–237.

Department of Health (2012a) *A Concordat between the Department of Health and the Telehealth and Telecare Industry.* London: DoH. https://www.gov.uk/government/uploads/system/uploads/attachment_data/file/155925/Concordat-3-million-lives.pdf.pdf (accessed 22 February 2015).

Department of Health (2012b) *The Power of Information: Putting All of Us in Control of the Health and Care Information We Need.* London: DoH.

Garg, A.X., Adhikari, N.K.J., McDonald, H. et al. (2005) Effects of computerised clinical decision support systems on practitioner performance and patient outcomes: A systematic review. *Journal of the American Medical Association* 293(10): 1223–1238.

Henderson, C., Knapp. M., Fernández, J.L. et al. (2013) Cost effectiveness of telehealth for patients with long term conditions (Whole Systems Demonstrator telehealth questionnaire study): Nested economic evaluation in a pragmatic, cluster randomised controlled trial. *British Medical Journal* 346: f1035.

HIMMS (n.d.) http://www.himss.org/ASP/topics_ehr.asp (accessed 14 November 2012).

Inglis, S.C., Clark, R.A., McAlister, F. et al. (2010) Structured telephone support or telemonitoring programs for patients with chronic heart failure (Protocol). *Cochrane Database of Systematic Reviews* Aug 4, CD007228.

Jaspers, M.W.M., Smeulers, M., Vermeulen, H. and Peute, L.W. (2011) Effects of clinical decision-support systems on practitioner performance and patient outcomes: A synthesis of high-quality systematic review findings. *Journal of the American Medical Informatics Association* 18(3): 327–334.

Koehler, F., Winkler, S., Schieber, M. et al. (2011) Impact of remote telemedical management on mortality and hospitalizations in ambulatory patients with chronic heart failure: The Telemedical Interventional Monitoring in Heart Failure Study. *Circulation* 123: 1873–1880.

Koppel, R., Wetterneck, T., Telles, J.L. and Karsh, B.T. (2008) Workarounds to barcode administration systems: Their occurrences, causes, and threats to patient safety. *Journal of the American Medical Informatics Association* 15(4): 408–423.

Latifi, R., Hadeed, G., Rhee, P. et al. (2009) Initial experiences and outcomes of telepresence in the management of trauma and emergency surgical patients. *American Journal of Surgery* 198: 905–910.

McLean, S., Nurmatov, U., Liu, J. et al. (2011) Telehealthcare for chronic obstructive pulmonary disease. *Cochrane Database of Systematic Reviews* July 6, CD007718.

Office for National Statistics (2011) Internet Access: Households and Individuals. Statistical Bulletin. http://www.ons.gov.uk/ons/dcp171778_227158.pdf (accessed 1 March 2015).

Purc-Stephenson, R. and Thrasher, C. (2010) Nurses' experiences with telephone triage and advice: A meta-ethnography. *Journal of Advanced Nursing* 66(3): 482–494.

PWC (2013) *A Review of the Potential Benefits from the Better Use of Information and Technology in Health and Social Care*. Final Report. London: PWC.

Scottish Government (2012) *A National Telehealth and Telecare Delivery Plan for Scotland to 2015: Driving Improvement, Integration and Innovation*. Edinburgh: Scottish Government. http://www.scotland.gov.uk/Resource/0041/00411586.pdf (accessed 22 February 2015).

Steventon, A., Bardsley, M., Billings, J. et al. (2012) Effect of telehealth on use of secondary care and mortality: Findings from the Whole System Demonstrator cluster randomised trial. *British Medical Journal* 344: e3874.

Timmins, F. (2006) Exploring the concept of 'information need'. *International Journal of Nursing Practice* 12: 375–381.

Young, C. and Wilkins, A. (2012) *Digital First: The Delivery Choice for England's Population*. http://digital.innovation.nhs.uk/dl/cv_content/32200 (accessed 22 February 2015).

Index